Lichen Sclerosis
Beating the Disease

Ginny Chandoha

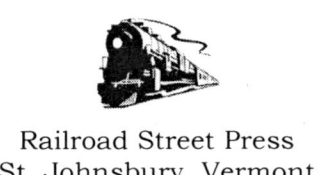

Railroad Street Press
St. Johnsbury, Vermont

Copyright ©2014 Ginny Chandoha

All rights reserved. No part of this book may be used or reproduced, stored in a retrieval system, or transmitted by any means, electronic, mechanical, photocopying, recording, or otherwise, without written permission from the author.

The scanning, uploading, and distribution of this book via the Internet or via any other means without the written permission of the author is illegal and punishable by law. Please do not participate in or encourage piracy of copyrighted materials. Your support of the author's right are appreciated.

Edited by Evelyn Fazio

ISBN 9781936711345

Railroad Street Press
394 Railroad Street, Suite 2
St. Johnsbury, Vermont, 05819

Disclaimer

This book is intended solely as a discussion of how the author healed herself of Lichen Sclerosis. The information herein is alternative, and not investigated, evaluated, or approved by any government regulation or agency. None of the recommendations, methods, therapies, or products discussed in this book are intended to treat, diagnose, or cure any disease or ailment.

The entire contents of this book are based solely upon the opinions of the author unless otherwise noted. The information in this book is merely intended as a sharing of knowledge and information gained from the experience and research by the author. It is hoped that the information provided will empower the reader to search for their own personal healing methodology. Liability for individual actions or omissions based upon the contents of this book is expressly disclaimed.

Neither the author nor the publisher is affiliated with any physician, health practitioner, company, service, or product.

Neither the publisher nor the author are medically trained physicians, and do not dispense professional or medical advice or service to the individual reader. None of the ideas, methods, therapies, products, or suggestions contained in this book are intended to diagnose, treat, cure, or act as a substitute for a one-on-one relationship with a qualified health care professional. The information herein is not intended as medical advice, and it is strongly advised that readers consult their healthcare provider before attempting to follow therapy of any type, or information presented in this book, especially anyone who is pregnant or breast feeding.

All matters regarding your health require decisions based upon your own research and discussions with a qualified health care professional. Neither the author nor the publisher shall be liable or responsible for any loss or damage allegedly arising from any information or suggestions in this book. Readers must assume full responsibility for their own health and how they choose to use the information presented in this book.

The publisher and the author expressly disclaim responsibility for any adverse effects resulting from any individual use of the information contained and described in this book.

Various chapters in this book describe the self-prescribed practices of the author as it exists at the time of publishing.

Manufactured in the United States of America

"And you may ask yourself, well, how did I get here?"
- Talking Heads

Contents

Acknowledgements   *i*
Foreword   *iii*
Introduction   *iv*

1 Rude Awakening 1

2 Toxic Topicals 14
    About Soap
    About Olive Oil
    Extra Virgin Olive Oil Nutrients
    Virgin Coconut Oil

3 Chemical Consumption 51
    Evolution and Food
    Food Defined
    Food Science
    Food Additives
    Artificial Sweeteners
    High Fructose Corn Syrup (HFCS)
    What's In That Fruit Juice?
    Chocolate
    MSG
    Honey
    Pesticides
    Pesticide Neutralizing Systems
    Genetically Modified Food (GMO)
    Labeling
    Irradiated and Microwaved Food
    Factory Farming
    Poultry
    Meat
    Processed Meats
    Meat Glue
    Fish
    Do Organic Fish Exist?
    GMO Fish
    Fish Fraud
    Milk
    Milk Substitutes

Infant Formula
What Else Could Be Hiding in Milk
  Products?
Water
Chlorination
Water Filtration Systems
Fluoride
Bottled Water
Air
Air Purification
Automobile Emissions
Heavy Metals Poisoning
Still Not Convinced?
How Does All This Relate to
  Lichen Sclerosis?

4 Diet & Exercise 217
  Diet
  Raw Food
  Cooking Oils
  Whole Butter vs. Margarine
  Sprouted Flour
  Exercise
  The Pedometer
  Electrolytes

5 The Missing Link? 248

6 Allopathic vs Alternative Medicine 253
  Over-the-Counter and Prescription Drugs
  Big Pharma's Influence on Doctors
  Allopathic Medications Side-Effects
  Problems Caused by Allopathic Medicine
    and Drugs
  How Allopathic Medicine Has Changed
  Vaccines
  Antibiotics and the Immune System

7 Disease Free 308

8 Preliminary Testing 314
  Body Composition Analysis
  Lyme Disease & Lyme Antibody Testing

Vitamin and Mineral Testing
　　　Heavy Metals Testing
　　　Cholesterol and Inflammation
　　　The Problem with Low Cholesterol
　　　Problems Related to the Use of Statins
　　　Hs-CRP
　　　Thickened Blood

**9　Vitamins, Supplements, and
　　Nutraceuticals** **327**
　　　Herxheimer Reaction
　　　Vitamin and Supplement Format
　　　Vitamins
　　　Homeopathic Rule of Thumb for Children
　　　Multivitamin
　　　B-Complex and B12 Vitamins
　　　Vitamin C
　　　Vitamin D3
　　　Vitamin E
　　　Calcium
　　　Supplements
　　　TPP Protease
　　　Probiotics
　　　Molybdenum
　　　L-Lysine
　　　Evening Primrose Oil (EPO)
　　　Omega-3 Fish Oil/Krill Oil
　　　Coenzyme Q10 (CoQ10)/Ubiquinol
　　　Detox Tea
　　　Healing Soaks
　　　Nutraceuticals
　　　Neuro-Antitox II™ Formulas
　　　Replacing Clobetasol with Organic
　　　　Extra Virgin Olive Oil

10　The Healing Protocol **386**
　　　Phase 1: Elimination of Toxic Topicals
　　　Phase 2: Elimination of Chemical
　　　　Consumption
　　　Phase 3: The Healing Protocol
　　　The Healing Protocol Outline
　　　First Quarter Schedule

Second Quarter Schedule
Third Quarter Schedule
Fourth Quarter Schedule
Beginning the Healing Protocol
First Two Weeks (Preliminary) Chart
First Quarter Chart
Second Quarter Chart
Third Quarter Chart
Fourth Quarter Chart

11 A Chapter Ends **405**
Spirulina
Chlorella
Olive Leaf
Vitamins and Supplements
Nutraceuticals
Healing Soaks
Detox Tea
Personal Care
Home Maintenance
Food
Cooking Materials
Household Cleaners and Disinfectants
Organic Fabrics
Air Purification
Water Purification
Bug Repellant
Capsule Filling Machine

12 The Politics of Health **428**

Appendices **445**
Appendix A: LS Case Studies	**447**
Appendix B: Non-LS Case Studies	**451**
Appendix C: Recommended Reading	**454**
Appendix D: Recommended Videos	**457**
Appendix E: Healing Protocol Products	**459**
Appendix F: Post Healing Protocol Products	**462**
Appendix G: Other Products	**463**
Appendix H: Organic Food Websites	**468**

Appendix I: Coupons and Discounts	**472**
Appendix J: Health Information	**474**
About the Author	475
Index	477

Acknowledgments

My deepest thanks and gratitude go to the following individuals and groups who, combined, have in so many ways helped me along the road to recovery.

Dr. Robyn Jacobs, my astute gynecologist, who didn't belittle my alternative approach and encouraged me to write this book.

Dr. Steven Coward, who answered my prayers and unknowingly set me on my path of discovery and recovery.

Denise Van Auken, who first suggested an alternative route to this doubting friend.

Kathy Byrd, whose organic products made the very first positive impact in my recovery, and she became a friend in the process.

I am truly indebted to Dr. David A. Jernigan, D.C., who continues to do brilliant and cutting-edge research and development in the field of biological medicine that changed my life forever.

My heartfelt thanks and love go to Carole, Erik, and their daughter, who unhesitatingly provided all the information that I asked for, offered wonderful insights, and bravely took a leap of faith as they stepped into unknown waters when the tide was against them.

Special thanks and love to Susan Winsauer, my dearest friend, confidant, and source of inspiration. Your words of encouragement always came at precisely the right moment and shone like a beacon in my darkest hours.

Evelyn Fazio, my friend and champion for so many years. Thank you for your expertise, guidance, and for helping me turn this monumental effort into reality.

My very special thanks and appreciation belongs to so many individuals and organizations who graciously gave permission to use their words, studies, statistics, articles, and insights. Without them, I could not have created this book.

My deepest love and appreciation goes to my husband, who has never ceased loving me through life's roller coaster ride, for his patience and for always supporting me, even when he may not fully understand me.

Foreword

"Ginny Chandoha hasn't just written a book about Lichen Sclerosis, it's also a book about what we in the naturopathic profession call "nature cure." If you remove the obstacles that prevent your body from working correctly, it will tend to fix itself. The mass of harmful substances that we put in and on our bodies is staggering. As Ginny points out, if you feed yourself well and quit dousing yourself in toxins, you will be well on your way to feeling better. And if you do have Lichen Sclerosis, read the entire book, because Ginny also provides details on how she cured herself using herbs and other therapies. In fact, I'm confident that her protocol will help people with many diseases, including other autoimmune issues.

This could literally be a text book in the naturopathic medical curriculum. Its content is vast, deep, and well-researched. Although I've been involved in natural medicine for twenty years, I still benefit from periodic reminders about how to live well. This book is a strong reminder. I improved my diet and cleaning products immediately upon reading it.

I thoroughly enjoyed this book, and read it again from cover-to-cover. It's one of those books every health care practitioner should read, and one that everyone would benefit from reading, and re-reading periodically."

       Steven Coward, ND
       Asheville Natural Health & Homeopathy

Introduction

Lichen Sclerosis is classified as a "rare" auto-immune disorder that has an unknown cause and for which there is no cure. There are different manifestations of Lichen, such as Lichen Planus, which typically forms lesions in the mouth or anywhere on the skin, including the genitalia. Lichen Sclerosus BXO afflicts the scrotum, foreskin, and/or glans of boys and men. The form of Lichen that affects females of all ages is Lichen Sclerosis et atrophicus. It affects the ano-genital area and the onset of the disease causes intense itching of the genitalia. Typically a corticosteroid cream is prescribed, to be used indefinitely.

In the early stages, white plaques, or spots, can appear anywhere in the ano-genital area, but typically affect the skin between the vagina and anus (the perineum). These white spots of flesh eventually wrinkle, and the skin thins until it tears and bleeds easily from the slightest pressure, often just from sitting down.

As the condition advances, the white plaques can spread over the entire genitalia to the anal area in what is described as a "figure eight" pattern. It can also occur inside the vagina. Vaginal skin can hemorrhage and appear as bruising; it can also form blood blisters. Labial skin can peel, leaving raw skin exposed, which makes urination excruciating. With thinning anal skin, simple bowel movements will tear the anus, causing intense pain and bleeding. The condition also may cause the genitalia to fuse together or be reabsorbed.

Surgery is not recommended unless fusion has caused blockage making urination or defecation difficult. Surgery is also rare because removal of affected areas will not stop the disease, and in 4 to 5 percent of cases, the disease evolves into vulvar cancer.

Lichen Sclerosis is an unbearably painful and hideously disfiguring disease. Marriages of sufferers have been ruined and lives destroyed. Because of the embarrassingly intimate nature of LS, it isn't readily discussed the way other conditions are, and because it is a rare disease, often it is misdiagnosed and treatment can be delayed as a result.

Rather than writing a medical primer on Lichen Sclerosis, it is assumed that the reader either already has received a diagnosis of this disease or else knows someone afflicted with it and thus already understands the specific details of the disease. Background information is available in print on the topic, along with numerous on-line references and websites devoted to Lichen Sclerosis that provide a great deal of information and discussion on the subject.

This book, by contrast, focuses on my personal journey from the moment of my diagnosis, where my research led me and how I reached my own conclusions about what caused my disease, my development and use of my specific healing protocol, and, finally, my medical discharge as a *former* Lichen Sclerosis patient.

During the four years I spent researching for this book, I tried to determine an actual, official number of cases of Lichen Sclerosis in the United States. But because many cases go undetected for years and others are misdiagnosed, the real number is difficult to pinpoint.

As if this disease of women isn't wretched enough when it affects adult women, the saddest cases involve extremely young children. While I haven't found any hard numbers, I did find these eye-opening figures: it is estimated that 15 percent of all cases involve children, and 5 percent of all pre-pubescent girls (ages 4-9) either have or will be diagnosed with Lichen Sclerosis. Today, even infants are being diagnosed with it, whereas it was previously typically found in menopausal women.

Based upon chat sites devoted to the disease and related disorders that I've visited in the course of my research as a sufferer, Lichen Sclerosis afflicts females in Australia, the UK, Sweden, Germany, and other European countries; reports of Lichen Sclerosis in the Middle East and Asia are also beginning to surface. Membership on these sites is in the thousands, with an average of 20 new members signing up per week. Clinical trials are in progress in the United States and Europe, mostly testing new topical creams.

Lichen Sclerosis was first diagnosed in 1887, when it was rare and only found in a handful of post-menopausal women. But now this "rare" disease affects young girls and women in all age groups and races around the globe.

As if the psychological and physical trauma of Lichen Sclerosis isn't unbearable enough, there is an even darker, and just as damaging problem that goes along with this disease, one that needs to be brought out into the open. The parents of my first case study will best describe their ordeal, both for the young girl with the disease, and how it affected her parents.

> *"My daughter always had really bad diaper rash. From 18 months onward she would rather walk or lay on her side than sit on her bottom because of the pain. I took her to the doctor many times, but was made to feel like an overprotective mother and was told not to worry about it, since it was only diaper rash and I should continue to apply diaper cream.*

When my daughter was two, she refused to wear a diaper any more. Toilet training went easily, but she still got sore, but now more localized around her labia and the opening of her vagina, which often made her vagina look bruised. There were purple spots with what looked like little white blisters and it must have itched because she often had her hands down her panties.

One day the daycare asked to speak to me about her behavior. They explained that my daughter was "playing with herself" during sleep time and relaxation time, and that when she wasn't playing, she would put her hands in her panties and rub herself.

Then they gave me a leaflet about child abuse, and had circled the part that reads 'often a child that has been abused would tend to play with their genital area a lot more than a normal healthy child.'

I dismissed that and took my daughter to the doctor. After examining her, he concluded that she had a yeast infection, it was nothing to worry about, and that the condition would go away with the cream that he prescribed. We went back every three to four months for a new prescription because her condition was not clearing up. The purple bruises and little white blister-like spots were still appearing and disappearing at different times.

One day the daycare called me and told me my daughter wouldn't come out of the bathroom and was screaming and holding onto herself. They told me to come as quickly as possible as she was in great distress.

When I arrived, my daughter was in a terrible state and the daycare teacher explained that she had tried to wipe my daughter after her bowel movement and that was when my daughter began screaming and wouldn't stop.

When I managed to calm my daughter down, she told me that the daycare teacher had really hurt her. I examined her and she was bleeding from her anus and her perineum, and her labia were inflamed and sore. I had examined her before she left home that morning and nothing had been out of the ordinary.

When I brought my daughter home, she needed to urinate. I will never forget her screaming while holding onto me so hard she drew blood with her fingernails.

My husband and I took her to the hospital. She was almost 4 years old by now and her pain was my pain; I felt every ounce of it as her mother. I was in tears because I felt there was no way I could help her.

At the hospital she was so desperate to urinate, she began screaming in the waiting room and the staff saw her right away. The doctor took one look at my daughter, left hurriedly, and came back with a pediatrician.

The pediatrician examined my daughter and asked me if she'd ever been abused that we knew of. I said no, not that we were aware of. Then he asked my daughter if anyone had hurt her. She told the doctor that the daycare teacher was always hurting her in the bathroom.

The doctor told me there were definite signs of abuse, especially the bruising, and he showed *me the tear at the entrance to her vagina that I had not seen before. I was asked if the clothes my daughter was wearing were the same ones she had worn to the daycare center, and when I confirmed that they were, they were taken, bagged, and marked as evidence.*

A nightmare was now unfolding before my eyes. The police and child services came immediately and I had to fill out and sign consent forms for them to conduct evidence testing on my daughter. They took swabs of her vagina for every possible kind of sexually transmitted disease. Then they took cotton swabs and wiped them all over my daughter's raw, sore skin, making her scream in pain. Nurses held her down as she screamed for me to help her while they took more samples from inside her vagina and anus. They performed a threadworm (tapeworm) test by placing tape across her anus and pulling the tape off, pulling away some of her skin with the tape, something I will never forget. Then they told me we could take her home and that the police and child services would contact us as soon as the results were in.

The following day I took my daughter to daycare as usual, but the police were there already, talking to the owners of the daycare center. My daughter's daycare teacher was also talking to the police, and they all looked at me as if I had committed some horrible crime. The daycare teacher had been immediately suspended from her duties, pending an investigation, and I was relieved the police and daycare center had acted so quickly.

But my relief was short-lived. Over the next eight months, my husband and I were both interviewed by the police and child services, as was the daycare teacher, and I was shocked to learn that she'd told them she'd thought we were abusing our daughter because she'd seen evidence of it at school. We even wondered about each other's possible guilt; I asked my husband if he had done anything to our daughter, and he was questioning my potential guilt as well.

My husband and I were taken into separate rooms for interrogation. We were terrified! Next, they interviewed our daughter, videotaping her testimony as evidence should the case go to court so she would be spared having to go through it again. We were upset, confused, and devastated. Were we going to lose our daughter? I swore that I wouldn't let that happen.

On the way home, our daughter asked us if we didn't want her anymore because she was sick. The child services interviewer had told her that she might have to stay with another family until she was better. Hearing this, we pulled over and I just held her tight, reassuring her that no one would ever be taking her away and that we wouldn't let her go anywhere without us.

The investigation was thrown out by the prosecution for lack of evidence aside from our daughter's "injuries," which weren't sufficient for a possible conviction. The daycare teacher was reinstated at the school.

Nothing was mentioned about our daughter's "injuries," but we were sent to a doctor specializing in child abuse. He was trained to ask specific questions to determine if a child had been abused, or if they had caused the injuries themselves. The doctor told us that our daughter had probably tried to insert a toy or other object into herself, and that had caused the bruises. He explained that the injuries were probably caused *by scratching herself, and that she had most likely caused her condition herself. Child services visited us on a regular basis, about once a month.*

Although our daughter's condition seemed to calm down for awhile, eventually she began to itch again, and the red, raw, sore skin reappeared, as did the bruising and the white spots. I took my daughter back to the hospital because she was in such incredible pain. We saw the same pediatrician as the previous time, who told us that the results of the previous visit's swabs had come back negative for semen or sexually transmitted diseases. He recommended a repeat treatment using the yeast infection cream.

Over the next few days, my daughter's condition became worse, to the point where I usually had to let her sit in the bathtub with the water running so she could urinate in less agony. The pain was so bad that her heart would beat rapidly, she would sweat profusely and, of course, she'd cry. It was horrific.

With this recurrence, I made an emergency appointment with my doctor, who examined my daughter while I explained the sequence of events to that point. Then he told me that she didn't have a yeast infection, but he suspected thread worms (tapeworms) because her anus was "on fire." Then I explained that she'd already been tested for them and the results were negative. Finally, at a loss for an explanation, my doctor referred me to a pediatrician.

My daughter was only 4 years old at the time and she had suffered so much that she began to refuse to drink anything to avoid urinating. We had to be careful that she didn't become dehydrated, and I tried to explain to her that it was important for her to consume liquids.

During all of this, I had been searching the Internet for diseases having my daughter's symptoms and found a website devoted to Lichen Sclerosis. The symptoms matched my daughter's and I printed every bit of information that I could find, then brought it with me to the appointment with the referred pediatrician.

I repeated my daughter's history and without even examining my daughter or telling her what I suspected, the doctor asked me if I'd ever heard of Lichen Sclerosis.

We were referred to a pediatric dermatologist, who confirmed that our daughter did, indeed, have Lichen Sclerosis. At last, we knew what it was.

We contacted child protective services, as well as the investigating officer in the abuse case against us, who took all of the information I'd discovered, even though the case was closed. I wanted our names to be cleared 100%. I wanted no doubt left in anyone's mind that we had hurt our child.

My daughter was put on Clobetasol, three weeks on, then one week off. Then it was reduced to two weeks on, one week off, and finally, then just once a week. Her skin was becoming transparent and it became a fight to apply the cream, which burned her skin badly, making her cry every time I put it on her. By now, she no longer trusted me, as everything I did to help her only hurt her, and she wasn't getting any better."

How many more little girls will suffer such terrible pain? How many more families will have to go through this kind of nightmare? For this disease to affect so many females of all ages around the world, there has to be a common link. Science has been searching for it, right down to our DNA, but perhaps the link is more common than anyone imagines.

This book has been developed to reveal that the link between auto-immune disorders in general and Lichen Sclerosis in particular is not the mystery the health care industry would have us believe. The cause is staring us in the face, and the cure is right in front of us. But instead of tackling the causes head on, we are instead examining minutia.

Instead of using allopathic creams and ointments that do nothing more than treat symptoms, suppress our immune systems, and keep us sick, in limbo, and on maintenance rather than returning to perfect health, I believe that it's time to take responsibility, be proactive, and reclaim our health.

While writing this book, at times I've been discouraged, especially when what I've accomplished in healing myself was dismissed by people not only in the medical profession but also by friends, family and even on blogs and discussion boards dedicated to LS. And yet, I've felt such joy and renewed motivation when someone encouraged me or explained how I've helped them. My husband has several times said to me, "If no one ever believes you, at least you have managed to cure yourself, and that's all that matters." But no matter what anyone thinks, the fact is that I cured myself of this disease, and if just one person reading this book understands what may be making them sick, discovers their own way to overcome this disease and takes control of their own health, then it has been worth it.

I'm living proof it can be done. And so is one brave little girl who I've never actually met. *Lichen Sclerosis: Beating the Disease* not only tells the story of my own journey from diagnosis to recovery, but also describes the progress of this child as she and her parents followed the protocol I used to heal myself. In addition, I include information about a gentleman who resolved his own health issues not involving Lichen Sclerosis by using the same healing protocol, which I explain in detail in this book.

It is my fervent hope that this book will help others to heal themselves, and I look forward to including their stories in future editions.

Chapter 1
Rude Awakening

On October 8, 2009, the life I'd known was changed forever. That was the day I was diagnosed with Lichen Sclerosis.

I was devastated by this news. How could this have happened to me? I'd done everything to stay healthy for my entire life. I'd taken my vitamins religiously, eaten only healthy foods, including lots of fresh fruits, vegetables, poultry and fish, and rarely ate red meats. Throughout the years I exercised regularly by biking, lifting weights, and running. How could I have acquired a "rare, incurable" disease? Where did I go wrong?

As I began looking for the causes of this disease, I realized that the human body is a wondrous thing and that I didn't really appreciate mine until it wasn't functioning properly. We are born with the self-protection our body needs. Our skin acts as our armor, protecting everything inside it from outside invaders. When we get a cut, our body bleeds to sterilize the wound, and then it forms a protective temporary scab while our body rebuilds itself, cell by cell. Our immune system stands like a sentry, always on guard. It sends in white blood cell warriors to fight off invasions of viruses and bacteria, and creates antibodies to recognize any of those marauders that may return. Old and damaged cells die, replaced by new ones, and there is a constant life-and-death struggle taking place inside us just beneath the surface. We are mostly oblivious to all of this, until our body's mechanisms aren't running smoothly. Our body communicates its difficulties to us, sometimes by pain, something we certainly notice. But sometimes one of the first indicators that something is wrong can be a skin condition, which we not only feel, but see.

In my case, my body began communicating its growing distress for most of my adult life. I can't really pinpoint when it began, but in my early adulthood I developed a tiny crack inside my left nostril. It would scab over, the scab would come off, and then the cycle would repeat. It was so miniscule and unnoticeable to anyone else; just something I lived with. Then, in my twenties, I developed tiny tan, raised, rough patches of skin a dermatologist diagnosed as harmless seborrheic keratoses that formed under my breasts where my bra rubbed against my skin. The dermatologist said they were benign and removed them, and in time a few grew back elsewhere. Knowing what they were, I ignored them, along with the message my body was sending me.

Then, within five years' time, another "minor" ailment appeared: a chronic condition called Blepharitis, which is an inflammation of the eyelids, whose cause is "unknown," and which has no standard cure. The ophthalmologist prescribed daily eye scrub pads. At around the same time, I developed my first ever eye infection, whose onset was sudden and inexplicable. My ophthalmologist accused me of not following his instructions for maintaining my contact lenses properly, but I protested that I'd followed everything to the letter and had not changed what I'd done for years with no problems. He prescribed steroid drops, which kept the infections to a minimum, but from that point on, I had at least two major infections per year. This would not be the last time I'd be blamed for my own illness. I had no idea why these eye conditions had suddenly developed and it never occurred to me that my body was sending me yet another message.

Not long after the eye infections began, I noticed that the skin around my mouth was becoming red, pale on some days, quite bright on others. The dermatologist diagnosed it as Rosacea and suggested I stay away from spicy food. Like my other ailments,

Rosacea is another chronic disorder that has no known cure and there is only speculation about the cause.

None of these conditions seemed related, but in hindsight, I believe that they were. What I didn't understand was that they represented an ever increasing alarm that my body was sounding to show me that something was going wrong.

And it didn't stop there. A few years later, I became allergic to elastic, or at least that's what I thought at the time, because within minutes of putting on a bra, the skin under my breasts would begin to itch and after a few hours, large, red, itchy welts would appear. If I scratched at the welts through my clothing, a red rash would radiate around the welts and the itching would nearly drive me mad. To try and calm the itching, I tried bathing the area, then applying talcum powder, but with no real success. Eventually the itching would subside on its own and the welts would slowly fade within a week, as long as I didn't wear a bra, or I reversed the bra so that cotton fabric, not the elastic, was against my skin.

About two years later, my ongoing minor annoyances stepped up their pace: my eye infections were becoming much more frequent, and instead of a bottle of steroid drops lasting for a few years, I was going through a bottle in a matter of months as those eye eruptions began showing up nearly every month or sooner. Then, the red welts formerly caused by wearing a bra began to appear simply from skin touching skin. I felt as if I was I getting older by the minute and falling apart, and fine lines became visible on my face. I decided that I quickly needed to do something to help myself and made up my mind that the next time I got a catalog offering sample skin care products, I'd try them. I liked how the product samples worked and I soon ordered most of the merchandise.

In the spring of that year I went jogging every day, trying to lose a few pounds. I was approaching my sixth decade, and did not want to be a fat old lady and wanted to stay attractive to my husband. In addition to shaping up, I bathed myself from head to toe in all the skin care products that now took up most of my bathroom closet space.

By the end of that summer, I'd developed an itch around my perineum, the area between the vagina and anus, but it didn't exhibit the symptoms of a yeast infection as it had no odor or discharge, and it didn't include a vaginal itch. I thought that sweat and irritation from jogging might have caused the problem, and my skin itched incessantly and the area looked inflamed. Showering didn't offer any relief, and I tried applying Vaseline, which seemed to help, but not much, and on some days it itched more than others. This went on for about a year.

As if all of this wasn't enough, one day I noticed something odd about my teeth when I checked them in the mirror after brushing. They seemed to have a line of demarcation halfway through them, and when I took a closer look, I was alarmed to see that they were disappearing! Our teeth are filled with dentine that is coated with enamel, and it is the dentine which gives our teeth that solid, opaque appearance. But the dentine in my teeth was missing from the bottom of the tooth to midway up. If I shone a light at my teeth and rubbed my tongue against the back of them, I could see my tongue right through my teeth. They were becoming transparent!

That winter, when I was watching The Oprah Winfrey Show, a doctor discussed how parabens are bad for us because they are hormonal disruptors that mimic estrogen, and can lead to breast cancer. I looked over all my bottles, jars, and tubes of skin care products and found that only a few listed paraben. I sadly set them aside, as they were some of my favorites. When the weather warmed up, I began jogging again when it suddenly occurred to me that the itching had stopped as mysteriously as it had begun. "Good riddance," I thought. But soon there was a new annoyance. The "allergy" to elastic had now spread to my bellybutton, right where the elastic on my panties touched my skin, making the skin crack and ooze slightly on either side. I put Vaseline on that, too, and it would heal, then crack again eventually. My bellybutton would be fine for weeks, but then it would flare up again.

We have been taught to expect that with age comes disease, aches, pains, discomfort, and things going wrong with our bodies, and consequently I attributed all of my minor problems to getting older. Another one of these age-related changes that I noticed was that my vagina seemed to be getting drier with each passing month, so I ordered a paraben-free lubricant, which was messy and inconvenient. To make matters worse, my perineum began to tear and bleed slightly when my husband and I engaged in intercourse, making intercourse painful.

One day while showering, I thought things just didn't feel right "down there," and I didn't remember my perineum feeling wrinkled in the past and my clitoris even felt smaller. "Drying up and shriveling up," I thought. My husband thought I was imagining things after I asked his opinion, and he humored me. My anus seemed to be drying up too, and would sometimes crack slightly and bleed during bowel movements, or from wiping too much or too vigorously. I purchased Vitamin E suppositories and cut them into tiny disks about 1/8 inch thick, and inserted one every night before bedtime. The extra lubrication, along with drinking more water, seemed to work, and I began using a separate Vitamin E suppository as a lubricant for my perineum, applying a coating by using the suppository the way one would apply lipstick. I thought the Vitamin E would help soothe, smooth, and strengthen the skin.

The following spring, I saw a program on bio-identical hormones. Because I'd had a breast cyst removed nine years earlier, I didn't think I was a candidate for hormone replacement therapy, and had heard about the link between HRT and breast cancer. But after seeing the program, I thought bio-identical hormones might be just what I needed. Finding a gynecologist who would prescribe bio-identical hormones proved to be difficult. After searching hospital rosters, the Yellow Pages, and asking friends for a referral, I decided to contact a nearby compounding pharmacy I found. I e-mailed the pharmacist and asked if he compounded bio-identical hormones, and requested a list of doctors who used his services for that purpose. He responded positively and we set up an appointment.

After my seeing the pharmacist and inspecting the compounding facility, I began making a list of the gynecologists who prescribed bio-identical hormones, I made an appointment with Dr. Robyn Jacobs, a certified obstetrician and gynecologist, who practices what she calls 'functional medicine,' which "looks closely at an individual's unique physiology and the role that environmental exposures (food, stress, toxins) play in the expression of health and disease."

I hadn't seen a gynecologist in years, and I told Dr. Jacobs about my vaginal dryness, the tearing of my perineum during intercourse, and then asked for bio-identical hormones. The doctor gave me a Body Composition Analysis, something I'd never experienced before. I had to lie still, without speaking with electrodes attached to my wrist and ankle. Then a low electrical current was coursed through my body, something I couldn't feel and which took only a matter of seconds.

The Body Composition Analysis revealed more about my insides than I ever wanted to know, including Weight, Fat Mass (FM), Fat Free Mass (FFM), Body Mass Index (BMI), Total Body Water (TBW), Extracellular Water (ECW), and Intracellular Water (ICW), also called Intracellular Fluids (ICF). Extracellular Water (ECW) refers to how much water your skin cells are retaining and Intracellular Water (ICW/ICF) indicates how much water your cells hold on a molecular level. About 99% of cellular molecules are water molecules, with water normally accounting for approximately 70% of the total wet-weight of a cell. Mine were reading 52.4%, and I was totally unaware of molecular cell structure, so the ICW/ICF numbers were meaningless to me. The only numbers that I focused on were for Fat Mass.

My physical examination was the first in a long time that a doctor had looked closely at my vaginal area. Dr. Jacobs told me that my vagina was inflamed, so she put a smear under the microscope to rule out a yeast infection. She prescribed estriol, a bio-identical hormone that regulates vaginal lubrication, in the form of a tiny, waxy-looking vaginal suppository to be used once a week.

She briefly discussed my perineum, telling me it looked "puckered," but before she could make a diagnosis, she needed to do a biopsy. She told me that the rest of my "architecture" looked pretty normal, except that my right labia minor had "re-absorbed," meaning it had shrunken to half its normal size and was very thin, not plump like the rest of my labia. I was unaware of it then, but it was a symptom of Lichen Sclerosis. After the exam, Dr. Jacobs ordered blood work, a mammogram, a bone density scan (DXA), and made a follow-up appointment in two weeks. As we walked back to our car, my husband asked how everything had gone. "Great," I said, "except for the biopsy." He hesitated, and then, in almost a whisper asked, "Of your breasts?" I explained everything Dr. Jacobs had said and done. Dr. Jacobs had not made an issue of anything, and I was sure some bio-identical hormones would fix me right up.

Two weeks later I returned to Dr. Jacobs' office for the test results and found that I have naturally high "good" cholesterol, and my vitamin and mineral levels met or exceeded the requirements for someone my age. She advised me to cut back on iron because I didn't need it, and that too much iron can contribute to illness. Her other advice was to increase my Vitamin D because I live in an area that doesn't get a lot of sun, especially in winter, and to split my calcium supplements between morning and evening. My bone density is fine, my mammogram was negative. I felt like I'd passed with flying colors.

But then she discussed the results of the biopsy and she said I had a condition called Lichen Sclerosis, which I'd never heard of. She prescribed a corticosteroid cream, Clobetasol Propionate, and said to apply it every day for two weeks, then to taper off to once or twice a week. She didn't say how long I should continue to use the cream, but I figured it would be like anything else: you apply it for a week or two, and that would be the end of that. "How long should I use the cream," I asked naively. She didn't really respond and an alarm sounded in my brain. "You mean, like forever!" I asked incredulously. "Well, yes," she said, and explained that it was an immune disorder. It could be from something I was eating, but because my case was so "mild," she didn't feel a food elimination diet was warranted. She then said that 4%-6% of cases turn into vulvar cancer, and she wanted to examine me every six months to keep an eye on my condition. I had suddenly gone from healthy to sick with a chronic illness that could lead to cancer! She examined me again, and I could hear the disappointment in her voice as she found another white patch between my left labias. She instructed me to rub a thin film of the Clobetasol cream on both sides between the labia, starting at the top crease at the clitoris, and all the way down to the perineum, on both sides. I left her office in disbelief and vowed to research the steroid cream and this unheard of disease as soon as I got home.

An auto-immune disorder? How could this have happened to me? It was embarrassing and unbelievable! How could my body have betrayed me? I'd done everything right. I'd been the picture of health!

The picture of health. It's amazing what we accept as health. If my body had an audible voice, I'm sure the conversation would have sounded something like this:

"*Hello!* Your nostril always had a crack and a scab. You ignored that, so I gave you seborrheic keratosis! You thought you had cancer. Scared you didn't I? Obviously not enough!

What do I have to do to make you hear me? I made your face turn red with rosacea! You stopped eating spicy food! Don't you get it? I'm sick!

I sent you another message! Blepharitis! Did you really think eye-scrubbing pads were going to fix it?

Hey! I told you that I was getting sicker by causing eye infections! You used steroid drops! You weren't listening!

Next it was itching red welts! I'm telling you there's something wrong with me! Couldn't you put it together?

You've ignored all of my warnings! Now it's Lichen Sclerosis. *Can you hear me now?*"

Loud and clear.

I Googled Clobetasol Propionate, the steroid cream that was prescribed for me, and discovered that all of the creams prescribed for Lichen Sclerosis suppress the immune system, and over time, have skin-thinning properties. I didn't think suppressing my immune system sounded like a good idea, and Lichen Sclerosis is already a skin-thinning disease, so why would I want to indefinitely apply to my skin a cream that also had those attributes? That would only be adding insult to injury. I had a sinking feeling.

My next search on the Internet made my heart pound and a knot grew in my stomach with every word I read about Lichen Sclerosis. "Unknown cause, no known cure, vulvar cancer, high morbidity" was the mantra. And then there were the photographs of advanced cases of the disease. I was terrified by the pictures of women with deformed genitals and turned to online chat groups and blogs devoted to the subject. They offered support and suggestions, but no solutions. Everyone seemed to be in a holding pattern of maintenance, waiting for the discovery of a cure. I turned away from the groups because reading all the horrible individual descriptions of symptoms only compounded my growing hysteria. I'd commit suicide before I ended up looking like what I saw in those photographs.

I'd always felt like I had led a charmed life, but not anymore. Now I felt nothing but fear, embarrassment, and isolation and was living in a Lichen Sclerosis vacuum. I could not bring myself to discuss it with anyone, except to say that I had a skin condition.

How did I get to this crossroad in my life? In desperation, I mentally examined the past years, trying to figure out what could have caused this disease. There had to be a cause. It just doesn't happen out of thin air, and for everything in nature, there is cause and effect. But my life is pretty mundane; I eat the same things and do the same things most of the time. What had I introduced into my life that was different? Was it food, as Dr. Jacobs had suggested, or something else?

After my diagnosis, I spent every waking moment researching Lichen Sclerosis. Because I couldn't sleep, I continued long into the night, looking at scientific evidence, and reading medical facts, statistics, theories, treatments, and clinical trials. And the more I read, the more distraught I became. After my diagnosis, I broke out in rashes, itched everywhere, and was utterly miserable just from stress.

My husband could not understand my panic and thought it was from reading all the bad news as I researched. "Leave it to you to come up with some weird disease," he commented and he blamed me for my disease. "You'd come back from running and wouldn't shower or change your clothes for hours," he'd say accusingly. I felt angry and frustrated because he couldn't seem to grasp the profound affect this disease had on me and would continue to have for the remainder of our lives. He thought I was obsessing over nothing and was irritated with me. He wanted to know why I couldn't just use the cream the doctor had prescribed and go on with my life? What was the big deal?

Despite my misgivings, I applied the cream once as instructed; not only did it not stop the itching and rashes that now seemed to be everywhere on my body, it also burned my tender genital skin and made matters even worse. I couldn't wash it off fast enough and found it completely unsatisfactory. And on top of the cream not working, nothing I read made any sense to me. Like my useless prescription, every suggestion I found online was for topical medications that only treated the symptoms. Nothing addressed the actual cause of the disease.

The effect of the diagnosis of LS was terrible for me. I could not sleep and could not stop thinking about the disease. I'd go to bed hoping to die in my sleep, but sleep was elusive as fear gripped my mind and visions of deformity encroached on every waking moment. I could think of nothing else except this horrible disease, but unlike other diseases, Lichen Sclerosis was much too personal and too awful to discuss with even my closest friends, and the stress was unbearable.

I knew that if I didn't get a grip on my life and my emotions, the effects of this stress would completely ruin my health. Feeling utterly alone and despondent, I reached out to the homeopathic doctor who was treating my brother. I emailed him and asked for his help, and he agreed to work with me. It was a huge weight off my shoulders to know I would no longer be facing this burden alone, and Dr. Steven Coward became the only light shining in my darkness. He had a calming and positive effect, and said several key things, the first being that "No disease is incurable," and the second, that "All diseases are organic in nature."

But there was one thing he said that really clicked in my brain. "Auto-immune disease means your immune system is inflamed." When Dr. Coward uttered those words, he not only turned my distress into determination; he also set me on the course that would end my nightmare.

What Dr. Coward said seemed to take away the mystery and scariness out of the term "auto-immune." Now it sounded conquerable, even though I felt like I was fumbling around in a dark room, trying to find the switch that had turned my immune system on full blast so I could turn it off again.

He also advised me not to use Clobetasol, and instead instructed me to take 1,000 mg of Omega-3 supplements four times a day, which would act as a natural anti-inflammatory. Although I hadn't been using Clobetasol, I felt fearful being told not to use it because it was the only medication available that might keep the disorder from progressing. I'd reasoned that if things seemed to be getting worse, I could always resort to using the Clobetasol, but now I felt like I was standing on a precipice. It was a leap of faith because I had no idea how this was going to turn out.

But despite this, eventually all the pieces began to fit in this auto-immune puzzle. My days and nights of constant research, along with something my doctor had said, and a suggestion made by a friend all helped make clear what had caused me to develop Lichen Sclerosis and then led to my recovery.

I started a daily journal, which proved to be valuable in tracking my journey to healing, and I also began a photo journal. Although they were intended to track the progression of the disease, they instead, recorded my recovery. Now, with my emotions in check, I was ready to get down to the serious business of finding a way to heal myself. I'd spent most of my working life in the computer industry so I was used to running diagnostics. I would apply those same skills to find what had corrupted my genetic software and damaged my physical hardware.

My mind replayed my life like a slide show, trying to find the moment my immune system went over the edge; as the images ran through my mind, each time it paused on the same frame. It was suddenly clear to me how this had all started.

Chapter 2
Toxic Topicals

"Chemicals have replaced bacteria and viruses as the main threat to human health....The diseases we're beginning to see as the major causes of death in the latter part of this century and into the 21st century are diseases of chemical origin."

Dr. Rick Irvin, Toxicologist, Texas A&M University

"Any type of control over the chemicals used in products would stifle innovation if manufacturers first had to prove their products were safe before bringing them to market."

Michael Walls, American Chemistry Council

The onset of my perineum starting to itch occurred several months after I'd begun using skin care products, something I had never done before. Could that be it? They were "natural," and full of "beneficial" botanicals and oils such as olive, jojoba, and others. But there were also a lot of other things included in these products, things I wasn't familiar with and had no idea why they were in the products.

In full investigation mode, I gathered up all the bars, jars, tubes, and bottles of soap, toner, moisturizers, facial scrub, facial mask, and cleanser, even the ones I'd put aside and had stopped using, and lined them up by my computer. I'd found the Environmental Working Group's cosmetics industry database Skin Deep, the most comprehensive compilation of ingredients used in every product found in supermarkets, cosmetics counters, and pharmacies, and began entering into the EWG's database the ingredients listed on all the skin care products as well as my shampoo, bars of soap, toothpaste, laundry and dish detergent, over-the-counter ointments such as hydrocortisone, and the Clobetasol.

Per the product insert, here is what Clobetasol contains: **Clobetasol propionate** - A *synthetic fluorinated* corticosteroid, in a base of:

- **Hypromellose** – A propylene glycol ether of Methylcellulose. Studies show gastrointestinal effects.

- **Propylene Glycol** – Provokes skin irritation and sensitization in concentrations as low as 2%. Linked to cancer, developmental and reproductive toxicity, immunotoxicity, organ system toxicity, cellular level changes, and neurotoxicity.

- **Mineral Oil** – Used as a skin protectant, it is a liquid mixture of hydrocarbons obtained from petroleum. Linked to cancer, immunotoxicity, organ system toxicity, and skin, eye and lung irritation.

- **Polyoxyethylene Glycol 300 Isostearate** – Used as a binder or lubricant, it is regarded as "safe" for use in cosmetics with limited exposure. It is *not considered safe to use on injured or damaged skin* (precisely what LS skin is). It is linked to organ system toxicity, as well as contamination with ethylene oxide, and 1.4-dioxane.

- **Sodium Hydroxide** – An inorganic base, it is linked to cancer, neurotoxicity, organ system toxicity. Studies show metabolic effects at very low doses.

- **Carbomer 1342** – Not assessed for safety. Carbomer is a term used for a series of polymers made from acrylic acid. Carbomers are white, fluffy powders but are used as gels in cosmetics and personal care products.

No wonder Clobetasol burns our skin, or that Lichen Sclerosis can evolve into cancer of the vulva! I was supposed to put this on myself indefinitely? I don't think so! After researching the ingredients in Clobetasol, I fully understood the product warning not to use it for long periods of time. It's not because it is so potent or effective, it is because it is so toxic.

I continued checking the ingredients in every product I'd been using, some of which I'd used only occasionally, some weekly, but most of which I used daily for most of my life, including shampoo, deodorant, toothpaste, talcum powder, hydrocortisone cream, and shaving gel. What I discovered was so distressing that I developed a full body rash from head to toe. My heart pounded, I had panic attacks, lost sleep and my appetite, and had a constant knot in the pit of my stomach. Why? Because I discovered that there are over 80,000 chemicals in our daily environment, with an average of 3,000 new chemicals added each year, including personal care products. Here is a sampling of the ingredients I found in my everyday products, along with their implications:

- **Ammonium Hydroxide** – Concerns about this ingredient include bio-accumulation, organ system toxicity, skin, eye and lung irritation, and cancer. This ingredient can be found in hair color and bleaching, moisturizers, toners, anti-aging formulas, mascara, acne remedies.

- **Benzoyl Peroxide** – There is strong evidence linking it to organ system toxicity, skin/eye/lung irritation, immunotoxicity, developmental and reproductive toxicity, and cancer. Products that may contain benzoyl peroxide include facial cleanser, bar soap, exfoliants, shaving cream, moisturizer, nail polish, facial mask, nail glue, and acne remedies.

- **Butylene Glycol** – Studies show growing evidence that this ingredient is linked to neurotoxicity, endocrine disruption, organ system toxicity, and developmental/reproductive toxicity. It can be found in moisturizers, foundation, anti-aging formulas, facial cleanser, eye cream, mascara, sunscreen SPF 15-30.

- **Ceteareth-20** – Linked to neurotoxicity, organ system toxicity, skin, eye and lung irritation at low doses, enhanced skin absorption, contamination concerns, and violation of industry recommendations. Deemed unsafe for injured or damaged skin.

- **Cocamidopropyl Betaine (Betane)** - It's an inner salt of the fatty acids derived from coconut oil. It doesn't sound as if it would be harmful but it is a known immune system toxicant, and is often contaminated with 3-dimethylaminopropylamine (an immunotoxicant), and nitrosimes (impurities linked to cancer, developmental and reproductive toxicity, immunotoxicity, allergies, endocrine disruption, organ system disruption, neurotoxicty, and cellular level changes).

- **Dimethicone** – Linked to organ system toxicity.

- **Disodium EDTA** – Studies as far back as 1956 show brain, nervous system, and behavioral effects at low doses. This ingredient is linked to endocrine disruption, neurotoxicity, organ system toxicity, enhanced skin absorption, developmental and reproductive toxicity, and cancer.

- **Disodium Ethylene Dicocamide PEG-15 Disulfate** – Used as a humectant for moisture retention, solvent, binder, emulsion stabilizer, and viscosity agent, it is deemed unsafe on injured or damaged skin. It is linked to organ system toxicity, as well as ethylene oxide and 1.4-dioxane contamination.

- **Fragrance** – Top prize goes to this concoction of chemicals. Research reveals repeated exposure to this ingredient can cause neurotoxicity, immunotoxicity, and allergies. According to USFDA regulations, "fragrance" is considered proprietary and a manufacturer does not need to reveal the contents. It can contain in excess of 20 chemicals. Fragrance is found in practically everything, including shampoos, conditioners, deodorants, moisturizers, makeup, bath soaps, bubble bath soaps, baby shampoo/powder/lotions/oils/creams, nail polish, polish remover, suntan preparations, bleaches, hair coloring, aftershave lotions, foot powders, feminine hygiene deodorants, nighttime skin preparations, perfumes, body washes, dish and laundry detergents. The list goes on and on.

- **Glyceryl Stearate Citrate** – Used as an emulsifier, the Cosmetic Ingredient Review Board assesses this ingredient to be safe only when used in prescribed concentrations, or limitations. Considered safe based on assumption of low absorption. The Cosmetic Safety Review Board is a self-regulating cosmetics industry panel that has provided no safety data. This assessment is based upon testing of a related chemical, not this one in particular.

- **Lauric Acid** – A fatty acid with many s̄ product uses, such as emulsifier, surfactu͏̄ and "fragrance" ingredient. Studies done as long as 40 years ago show brain, nervous system, and/or behavioral effects at low doses. This ingredient is linked to cancer, neurotoxicity, organ system toxicity, and skin irritation.

- **Magnesium Aluminum Silicate** – This ingredient shows strong evidence of neurotoxicity, organ system toxicity, developmental and reproductive toxicity. High levels of aluminum in the brain have been linked to dementia diseases such as Alzheimer's. Found in deodorants.

- **Methylparaben** – One of several chemicals in the paraben family, research shows exposure to this ingredient can cause neurotoxicity, biochemical or cellular level changes, endocrine disruption, organ system toxicity, immunotoxicity, cancer. Products containing this chemical include facial moisturizer, foundation, anti-aging formulas, eye shadow, mascara, hair color and bleaching, facial cleansers, conditioners.

- **Niacinamide** – In vitro tests show positive cell mutation. One or more animal studies show endocrine disruption at moderate doses, blood and liver effects at very low doses. Other studies show biochemical changes at very low doses that are not yet understood how human health is impacted.

- **Nitrosamines** – This impurity lights up the hazard board with great concerns about neurotoxicity, endocrine disruption, organ system toxicity, biochemical/cellular level changes, immunotoxicity, developmental and reproductive toxicity and cancer. Products that can contain this impurity include, moisturizer, shampoo, body wash, facial cleansers, anti-aging formulas, mascara, nail polish, hair color and bleaching, foundation, conditioner, styling gel, hair spray, sunscreen SPF 15-30, acne remedies, lipstick, eyeliner, eye cream, eye shadow, dandruff/scalp treatment, shaving cream, concealer, bubble bath, toners, facial masks, toothpaste, lip balm, after shave, bar soap, lip gloss, baby shampoo, tooth whitening, makeup remover, anti-itch/rash creams, blush.

- **Panthenol** – This ingredient can come from plant or animal sources, or may be a synthetic. Animal studies indicate broad systemic effects at high does. There is little to no toxicity information available.

- **Paraben** – Parabens are known neurotoxins, endocrine disruptors, linked to organ system toxicity, developmental/reproductive toxicity, and cancer. Paraben is found in shampoo, conditioners, deodorant, makeup remover, tanning oils, exfoliants, shaving cream, hair relaxer, and sunscreen, as well as many other commercial products, including hydrocortisone cream, even "natural" products like calendula gel.

- **Propylparaben** – A member of the paraben chemical family, there is strong evidence pointing to endocrine disruption, organ system toxicity, immunotoxicity, developmental and reproductive toxicity, and cancer. It can be found in moisturizers, foundation, lipstick, eye shadow, mascara, anti-aging formulas, sunscreen, makeup, lip gloss, and facial cleansers.

Why are parabens (including methylparaben, butylparaben, isobutylparaben, ethylparaben, and propylparaben) found in nearly every topical cream, cosmetic, or over-the-counter ointments? The compounding pharmacist explained to me that parabens act as a preservative, giving products a longer shelf life. As if putting this poison on us isn't bad enough, we may be eating it too. Recently I found parabens and methylparaben listed as ingredients on a package of donuts!

In a recent study, tissue samples taken from 20 mastectomy breast tumors were found to have one or more concentrations of different parabens in 99% of the samples. Over 60% of the tissue samples had concentrations of all five parabens. The concentrations in nanograms per tissue sample were:

1. propylparaben – 16.8
2. methylparaben – 16.6
3. butylparaben – 5.8
4. ethylparaben – 3.4
5. isobutylparaben – 2.1

- **Pentylene Glycol** – One or more animal studies show brain, nervous system, or behavioral effects at high doses. It is linked to neurotoxicity, organ system toxicity, and skin/eye/lung irritation.

- **Propylene Glycol** – This ingredient hits the jackpot in possible hazards. It is considered "non-toxic" when taken orally, but provokes skin irritation and sensitization in humans at concentrations as low as 2%. Industry products can contain up to 50%. It is linked to cancer, developmental and reproductive toxicity, immunotoxicity, enhanced skin absorption, organ system toxicity, neurotoxicity, and cellular level changes. It's an ingredient used in anti-freeze and is found in hair color and bleaching, moisturizers, anti-aging formulas, conditioner, foundation, styling gel, shampoo, mascara, facial cleansers, is an ingredient in fragrance, and as previously mentioned, used in Clobetasol to treat Lichen Sclerosis.

- **Red 33** (CI 17200) – Linked to cancer, it is a colorant used in lipstick, makeup remover, bath products, and moisturizer.

- **Red 40** (CI 16035) – FD&C colors are bituminous coal or petrochemical derivatives and are continuously animal tested due to carcinogen properties. This colorant is linked to cancer, developmental and reproductive toxicity, and organ system toxicity.

- **Sodium Hyaluronate** – Studies show neurotoxicity, organ system toxicity, developmental/reproductive toxicity, and skin/eye/lung irritation at moderate doses.

- **Sodium Hydroxide** – Its common name is lye, or caustic soda, and is approved by the FDA for use as a food additive. The cosmetics industry uses it as a pH adjuster and buffering agent. It has not been assessed for safety by the industry cosmetics panel. It is linked to neurotoxicity at very low doses, as well as skin/eye/lung irritation, and cancer.

- **Sodium Lauroyl Isethionate** - It acts as a surfactant. Surfacants are abrasive chemical ingredients found in most commercial cleansing products. In vitro tests on mammalian cells show positive mutation.

- **Sodium Palmitate** - Used as a surfactant, the sodium salt of palmitic acid. It is also u as a food additive! Studies indicate cell mutation, and bio-accumulation, which means our body cannot readily degrade or easily eliminate it, thus it is stored in every cell of our body. Over time, the accumulation in our body becomes toxic overload.

- **Sodium Silicate** - It is the sodium salt of silicic acid and is linked to allergies, immunotoxicity, organ system toxicity, and skin irritation.

- **Sodium Stearate** - The sodium salt of stearic acid is used as a surfactant, viscosity agent, and emulsifier. Very early studies show broad systemic effects at moderate doses. Aside from being an environmental concern, it is linked to organ system toxicity. It is an ingredient in deodorants, soaps, eye shadow, shaving cream, moisturizer, body wash, and exfoliant scrubs.

- **Sorbitol** – It is a sugar alcohol that acts as a humectant for moisture retention and thickening. Not only is it used by the cosmetics industry, but it is also used in the pharmaceutical and food industries as a sweetener and gelling agent. In vitro tests show positive mammalian cell mutation. Sorbitol is linked to organ system toxicity, and cancer. It's an ingredient used in mouthwash and toothpaste.

- **Stearic Acid** - It acts as a surfactant, as well as an emulsifying agent. It is also an ingredient in the blanket term "fragrance." It is linked to cancer, neurotoxicity, organ system toxicity, and skin irritation.

- **Tetrasodium EDTA** – It's a chelating agent that allows for enhanced skin absorption and is linked to organ system toxicity and skin irritation. It is found in shampoo, bar soap, body washes, facial moisturizers, foundation, eye shadow, and hair coloring.

- **Tetrasodium Etidronate** – It is a diphosphonic acid derivative, and acts as a chelating agent, emulsifier, and viscosity controller. Linked to organ system toxicity, studies show kidney or renal system effects at moderate doses. Found in detergents and other cleaning agents, cosmetics, and swimming pool chemicals.

- **Triclosan** – This chemical is found in anti-bacterial soaps as the active ingredient. It is linked to liver and inhalation toxicity, and even low levels of triclosan may disrupt thyroid function. The American Medical Association recommends that triclosan not be used in the home, as it may encourage bacterial resistance to antibiotics.

- **Titanium Dioxide** (CI 77891) – A colorant with low skin absorption properties on its own, but studies have not been conducted to trace the effect when coupled with other skin absorbing agents. The concern is when the ingredient is inhaled. It is carcinogenic and linked to immunotoxicity, cancer, organ system toxicity, cellular level changes, and skin, eye, and lung irritation.

- **Yellow 5** – A colorant found in personal care products, it is linked to cancer, developmental and reproductive toxicity, neurotoxicity, organ system toxicity, and bioaccumulation. Studies show effects at very low doses.

- **Yellow 6** – A colorant linked to cancer, developmental/reproductive toxicity, neurotoxicity, organ system toxicity.

- **Sodium Lauryl Sulfate/Sodium Laureth Sulfate** (referred to as SLS/SLES)

  I link these two ingredients together because they are often combined in products. Combined, or individually, I consider them to be some of the most hazardous and frightening of all ingredients, which is why I'm devoting so much space to these two chemicals.

  Also known as sulfuric acid monododecyl ester sodium salt, SLS is commonly contaminated with dioxane. Concentrations of SLS as low as 0.5% can cause irritation, 10-30% concentration can cause severe irritation, and skin corrosion. Some soaps contain as much as 30% SLS. SLS is usually the number one active ingredient in all soaps, shampoos, toothpastes, cleansers, laundry detergents, dish detergents, and just about everything that has a foaming action.

  Thanks to "deep penetrating" chemicals in personal care products, SLS enters the body through the skin. Because these are synthetic chemicals, the liver cannot break down and eliminate them, and residual levels remain in the heart liver, lungs, and the brain.

  Once in the body, the SLS molecule attaches to estrogen hormone receptors, mimicking the effects of estrogen in various systems. The result is that the body cannot distinguish between estrogen our body makes (endogenous), and SLS, which affects normal endocrine functions.

SLS also contains protein denaturing properties. Our cells are made from protein and our bodies are continually producing new cells to replace old and damaged ones. SLS forms a chemical bridge between fat-soluble and water-soluble parts of the protein molecule, which disrupts the hydrophobic process needed to maintain a cell's protein structure. The end result is that existing proteins are damaged, and new proteins under construction can be damaged as well. In other words, the cellular template has been damaged, which causes us to reproduce imperfect cells. This denaturing effect on cell reproduction is *usually irreversible*, and can also lead to early stage skin cancer.

On websites devoted to Lichen Sclerosis, I'd find references to using "milder" soaps, such as Dove or Cetaphil. I researched the ingredients of those products as well and the results were not encouraging. Let's take a look at what these "mild" soaps contain.

ABOUT SOAP

Dove Cream Oil Ultra Rich Velvet Beauty Bar
Ingredients: Sodium Lauroyl Isethionate, Stearic Acid, Sodium Tallowate or Sodium Palmitate, Lauric Acid, Sodium Isethionate, Water, Sodium Stearate, Cocamidopropyl Betaine, Helianthus Annuss (Sunflower) Seed Oil, Sodium Cocoate or Sodium Palm Kernelate, Fragrance, Sodium Chloride, Propylene Glycol, Tetrasodium EDTA, Tetrasodium Etidronate, Red 33 (CI 17200), Red 40 (CI 16035), Titanium Dioxide (CI 77891).

Dove Nourishing Care Shea Butter Beauty Bar
Ingredients: Sodium Lauroyl Isethionate, Stearic Acid, Sodium Tallowate or Sodium Palmitate, Lauric Acid,

Sodium Isethionate, Water, Sodium Stearate, Cocamidopropyl Betane, Sodium Cocoate or Sodium Palm Kernelate, Fragrance, Butyrospermum Parkii (Shea Butter), Sodium Chloride, Tetrasodium EDTA, Tetrasodium Etidronate, Titanium Dioxide, Yellow 5, Yellow 6.

Dove White Beauty Bar
Ingredients: Sodium Lauroyl Isethionate, Stearic Acid, Sodium Tallowate or Sodium Palmitate, Lauric Acid, Sodium Isethionate, Water, Sodium Stearate, Cocamidopropyl Betaine, Sodium Cocoate or Sodium Palm Kernelate, Fragrance, Sodium Chloride, Tetrasodium EDTA, Tetrasodium Etidronate, Titanium Dioxide (CI 77891).

Cetaphil
Ingredients: Water, Glycerin, Caprylic/Capric Triglyceride, Helianthus Annuus (Sunflower) Seed Oil, Pentylene Glycol, Butyrospermum Parkii (Shea Butter), Sorbitol, Cyclopentasiloxane, Cetearyl Alcohol, Behenyl Alcohol, Glyceryl Stearate, Tocopheryl Acetate, Hydroxypalmitoyl Sphinganine, Niacinamide, Allantoin, Panthenol, Arginine, Disodium Ethylene Dicocamide PEG-15 Disulfate, Glyceryl Stearate Citrate, Sodium PCA, Ceteareth-20, Sodium Polyacrylate, Caprylyl Glycol, Citric Acid, Dimethiconol, Disodium EDTA, Sodium Hyaluronate, Cetyl Alcohol.

Glycerin Soap

It is rare for real soap makers to actually "make" glycerin. For commercial use, glycerin soap is referred to as "melt and pour" soap. The only way a soap base can be melted and poured is if it has propylene glycol added to it. What makes it clear is that alcohol is added. A manufacturer simply buys pre-made glycerin base, melts it, adds dyes (chemical) and fragrance (chemical scent, not essential oils), and pours it into molds. Do not think for one minute that glycerin soap is any better than any other commercial soap. And don't be fooled into thinking that liquid glycerin soap is a safe alternative. In order for it to remain liquid, it is usually combined with several other toxic chemicals such as sodium lauryl sulfate. The only soap you can be certain that does not have chemicals, dyes, or fragrance is 100% organic soap.

When researching the ingredients of various products, I found it quite interesting when visiting manufacturer websites. Rarely could I find a list of actual ingredients. Instead, the sites were filled with *puffery*, a legal term used in the advertising industry to exaggerate the quality of a seller's product, the validity of which cannot be precisely determined.

The personal care industry claims these ingredients are not harmful in such small amounts. Keep in mind that industry is self-policing, and therefore companies can claim anything they want about the safety of their products. While these ingredients alone might not be harmful in small amounts, there are no studies on the effects of these ingredients when combined. Many have not been tested or assessed for safety whatsoever. They are assumed safe on the assumption of low skin absorption, yet they are combined with chemicals that enhance skin absorption.

Why should we assume that any chemicals are safe, no matter how much or how little is used? At what level is repeated exposure to small amounts of lead considered safe? How much mercury is safe? How much arsenic? We now know that no amount of exposure to any of those three compounds is safe. Would we knowingly rub lead, mercury, or arsenic on ourselves? I doubt it, but we may be doing exactly that by using many products we keep in our homes. Why do we readily accept daily doses of so many chemicals found in our everyday personal care products?

After investigating all those ingredients, I began thinking long and hard about how every single product in our house contained one or more of the hazardous chemicals listed above. How could I not come to the conclusion that these chemicals were responsible for my skin and other conditions? After all, our skin is not only the largest organ of elimination; it's also the largest organ of absorption, making chemicals absorbed through our skin more toxic than if we'd eaten them. And these toxins were in the soap I'd bathe with. No wonder I'd itch right after a shower! They're also in the shampoo, the conditioner, and the deodorant. There's fragrance in talcum powder, too. These toxic chemicals are in moisturizers and skin creams, dish detergents, laundry detergents, and even the most "natural" toothpaste on the market.

After coming to this realization of the toxic overload surrounding me, one day, I went through the house and emptied our shelves of every personal care product we owned, much to my husband's chagrin. Next I thought about our laundry. Clothing is washed in detergent containing toxic chemicals, which make our clothes stiff and rough. Another chemical, "fabric softener," is required to make clothes feel soft, and then, yet another chemical-laden product is used in the dryer to avoid static cling.

The result of all this is that the body is bathed in chemicals and our clothing retains the laundry detergent chemicals no matter how many times they are rinsed. Even laundered bedding is full of it, and it's appalling to think that our bodies are surrounded by these toxins 24 hours a day as we bathe in them, wear them, and sleep in them.

We even brush our teeth with SLS. While many products contain skin penetrating chemicals, SLS in the mouth has a much faster point of entry: sublingual. *Sublingual,* from Latin, literally means "under the tongue." It is a pharmacological route whereby drugs, enzymes, or chemicals can enter directly into the bloodstream via absorption under the tongue. Sublingual absorption is efficient at a rate of 3 to 10 times greater than swallowing, and is surpassed only by hypodermic injection. When SLS is introduced in the mouth via toothpaste, it can be quickly absorbed into the blood stream and carried to every tissue, every organ of the body, including the brain.

Maybe all of these chemicals by themselves seem harmless. For instance, potassium nitrate, sulfur, and charcoal aren't deadly by themselves. But mix them together and you've created an explosive. The cocktail of chemicals being combined in our everyday products have created a toxic time bomb within our bodies and we are developing "rare" and "incurable" diseases as a result.

I felt sick after reading about all the poisons in the products I was using, and I also felt betrayed and angry that my body had been damaged beyond repair! Maybe I couldn't change what had already happened to me, but I certainly wasn't going to allow more damage to occur by continuing to use these dangerous products.

I searched the Environmental Working Group's website for toxin-free soap. Sadly, of thousands of manufacturers, only a handful popped up whose products were rated toxin-free. Out of the shockingly brief list, I picked one that appealed to me because of the name: Soap for Goodness Sake. A lovely lady, Kathy, makes organic, toxin-free soap in her Oklahoma kitchen. Browsing her website, I was delighted to learn that she uses only organic ingredients and high-grade essential oils.

One thing to bear in mind is that not all essential oils are created equal. The essential oils used in most soaps and detergents, including many "handmade" soaps found in health and specialty shops, are cheaper oils achieved through chemical processing, and contain hexane. Hexane is a chemical derived from crude oil, and is used as a solvent. High grade essential oils are organic and achieved by extracting plant oils through cold pressing, or steam distillation, making them more expensive. Most commercial products merely contain fragrance, which we know is nothing more than a concoction of more chemicals.

In addition, just because a product lists olive oil as an ingredient, it doesn't make it good. Unless it is labeled as organic extra virgin olive oil, it is actually pomace olive oil, which is made from the last pressing of any possible remaining oil from olives that have been previously repeatedly pressed. To get every last drop, a chemical such as hexane is added to force the last bit of remaining oil to depart from the fruit. That inevitably leaves traces of hexane in the oil, which then ends up in products made from it, including supposedly high quality soap.

On the Soap for Goodness Sake website I was delighted to find organic unscented soaps without a long list of unpronounceable ingredients. There are many soap products to choose from, but I wanted soap with the least amount of ingredients. My skin tends to be on the dry side, thus my personal favorite is saponified organic extra virgin olive oil soap, which I still use. The two ingredients are organic extra virgin olive oil, and water, period. Saponification occurs when an alkali (lye) and acid (vegetable oil such as extra virgin olive or virgin coconut oil) are combined. A chemical reaction occurs, and the outcome is what we know as soap.

Because Lichen Sclerosis skin has been damaged and sensitized, for people with LS, and for even those who do not have the disease, *less is more*. We have been programmed to believe we need more lather, more scent, and more of everything. But our skin is already permeable, and "skin penetrating" and "deep penetrating" chemicals in personal care products make it even more permeable, allowing it to be infiltrated by a multitude of chemicals and microorganisms that damage us on a cellular level. So forget the "rich lather," forget the multitudes of "essential oils" (are they really essential oils that have been steam distilled or cold pressed?), and forget the rest of the long list of ingredients found in most commercial soap products. If we are going to get well, we must break that mindset and live by that code of *"less is more."*

I ordered my first bars of organic, unscented, toxin-free soap, organic shaving soap, and toothpowder fourteen days after having been diagnosed with Lichen Sclerosis. I went throughout the house, boxed up every commercial product, and put it aside for the local food pantry. Yes, I felt guilty for passing on poison products, but, sadly, most people do not believe that these things are harmful, and are more than happy to receive them for free, no matter how toxic they are to them.

This purging of the house was my first step toward becoming healthy, and it didn't come easily. My husband didn't readily accept that I was tossing out new, unused packages of toothpaste, soap, shampoo, moisturizers, and shaving gel. He scoffed at the concept and couldn't imagine how any of this would make a difference. Most of all, he was angry to see many dollar's worth of products being given away.

But after only a couple of days of bathing and washing my hair with the organic soap, I noticed that I no longer was itchy after showering. There were other unexpected benefits from using the organic soap. With commercial products, the shower stall would always form soap scum. I've come to realize that soap scum is nothing more than a collection of synthetic chemicals found in commercial products. It would take harsher and harsher cleansers to get the crusty film off, and within days of cleaning the shower, the film would start to build again. With the organic soap, the shower stays clean and my bath sponge rinses clean. With commercial soaps, the sponge would become slimy after awhile, and it would never rinse clean of suds. Another advantage to using this organic soap for bathing and washing my hair was that it eliminated the need for using two separate products.

The Soap for Goodness Sake tooth powder consists of baking soda, xylitol (a sweetener derived from the fibers of fruits, vegetables, and birch trees), saponified coconut oil, and spearmint oil, which I purchased to replace regular toothpaste. My husband grudgingly gave it a try, insisting that we keep at least one tube of regular toothpaste just in case. We both found that the tooth powder gets our teeth very clean, leaves us with a nice fresh, minty taste in our mouths, and is very handy for traveling. After a couple of months using the tooth powder he decided to give the previous "natural" toothpaste another try, just as a comparison, and found that it burned his mouth and made his gums and lips sore. Needless to say, the final tube of commercial toothpaste bit the dust. Not only that, but he'd always had a problem with gingivitis, but since switching to the new tooth powder, his gums have cleared up.

Next, encouraged by my body's quick positive response to this non-toxic soap, I toyed with the idea of using the organic soap to replace my laundry detergent. A flurry of emails back and forth to the owner of Soap for Goodness Sake was disappointing. There was no laundry detergent available, but Kathy suggested I try grating the soap into flakes and using it. I chose, and continue to use, Soap for Goodness Sake's "Eco Goodness" Saponified Organic Extra Virgin Coconut Oil Soap as my laundry detergent. It contains only two ingredients, 100% organic extra virgin coconut oil, and water.

Because I use it as laundry detergent, I purchase it in bulk and buy "seconds" when they are available, which means only that the bars didn't come out of the soap mold properly and are slightly misshapen, and they don't have labels. Who cares? To grate the soap, I cut the bars into three pieces and run them through the Cuisinart. In about 15 minutes, eight "seconds" bars become enough laundry soap to last 3-4 months. A full load of laundry takes approximately ½ cup of grated soap, and of course the Cuisinart cleans up like magic.

Just as with using the organic soap for bathing and shampooing, I found unexpected positive results from switching to this organic laundry soap. Aside from no longer wearing toxin-laden clothing or sleeping in toxin-soaked bedding, the laundry washed in the organic soap is soft, even without fabric softener or dryer sheets. Denim jeans come out of the dryer so soft, they feel like they've been stone washed a billion times. Best of all, the agitator in the washing machine, which would become grey and dingy if I didn't scrub it regularly, is now self-cleaning because there is no chemical residue left behind from the organic soap.

Once I began using the organic soap for my laundry, I emptied our clothes closet, drawers, and linen closets, and then spent two weeks washing and drying everything that would touch our skin. Repeated washings (it can take up to 5) in this 100% organic soap removed the chemical buildup left from commercial products. You can tell when synthetic chemicals have been fully removed because clothes laundered several times organically will no longer create a lot of suds, and they will rinse clean with only one rinse. Because the fabric absorbs some of the natural oil in the soap, another "side effect" of using organic laundry soap is no static cling, no matter how long the clothes are "fried" in the dryer.

We don't think of our clothing or linens as being poisonous or dangerous to our health, but in reality, they are. Not only are they full of the chemicals we launder them in, they're also full of chemicals from manufacturing. Cottons that are not organic come from genetically modified cotton. The cotton plants have been modified not only to generate their own internal pesticide, but they are sprayed with a toxic herbicide. These chemical residues remain even after manufacturing.

Chemicals are also used so clothes retain a pristine appearance, are flame retardant, and stain resistant. Case in point: a friend of ours who had purchased a new pair of pants wore them on a rainy day and the pant legs got very wet, clinging to his legs until the fabric dried. Shortly afterward, he developed a very nasty rash on his legs that required a visit to the doctor and several weeks of medication before this mysterious rash went away. That's another reason I never wear new clothing without first having laundered it several times in my shredded organic extra virgin coconut oil laundry soap.

Resorting to simple organic soaps for bathing and laundry, I was stepping back in time. My husband had joked that the next thing I'd suggest would be to take our clothes down to the stream and beat them with a rock, but even my skeptical husband could not deny how much I was improving, with physical changes taking place before his eyes. My scarlet welts and rashes began to dissipate, unlike when I used commercial products. After switching to the organic soap, the rashes and welts not only became less frequent, but their healing time became shorter, and within four months, all occurrences of the rashes and welts had ceased. Now I can wear a bra all day and I never break out into a welt or rash.

I now use the organic extra virgin coconut oil soap to clean everything, even my toilet bowl, and use it as hand soap. In my purse I carry a small section of the organic soap for washing my hands when I use a public rest room.

The mother of the child whose story appears as a case study in Appendix A reports that the organic extra virgin coconut oil soap is also good for use in the dishwasher, and that it cleans shoes and removes magic marker. I've found that it also removes stains and cleans carpeting very effectively. In addition, I switched to plain white vinegar instead of expensive dishwasher rinse products. A gallon of white vinegar costs far less than commercial dishwasher rinse agents, is non-toxic and it also rinses dishes and glasses crystal clear, with no residue left behind, and it doesn't etch glass or silverware. This is just one more example of how easy and inexpensive it is to replace toxic commercial products.

Plain organic coconut oil soap (or any plain organic soap for that matter) will kill 99.9% of germs on contact. I wash my kitchen countertops with the organic soap, and then wipe them down with white vinegar. Studies have shown that there is no difference using plain soap versus anti-bacterial soap when it comes to killing germs. What's more, antibacterial soaps contain triclosan, which has been linked to the development of antibiotic resistant bacteria such as MRSA. But even worse, studies show that triclosan has been linked to:

- Destruction of human cells
- Endocrine disruption
- Destruction of both good and bad bacteria

We are surrounded by "germs" at all times, including bacteria and viruses. It is impossible to eliminate them from our lives, no matter how much we clean and scrub. Our bodies are covered with beneficial germs designed to eliminate the pathogenic kind, and the overuse of chemicals actually weakens the immune system. And we actually benefit from being exposed to germs because they stimulate our immune system to produce antibodies. If we were to live in a germ-free bubble, our immune system will not be exposed to microbes, which means it will not produce antibodies; this actually makes us more prone to illness. Even when it comes to cleaning, once again, *less is more.*

Someone remarked to me that using the Soap for Goodness Sake products is too expensive and too time consuming for a busy household. And yet we can find time to be on the computer, update our Facebook page, use Twitter, talk and text endlessly on our cell phones and watch television. But we're too cheap or too busy to take control of our health? That doesn't make sense.

I think of it this way: all of this toxic soap, shampoo, bathroom scrubs, laundry and dish detergent, fabric softeners, and anti-cling cloths have been replaced by a single organic soap. A variety of toothpastes have been reduced to a single small bottle of tooth powder. Just three items have replaced a multitude of chemical loaded products.

But what about deodorant? Moisturizers? Facial scrubs? As with most personal care products, no matter who the manufacturer is, what they are selling is convenience at a high price. Anyone can create organic, non-toxic personal care products right off the pantry shelf at a fraction of the cost. It simply takes a change in mindset and willingness to simplify all that bathroom clutter.

Truthfully, I haven't yet found a deodorant that I'd want to use, no matter how "natural" or "organic" they are purported to be. Instead, after showering I apply organic white vinegar, which acts as an astringent, to my armpits, allow it to dry (do not use immediately after shaving armpits), then wipe with a slightly damp cloth to eliminate the vinegar smell. Next I dust organic GMO-free cornstarch onto my armpits. It is a good substitute not only for deodorant, but also for talcum, baby powder, or foot powder. Buy a new powder box and puff from a powder/cosmetics distributor and be sure to never use a powder puff or powder box that previously held commercial powder. I simply put organic corn starch in the powder box and apply it under my arms with a powder puff. The corn starch is absorbent; a light application quickly becomes invisible and it doesn't leave marks on clothing.

For a facial scrub/exfoliant, I lather my hands with organic extra virgin olive oil soap, apply about a tablespoon of organic corn meal to the lather, and wash my face with it. It leaves my skin smooth and rejuvenated.

ABOUT OLIVE OIL

Finding a good moisturizer has been a process of experimentation and elimination, but I now have two perfect solutions that work for my skin type. The first is Olio Beato 100% organic first cold pressed, unfiltered extra virgin olive oil. Not only is it good as food, it's also great on my skin. It's light in texture and has a faint, fruity scent. When I buy a big bottle for cooking, I pour a small amount into a dark glass bottle that has an eyedropper top. Because a little olive oil goes a long way, it's best to rub a drop or two into the skin until it's smooth but not oily. Other organic extra virgin olive oil will work just as well as the Olio Beato brand, but it must come in a dark bottle and must be 100% organic first cold press. Anything other than organic extra virgin olive oil has been heated, processed and refined by machine or chemical such as hexane, thus destroying its nutritive value, and it potentially contains a contaminant.

If an olive oil has between 0.9% and 2% acidity, it is designated Virgin olive oil. If it has between 2% and 5% acidity, it is simply labeled as olive oil. Olio Beato always has an acidity content of below 0.5%, which means it is extra virgin olive oil. Why insist on organic extra virgin olive oil? Because organic extra virgin olive oil contains only the best that nature has to offer, even though it costs more than other olive oils. But consider this before you make the wrong decision: There are so many versions of olive oil on the shelves. The only one you can be 100% sure is pure and safe is organic extra virgin first cold pressed.

Extra Virgin Olive Oil is considered to be the finest grade of olive oil, and has the maximum nutritional value. Organic assures there are no impurities, and extra virgin means that the olives first were stone crushed, then the paste is put onto trays that are inserted into a manual or expeller press. Virgin olive oil is lower quality oil and has a higher acidity. It is made by pressings *after* the initial press for Extra Virgin olive oil.

In a recent study, researchers tested 134 samples of top non-organic name brand extra virgin olive oils and nearly three quarters of the oils failed the purity test. Those that failed had been mixed with canola, soybean, nut, or seed oils.

Olive oil blends include both refined and unrefined virgin olive oils and is the bulk grade that most people consume all over the world. The refining process consists of treating bad virgin olive oil, which is olive oil with severe defects such as high acidity caused by using bad fruit or from improper handling and processing. In treating the bad oil, sodium hydroxide is used to neutralize acidity. The oil may be heated to as high as 430°F under a vacuum to remove the volatile components. Then it is combined with virgin or extra virgin olive oils for color and flavor. In the US, grades labeled as "Extra Light" fall into this category.

Pomace Olive Oil is made by soaking the remains of olives in baths of hexane after all the other pressings are done. Hexane, as explained earlier, is a solvent derived from petroleum. It forces the last remains of oil out of the olives and the oil is deemed unfit for human consumption; it is sold for use in the cosmetics industry, used as a solvent, or as wax. This is the type of "olive oil" used in commercial soap, shampoo, and other personal care products.

This scenario holds true for every kind of oil used in the personal care industry, so when you see ads for commercial products touting olive oil, jojoba oil or "botanicals," what they include is the bargain basement, bottom of the barrel, unfit for human consumption, cheapest grade oil. Doesn't this make you want to rush right out and buy those products? This is only one of the dirty little secrets that commercial personal care manufacturers don't want you to know about.

Don't be fooled into thinking that "natural" or "handmade" soaps are any better. Unless the soap maker can tell you that the oil being used is organic and extra virgin, most likely it is nothing more than pomace olive oil, or an equally low grade type of other vegetable oil, or else a mixture of oils readily available to the soap trade.

For anyone with LS, the skin is sensitized and it's important to refrain from any soap containing any other type of oils, no matter how "skin loving" they are supposed to be. Also, some "natural" and "handmade" soap manufacturers use oxides to create colors in their soaps. Oxides are minerals found in the earth's crust, and to be used in soaps, they must first be processed and refined, and this can mean they contain unwanted minerals. Colored soaps may look pretty, but colorants serve no other purpose than eye candy and can cause problems for someone with LS. Keep it simple, and remember; *less is more*.

When you're buying olive oil, keep in mind light and air are the worst enemies of olive oil, must be kept in a cool, dark place and tightly sealed. Oxygen promotes chemical changes in the oil, and the Omega-3's in it are fragile and prone to rancidity. Always pick an olive oil that comes in a bottle made of dark glass, and look for one that's on a shelf that's away from light. Also try to buy from a store where turnover is brisk because organic extra virgin olive oil has a short shelf life of only 6 months. A good way to keep track of freshness is to add the purchase date to the label and be sure to use it within six months.

EXTRA VIRGIN OLIVE OIL NUTRIENTS

- **Tocopherols** - Vitamin E, Vitamin A, Vitamin K

- **Vitamin E** is number one in protecting the skin's cell membranes from free radicals.

- **Vitamin A** is comprised of retinoids (retinal, and retinoic acid), which are essential for vision, skin health, and bone growth. Absorbed through the skin, Vitamin A increases the rate of new skin cell growth and increases collagen.

- **Vitamin K** is essential as a calcium binder to a small number of proteins involved in the process of blood clot formation and it helps regulate cellular growth.

- **Chlorophyll** – It promotes the healing of skin conditions and wounds.

- **Flavonoids** – Also collectively known as Vitamin P and Citrin. Experimental evidence shows that these act as biological "response modifiers" and help control allergic, inflammatory, microbial reactions and cancer.

- **Oleocanthal** – A non-steroidal anti-inflammatory and antioxidant, and it also relieves inflammation and pain.

- **Phytosterols** – Phytosterols inhibit the intestinal absorption of cholesterol and reduce cancer risk. There is evidence to suggest that phytosterols improve urinary tract symptoms and symptoms related to an enlarged prostate, or benign prostatic hyperplasia.

- **Polyphenols** – (Oeuropein & Tyrosol) Anti-inflammatory, antioxidantal and anti-coagulant. Polyphenols help to neutralize free radicals and repair damage to cell membranes.

- **Squalene** – Squalene helps regulate sebum, which is produced by the sebaceous glands in our skin and is secreted through our pores. It forms a coating on the skin that acts as a barrier, inhibits the growth of micro-organisms, and lubricates our skin and hair.

- **Betaine** - Betaines are substances synthesized by cells for protection against environmental stress.

- **Calcium** – Calcium is the most abundant mineral in the body and is required for muscle contraction, blood vessel expansion and contraction, secretion of hormones and enzymes, transmission impulses throughout the nervous system, plus maintenance of constant concentrations of calcium in blood, muscle, and intercellular fluids.

- **Iron** – An essential mineral for the human body, iron functions primarily as a carrier of oxygen in the body, both as part of hemoglobin in the blood, and myoglobin in the muscles. It also aids in immune function, cognitive development, temperature regulation, energy metabolism, and work performance.

- **Potassium** – Potassium is a very important mineral for proper function of all cells, tissues, and organs in the human body. In addition, it is also an electrolyte that conducts electricity in the body and plays a key role in muscle contraction.

- **Omega-3 Fatty Acids** – Omega-3 Fatty Acids are essential fatty acids necessary to human health, but our bodies can't make them. They play a crucial role in brain function, normal growth and development, as well as acting as an anti-inflammatory. Studies show a connection between Omega-3 Fatty Acids and the reduction of skin disorders, high cholesterol, high blood pressure, diabetes, rheumatoid arthritis, heart disease, systemic lupus, depression, bipolar disorder, osteoporosis, schizophrenia, ADHD, IBD, asthma, macular degeneration, breast, colon, and prostate cancers.

- **Omega-6 Fatty Acids** – Omega-6 Fatty Acids are also considered essential fatty acids that are necessary to human health, and like Omega-3s, our bodies can't produce them. They help stimulate skin and hair growth, maintain bone health, regulate metabolism, and maintain the reproductive system. Gamma-linolenic acid in particular helps fight inflammation; Omega-6 Fatty Acids, when combined with Evening Primrose Oil, was found to reduce symptoms of Eczema, as well those of PMS, MS, osteoporosis, menopause, high blood pressure, breast cancer, ADHD, allergies, rheumatoid arthritis, and diabetic neuropathy.

Used as a moisturizer, organic extra virgin olive oil is beneficial because all of these nutrients, when absorbed through the skin, can only help. And which would you prefer to be absorbed through your skin? These wonderful nutrients, or one of the items on that long list of dangerous chemicals such as Lauric Acid, or Propylene Glycol?

Whenever I broke out in rashes and welts from wearing a bra, applying a few drops of the olive oil to the affected area was soothing, the itching would stop, and the rash and welts would heal. As a precaution, I began applying a thin coat of organic olive oil to my skin each day before putting on a bra, but now that I no longer get rashes and welts, this step is no longer necessary.

After I began using the organic extra virgin olive oil, I discovered that applying some of the oil to LS affected areas not only helped soothe the itching, inflammation, and cracking, but it also had a healing effect, making the crinkled skin stronger and more elastic. Given the choice of whether to use organic extra virgin olive oil on my LS-affected skin, or Clobetasol, it was a no-brainer to go with the olive oil.

VIRGIN COCONUT OIL

My other favorite moisturizer is also right out of the kitchen. Not only do I use Nutiva organic virgin coconut oil for cooking, but I generously apply it to all areas of my body for a smooth and young-looking skin. It is especially beneficial when applied to dry, itchy, or sunburned skin, and is an excellent replacement for petroleum-based products like Vaseline. (Nutiva has removed "extra" from their label.)

Organic virgin coconut oil is a whole food and contains lauric acid, which is a medium-chain fatty acid with anti-fungal, anti-viral, and anti-bacterial qualities.

On the other hand, the lauric acid used in commercial moisturizing products has been isolated and neutralized with the addition of sodium hydroxide. As discussed previously, this form of lauric acid is toxic.

Today, there are over 80,000 chemicals used all over the world, with more being developed every day; yet only about 200 have been tested for safety. The rest we're all testing on ourselves in the products we use. In the United States, chemicals have been deemed safe until proven otherwise. But things are starting to change. For the first time, the twenty-seven countries of the European Union have placed the burden of proof on the manufacturers, assuming the chemicals in products are *unsafe* unless proven otherwise. By the end of 2010, manufacturers in the EU were required to bring their products to government-approved independent laboratories for testing under a new law, which is called REACH, for Registration, Evaluation, Authorization, and Restriction of CHemicals. As a result, many harmful ingredients have been removed from products in the EU, or replaced with truly "natural" ingredients, making those long lists of ingredients much shorter—and safer to use.

Alas, many chemicals banned in Europe can still be found in products in the United States. You won't find Dibutyl Phthalates, which are known hormone disruptors, in European products, but you'll find them in U.S. products such as nail polish. You also won't find petroleum distillates in European lipstick or mascara, but you'll find these carcinogens in cosmetics in the U.S.

Why aren't people in the United States being protected from these dangerous substances? Why doesn't the Food and Drug Administration or the EPA ban these harmful chemicals? It's because the EPA has little or no authority or control over chemicals used in the U.S. unless they've caused pollution, or were in an environmental catastrophe such as an oil spill. In 1976, Congress passed the Toxic Substances Control Act (TOSCA), giving the EPA authority to control all new and existing chemicals. There are only about 300 chemicals on the EPA's "Chemicals of Concern" list, which somehow has not been updated since 1976.

During President George W. Bush's administration, the EPA was stripped of any authority to investigate and ban chemicals it found hazardous. In 2010, a bill was created and brought before Congress by the Environmental Working Group, calling for a program in the U.S. that is similar to the REACH program in Europe. Only Congress can pass this bill, and only Congress can approve funding for the EPA to undertake such testing. But with the fiscal crisis, budget cuts, chemical industry lobbyists loudly predicting a further downturn in the economy if manufacturers have to prove that their products are safe, and with manufacturers contributing heavily to campaign coffers, now that corporations are allowed to do so under the recent Supreme Court decision in the Citizens United Case, my guess is that it will be a long wait before that bill is passed by Congress.

Because there is so little product safety testing done by the FDA, the personal care industry sets up its own panel to decide what are "safe levels" of chemicals in their products, and the Food and Drug Administration uses those findings to determine how much risk is posed to the public compared to the economic hardship to the multi-billion dollar industry if those products are not allowed on the market. If revamping a product for safety reasons is deemed "too costly," it is not withdrawn from the market and to my knowledge, no personal care products have ever been withdrawn because of danger to the public.

But if you think about it, why should any level of a chemical be considered "safe" for our bodies? A case in point is lead, which used to be considered to have "safe" levels. We now know there are *no* safe levels of lead, just like there are no "safe" levels of mercury or arsenic, and we wouldn't dream of knowingly using products containing those ingredients. So why, then, do we accept "safe" levels of other chemicals if we don't have to? The personal care industry studies us intensely, asking us to participate in surveys so they can study our buying habits; they use focus groups to find out what makes us choose one product over another, and they also know that if they include a long list of ingredients in very tiny print, we're probably not even going to finish reading the list—if we can even see it. They know we're more impressed with glitzy packaging and seductive advertising than we are in researching exactly what goes into that product and what all those ingredients really are. They know that we prefer convenience to research and that we're not going to go through all the trouble to find out if every ingredient is safe, at least not until there's a crisis.

Despite what I believe, in truth there is no scientific data currently available that can prove conclusively that products I used for my entire life until recently caused me to develop Lichen Sclerosis. But after reading studies showing that the chemicals used in these everyday products cause endocrine disruption, neurotoxicity, skin irritation, cell mutation, bioaccumulation, and that I developed Lichen Sclerosis only months after introducing new skin care products into my life, I have no doubt these toxic topicals are major contributors to not only my disease, but many other auto-immune disorders that are widespread in our population.

Within four months after removing all commercial products from my home in favor of organic or non-toxic ones, my overall body itching, welts, and rashes were subsiding, and my LS flare-ups were becoming less frequent. No fabrics other than those washed with the organic extra virgin coconut oil soap touch my body, and I only bathe and wash my hair with organic extra virgin olive oil soap. Whenever I urinated, or had a bowel movement, I gently washed myself with a soft cloth moistened with nothing but hot filtered water and afterward I generously applied a new film of organic extra virgin olive oil, none of which I need to do now.

I cannot stress enough that anyone diagnosed with Lichen Sclerosis must adopt the mindset that less is more: less ingredients, less essential oils, less toxins, less everything. Keep it simple, and don't be seduced by glitzy advertising. Recently I saw an ad for a shampoo claiming to be rich in "essential oils and botanicals." But my response would be, "But what about all the other toxic crap? How come nobody mentions those ingredients?"

During my LS ordeal, it began to dawn on me that toxins were hidden in everything I touched. As my veil of ignorance was lifted, I went on high alert, carefully examining the ingredients of every single thing before I allowed it into my life. Any long list of ingredients sent up a red flag, and if there were ingredients I couldn't pronounce and had no idea what they were, it sent up a flare. I became something I'd never been before: a toxinophobe. And being a toxinophobe means that I know enough to be suspicious of everything, to read the labels, and to scrutinize ingredients before I purchase anything. I cannot possibly remember all 80,000+ chemicals used in personal care products, so I rely on a very simple rule of thumb in the form of a question: Is it organic? Does it grow in nature? If it's a name I've never heard of, can't pronounce, and it doesn't grow in nature, then I'm positive I don't want it anywhere near me, let alone on my skin.

Chemical Sources:

Federal Trade Commission Policy Statement on Deception, 103 F.T.C. 174 (1984), appended to Cliffdale Assoc. Inc., 103 F.T.C. 110 (1984), http://www.ftc.gov

U.S. Department of Health & Human Services, Household Products Database, http://householdproducts.nlm.nih.gov

Abedin, Shahreen et al, RxList Inc. March 19, 2008, http://www.rxlist.com

Adamson, Brian, "Sodium Lauryl Sulfate (SLS) and Sodium Laureth Sulfate (SLES): The Killers in Your Bathroom?" http://www.natural-health-information-centre.com. Accessed April 25, 2010.

Adamson, Brian, "The Potential Implications of SLS and SLES on Human Health." http://www.natural-health-information-centre.com. Accessed April 25, 2010.

Center for Environmental Health (CEH), "Lawsuit Launched to End Mislabeling of 'Organic' Personal Care Products," Press Release, June 16, 2011. http://www.ceh.org/making-news/press-releases/29-eliminating-toxics/528-lawsuit-launched-to-end-mislabeling-of-organic-personal-care-products-

Environmental Working Group, Skin Deep® Cosmetics Database. http://www.ewg.org/skindeep/

Fitzgerald, Randall, *The Hundred-Year Lie*. Plume, 2007

Gupta, Dr. Sanjay, "Toxic America." CNN, June 2, 2010

Gupta, Dr. Sanjay, "Toxic Childhood." CNN, June 3, 2010

Mercola, Dr. Joseph, "The Soap You Should Never Use—But 75% of Households Do," August 29, 2012. http://articles.mercola.com/sites/articles/archive/2012/08/29/triclosan-in-personal-care-products.aspx

Mercola, Dr. Joseph, "The Four Most Dangerous Myths About Washing Your Hands, February 25, 2011. http://articles.mercola.com/sites/articles/archive/2011/02/25/myths-about-hand-hygiene.aspx

Soap For Goodness Sake LLC. http://www.soapforgoodnesssake.com

The Good Human, "Wearing Makeup Puts 5 Pounds of Chemicals Into Your Body...Per Year," July 17, 2007. www.thegoodhuman.com

Paraben Sources:

Breast Cancer Fund, "Parabens." www.breastcancerfund.org/clear-science/chemicals-glossary/parabens.html

Darbre, P.D. et al. "Concentration of Parabens in Human Breast Tumors." Journal of Applied Toxicology. 2004 Jan-Feb;24(1):5-13. http://onlinelibrary.wiley.com/doi/10.1002/jat.1786/pdf

Mercola, Dr. Joseph, "99% of Breast Cancer Tissue Contained This Everyday Chemical (NOT Aluminum)," May 24, 2012. http://articles.mercola.com/sites/articles/archive/2012/05/24/parabens-on-risk-of-breast-cancer.aspx

Yard, Delicia Honen, "Parabens Found in Breast Tumor Tissue of Nonusers of Underarm Products," Oncology Nurse Advisors, January 30, 2012. http://www.oncologynurseadvisor.com/parabens-found-in-breast-tumor-tissue-of-nonusers-of-underarm-products/article/224385/#

About Olive Oil Sources:

Amazing Olive Oil, "Nutrients in Olive Oil." http://www.amazingoliveoil.com/nutrients-in-olive-oil.html

Amazing Olive Oil, "Olive Oil Grades and Ratings." http://www.amazingoliveoil.com/olive-oil-grades-and-ratings.html

Amazing Olive Oil, "Shelf Life and Storage." http://www.amazingoliveoil.com/olive-oil-shelf-life.html

Bardot, J.B., "The Great Olive Oil Fraud – Why Your Extra Virgin Olive Oil May Not Be Virgin At All," Natural News, July 18, 2012. http://www.naturalnews.com:80/036509_extra_virgin_olive_oil_fraud_bottle.html

Coates, Dr. Paul M., et al. National Institute of Health, Office of Dietary Supplements, July 7, 2010. http://www.ods.od.nih.gov

Drake, Victoria J., Ph.D., "Essential Fatty Acids," Linus Pauling Institute, Oregon State University, April 2009. http://lpi.oregonstate.edu/infocenter/othernuts/omega3fa/

Olivus, "Health Benefits." http://www.olivus.com/products_olivus.htm

Pietro DeMarco, "How Olio Beato Olive Oil is Made." http://www.organicoil.com

Chapter 3
Chemical Consumption

There are some basic disturbing facts about Lichen Sclerosis, as well as about toxic chemical overload that aren't commonly known. For example:

- *It is estimated that 5% of all pre-pubescent girls, ages 4-9, have been, or will be diagnosed with Lichen Sclerosis.*

- *It is estimated that 15% of all Lichen Sclerosis cases involve children, and that percentage is rising.*

- *A 2009 study of the cord blood of 10 newborns showed them to have an* **average of 232 chemicals** *already in their systems. The term for this is "pre-pollution."*

- *In a landmark 12-year study of air pollutants breathed in by pregnant women, Dr. Frederika Perera, Columbia University Center for Children's Environmental Health, found that 100% of the women tested positive for detectable levels of pesticides. Of the babies born to these women, 15% have shown chromosomal abnormalities and developmental problems.*

Having ended what I call Part 1 of my overall healing strategy by removing toxic commercial personal care products from my environment, I next began to zero in on food. My gynecologist had mentioned a food elimination diet to find out if something I was eating was stressing my immune system. At the time, she thought it was unnecessary to go through the elimination diet because my case was mild. But her comment stuck in my mind.

Just as I'd become suspicious of all the ingredients I was putting *on* my body, I began to suspect there was something in the foods I was eating. But I already made nearly all of our food from scratch, and didn't believe I purchased a lot of processed or pre-packaged foods. We also made healthy fresh salads every night, so I thought we were ahead on those counts. But now, a closer examination of the ingredients in the everyday products on my kitchen shelves, in my refrigerator, and freezer gave me pause.

We long knew about the dangers of high fructose corn syrup (HFCS), and had avoided most things that included it. I say most "things" because food manufacturers had discovered that high fructose corn syrup was a cheap substitute for cane sugar, and have put it in nearly everything that needs any type of sweetening. Scrutinize your ingredients labels and you'll find HFCS lurking in the oddest foods, including ketchup, mustard, cereal, bread, fruit juice, the list goes on and on. It made me wonder what else was hiding in my pantry, cupboards, and refrigerator?

I've always thought I've eaten healthy fresh foods and we are constantly pushed to eat more fruits and vegetables, to eat whole grains for fiber, and to eat more fish instead of red meat as a source of protein; each of these foods is promoted as being beneficial to our health and well-being, and as the major components for life's building blocks. I happen to like fruits and vegetables. Every night I eat a large freshly made salad. Dessert consists of some type of fruit, be it melon, berries, grapefruit, apple, or orange, or a combination of fruits. During the day I'd have a banana, strawberries, or whatever other fruit we had in the house. Nuts or homemade popcorn are my favorite snack food and we'd almost always have freshly made organic brown rice with our meals. Eating an organic Greek yogurt with fresh strawberries is like eating ice cream. This has been my diet of all the right stuff for nearly a lifetime. With all the nutrients I've been feeding myself, how could my immune system end up so inflamed? How could I possibly be sick?

But I wasn't eating as healthy as I'd once thought.

Yes that yogurt was organic, but it was also made from pasteurized milk. While I believed that I had made our food "from scratch" the way my mother did because I didn't buy the mass produced knockoffs like instant mashed potatoes, in hindsight I realized my mother had never used ready-made, packaged ingredients. Buying a jar of pasta sauce and adding ready-made seasoning from a jar, fresh onions, and pre-packaged Italian sausage doesn't make it "from scratch." Whipping together a meal combining fresh ingredients with processed ingredients from a jar, box or bag doesn't make it "homemade" either. And fresh ingredients doesn't necessarily mean healthy. Unknowingly my poultry, meats, fruit, and vegetables, had all come from factory farms where they had been produced in the cheapest, most expedient way possible.

Those beautiful, green, leafy vegetables look so innocuous. Red ripe tomatoes, loaded with lycopene, are supposed to be good for us, aren't they? An apple a day keeps the doctor away, or so the saying goes. Now we can have grapes all year long, instead of only when they are in season here, thanks to imports from other countries. And they look so appetizing. But had I been eating a healthy diet? Think again!

I'd begun feeling like I was coming down with a cold soon after eating yogurt or nuts. I'd develop a sore throat and just feel sick for about an hour afterward. It occurred to me I might have developed an allergy to milk products and nuts, so I stopped eating them.

My ever increasing suspicion about what was in foods containing the blanket terms "spices" or "seasoning" not only drove me to further research, but I made the snap decision to avoid eating anything that listed those ingredients.

If it had been hard for my husband to watch cartons of personal care products be given away, seeing me suddenly refuse to eat things I'd been devouring for years infuriated him. We had more harsh words and these sudden changes in everything we'd used or eaten were more than he could stand. He threatened to walk out the door and not look back, and he couldn't understand how everything I'd been doing all my life, everything I'd been eating all my life, had suddenly become my enemy. To him, my actions seemed sudden and ridiculous. When I'd point out the mysterious "spices" or "seasoning" on a product label, he'd snarl, "That's not it!" meaning those ingredients hadn't caused my LS. But if they weren't "it," then what was?

If the commercial topical products I had been using had caused welts, rashes, and skin irritations that stopped when I switched to simple organic soap and organic extra virgin olive oil, then what about the ingredients I was eating every day? The more research I did on food ingredients, the more I began connecting the dots. Here's just a bit of what I found out:

- Over 3,000 chemicals are added to our food supply in the form of herbicides, pesticides, insecticides, and fungicides. More than 10,000 chemicals in the form of preservatives, emulsifiers, and solvents are used in processing and storing all foods.

- Current studies reveal that many people have between 400 and 800 foreign chemical residues stored in their body's fat cells.

And that's just the tip of the toxic iceberg. In a collaborative study by Mount Sinai School of Medicine in New York, the Environmental Working Group, and Commonweal, researchers at two major independent laboratories found an average of 91 industrial compounds, pollutants, and other chemicals in the blood and urine of nine volunteers, with a total of 167 foreign chemicals found in the group. Like most of us, the nine volunteers tested are not in contact with job-related chemicals, and they do not live near industrial facilities.

Scientists refer to this contamination as a person's toxic body burden. Of the 167 chemicals found in these nine individuals, 76 cause cancer in humans or animals, 94 are toxic to the brain and nervous system, and 79 cause birth defects or abnormal development. The danger to human health from these chemical combinations has never been studied.

How can we have so many foreign chemicals in our bodies, and what are they doing to us?

There are chemicals in the air we breathe, spewed from manufacturing facilities, automobiles, the sprays used in the home to clean, disinfect, paint, and even provide the home with that "fresh scent." Chemicals in herbicides are used indiscriminately to kill off everything we don't want, from crab grass to dandelions. "Poisoned lawns" a friend calls them. Our water is becoming more and more polluted with pharmaceuticals that are washed off of us, excreted from us, or dumped down the drain by us. And our food chain is bombarded with pesticides, herbicides, food additives in the forms of dyes, chemical taste and texture enhancers, anti-caking agents, and chemical preservatives.

The more I researched how Big Food grows and produces what we eat, the more disgusted and enraged I became. Just as cartons and cartons of personal care products had been taken to the local food pantry, I set about emptying our home of every non-organic food item we had. I emptied every spice rack, shelf in the pantry, closet, refrigerator, and freezer of anything that was not organic. That left pretty much nothing in the house to eat, and watching thousands of dollar's worth of "perfectly good food" being given away nearly sent my husband over the edge.

I spent a solid month searching for organic replacements for everything. I joined a food co-op that is nearly 50 miles from my home because it has a large selection of locally grown organic produce, meats, and other items that our local grocery store doesn't carry. Near the food co-op is a health food store that carries or will order bulk organic items that I use frequently, as well as stocking a large selection of organic food items not found at the food co-op. The health food store owner has a membership program as well, and for a mere $25 a year, each member gets a 10% discount on every single item purchased, plus monthly member specials that have a 20% discount. When I order something in bulk, I get an automatic 15% discount, and I recouped my initial $25 membership fee within two weeks. It was also gratifying to find that the big chain supermarket now had an impressive "organic foods" section. Just 10 years ago, that section consisted of only two short aisles, but it has grown to a substantial department of its own, with many aisles, freezers, and a fresh produce section. Even in the regular meat department of the store, I was thrilled to find packages of organic, grass-fed ground beef, as well as grass-fed ground bison, which are never allowed to be given growth hormones or antibiotics. In a neighboring state, I joined a food co-op that is the size of a mega-supermarket, and it carries more organic foods and products than all of my other sources combined. Since it is 100 miles away, I only get there about once a month.

What I couldn't find in my "local" organic stores, and "local" meaning further than 100 miles round trip, I bought online. I spent a month or more searching for, comparing prices of, and ordering things as obscure as an organic replacement for Bisquick, which I did find. UPS and FedEx were at our door every day, and soon every shelf, cupboard, the refrigerator and freezer were filled with everything organic, from chicken, to bell peppers, to salt and pepper.

Sometimes I couldn't find an organic version of something I'd used for years, such as a specific poultry seasoning, which not only was it not organic, but it contained the dreaded blanket term "spices," along with an anti-caking agent, so alas, it had to go. But before tossing it, I read the ingredients list and began to experiment with making my own organic version of the seasoning, minus the "spices" and anti-caking agent. It took a lot of taste testing, but I finally perfected it to the point that people now ask me what it is that I use and how I make it.

My husband's anger over the loss of "perfectly good food" quickly changed to delight as food began tasting better than it had in a long time. For years we had complained that oranges were so bland, tasteless, and sour, that they no longer tasted like oranges. Now, every organic orange we bite into is juicy, sweet, and deeply flavorful. Organic grass-fed ground bison is not only really beefy in taste, but the meat is full of natural juices and isn't dripping with fat. For years I'd complained about eggs, which were getting smaller, paler, and more tasteless, and with such thin shells that they'd practically crush instead of cracking open. Organic food, aside from being more nutritious, simply tastes better. But why is that?

EVOLUTION AND FOOD

First we need to understand how we and our food have evolved. Originally we were hunters and gatherers who ate whatever we could catch, and whatever grew around us. We learned how to raise the animals we caught so we no longer had to hunt for them, and we learned how to grow our food so we no longer had to forage for it. We changed from hunters to farmers, and the food we raised and grew was raw, pure, and didn't contain pesticides, herbicides, growth hormones, preservatives, food coloring, chemical flavor enhancers, or anti-caking agents.

Early man explored and migrated to other parts of the world, bringing with him meat, vegetable, and grain crops in order to provide sustenance in an unknown land. He planted seeds and raised animals in places where they weren't indigenous, and the wild, indigenous, and non-indigenous food groups grew and mingled together by wind, insect, and mating. Nature understood combining only similar genetics, and new and stronger strains and species evolved. It is natural selection and survival of the fittest. The food that we raised sustained us and we evolved into healthier human beings. Each new generation grew bigger, stronger, smarter, healthier, and lived longer than the previous generation.

Fast forward to 2004, when Eric M. Bost, then Undersecretary of the Food, Nutrition and Consumer Services (FNCS) testified before the House Committee on Government Reform and the Subcommittee on Human Rights and Wellness. In his testimony on obesity, he stated that "If we do not stem this tide, many children in this generation will not outlive their parents." How did we go from being a robust nation only a generation ago to a nation that comes in at 29th on the World Health Organization's list of countries ranked by the health of their population?

Before the Industrial Revolution, we were a nation of farmers who raised their animals and grew their crops in a sustainable manner, meaning current and future needs are met without damaging the environment. Farmers planted the biggest and best seeds that they saved from the previous year's crops. They preserved the nutrients in the soil by rotating crops, meaning one year a crop would be grown in a certain section, while other acres rested and were reconstituted by cover crops. Beans would be planted with corn so that the corn stalks supported the bean climbing tendrils. Tender vegetables were grown in the shade of big, leafy vegetables. Animals grazed in pastures, and their manure was used to fertilize the soil. Farmers raised free-range chickens, milked their cows and drank the milk raw, and allowed their animals to grow and fatten naturally. The biggest and strongest were used to ensure propagation of sturdy future generations.

Farming was labor intensive, lasting from dawn to dusk. Not only was there manual weeding, watering, tilling, and fertilizing, but there was harvesting the crops, butchering the livestock, and canning or salting of foods for a winter's supply. It was, and always will be, hard work, and at the mercy of Mother Nature. Floods, drought, hurricanes, tornadoes, pests, or animal sickness could wipe a farmer out. But with the dawn of the Industrial Revolution, growing food in America changed and set us on the path to today's environmentally-borne illnesses.

With the invention of automobiles came mechanized methods for tilling fields instead of using horses or oxen, and a farmer following behind on foot with a tiller tethered to the team. A machine could bale hay in a day instead of requiring several farm hands days to manually cut, rake, and roll the hay. With the aid of machinery, farmers could plant more crops.

The food industry was in its infancy, but with the arrival of automobiles and refrigeration, giant food corporations such as Dole, Green Giant, and others saw a way to bring food to the masses. These food corporations and the U.S. government paid farmers to grow crops not for themselves, but for the corporations. This was seen as a win win situation for all at the time, but what started out as a great idea, has ballooned way out of the farmers' control as time passed, to the point where they are now owned by the corporations, and have no say in what they grow or how they grow it. Farmers with corporate contracts no longer have the ability to rotate crops, replenish the soil with cover crops, or even save their best seeds from the previous year's crop. That's because every year they must now buy genetically modified seeds, and use increasingly stronger herbicides and pesticides to kill increasingly resistant weeds and crop pests.

Instead of allowing animals to fatten naturally, they are given growth hormones and fed synthetic and unnatural diets to fatten them up in half the time. Instead of gathering eggs from chickens roaming the farm or slaughtering them, chickens are now factory farmed.

FOOD DEFINED

What is food? It is live, nutritional matter that has been on earth since before the dawn of humans. Humans evolved eating what nature provided, and did not invent food. The only thing humans do is rearrange, modify, and manipulate what is already here.

Dr. Randy Wysong's definition of food is one of the best I've read:

"Food is that which nourishes and sustains life. Food is not technology; it is the living material that has sustained animal life from its beginnings. Natural real foods are inextricably linked to the life they support. All life from the beginning of time has been sustained by eating the fresh raw natural foods from the natural environment.

There are subtleties in apples, carrots, and meats that we only begin to understand. A simple potato contains over 150 chemically distinct entities, not just starch. Life forms have spent eons adapting to natural foods, thriving on the subtleties of their nutrients, and developing protective mechanisms against natural toxins. To suddenly consume the new modern processed concoctions presents to the body new chemicals, toxins, and altered nutrients to which life is not adapted.

New forms of "synthetic" foods, from a geobiologic perspective, do not fit the definition of food. By submitting to technology rather than nature, we become...unwitting participants in a giant experiment. So far this has resulted in the plethora of degenerative diseases, but the full consequences will only be known by our grandchildren."

When I became suspicious of everything I put into my mouth, my family and friends were not only perplexed; they were, and continue to be, annoyed, to put it mildly. At the time I changed my eating habits I bore, and still bear, the brunt of their ridicule. I continuously suffer their unenlightened comments, such as, *"But you've been eating this food all your life and it didn't make you sick."* Or, smug remarks like, *"Everything in moderation."* By now, even you, the reader, may be agreeing with them. But to all who think I've gone totally overboard in my refusal of non-organic food and who have made these comments, I offer some sobering statistics:

- Wearing makeup every day for one year will contribute to 5 pounds of chemicals absorbed into your body through your skin. This does not include chemicals from soaps, shampoo, perfume, hair colorants, moisturizers, or gels/mousse.

- The average soda drinker consumes 50 pounds of artificial sweetener in one year.

- The average American consumes 220 pounds of beef per year. If the majority of that is in the form of ground beef, they will also ingest approximately 55 pounds of ammonia hydroxide via a ground beef filler (aka pink slime) used to kill e-coli bacteria.

- The average American eating a non-organic diet will consume, on average, 61 pesticide residues per day. That amounts to 1.65 ounces of pesticides per day, which works out to 37.64 pounds per year.

- It is estimated that the average person ingests, from *all* sources (air, water, food, personal and household care products, smoke, automobiles, carpeting, household fabrics, clothing, plastics, aluminum foil, non-stick cookware, and so on), approximately *one ton* of chemicals per year.

The worst part is that there are absolutely zero studies done, or being conducted, to find out how this concoction of chemicals in our bodies is affecting us. But it's not rocket science. We are all walking lab rats who have been testing chemicals for 20, 30, 40, 50 years. Sadly, some of us are testing them right in the womb. All anyone has to do is look around. Fifty years ago, before high fructose corn syrup was introduced into the food system, obesity was not an issue. When I was growing up, there weren't many fat children. Diabetes in adults was minimal, and in children it was relatively rare. Other diseases, such as autism and fibromyalgia were rare or unheard of, but now according to the Centers for Disease Control, one in every 55 children is autistic. Childhood cancers have increased 300%, and according to the World Health Organization, despite the United States taking first place in health care costs compared to the rest of the world, we rank 29th in the health of our population.

To those who think otherwise, I haven't been eating *"this food"* all of my life. What we eat has changed more in the past 50 years than it has since the dawn of humans. I grew up in the 1950's and 1960's, when food was still pretty much real food. My mom cooked every meal from scratch, fruits and vegetables were seasonal, except those that were frozen, canned, or jarred. She went to the local butcher, who would have sides of beef, lamb, and pork hanging in a freezer, and had him carve the exact cuts of meat she wanted. If we wanted turkey, we went to the local turkey farm, where the turkeys were free roaming and would be slaughtered the day you wanted it. Chickens were raised and handled pretty much the same way, and I remember my mother rotating a whole chicken over the gas stove to singe the little feathers off. Potatoes were washed, peeled, boiled, and mashed. Eggs were large, with very hard shells. We made cakes and pies by hand and baked with fresh ingredients, rather than something dumped out of a box, can, or jar. We did have ice cream and soda on occasion, the former of which was made with real ingredients such as milk, eggs, cream, sugar. Soda was also made with pure cane sugar. And on those rare occasions when we went out to eat, it was at a restaurant, not a fast food chain.

Flash forward to today, where everything mentioned above is mass produced with the cheapest ingredients made of chemicals that artificially mimic the taste, texture, and smell of the real nutritional ingredients they are replacing. And now there's the added bonus of preservatives.

I equate eating *"this food"* these past 20 to 30 years with smoking cigarettes. With each puff, over 7200 chemicals are inhaled into the body. If you smoke one cigarette, or even one pack of cigarettes, you cannot expect to have a black spot on your lung, emphysema, COPD, or some other respiratory disease within a day, week, month, or even a year. Yet 20, 30, 40 years later, when a diagnosis confirms one of these diseases, not one single person would dispute or refute the link to smoking as the cause.

And yet, so many people find it inconceivable that *"this food,"* laden with synthetic sugar, pesticides, herbicides, fungicides, preservatives, chemical additives and colorants that they've been eating for 20, 30, 40 years could possibly make them sick. Why is that? Is it because a bite into a pesticide-laden piece of lettuce doesn't give off an ominous cloud? Is it because the chemicals used in food products have "clean" names for labeling purposes so as not to sound too offensive? After all, enriched flour sounds a lot more appetizing than "paste" made from the milling waste of whole grains (which I think of as "floor sweepings"). Because high fructose corn syrup has received the bad reputation it deserves and some people have become aware of its dangers, making some of the public shy away from it, the Corn Refiners Association tried unsuccessfully to petition the FDA to change high fructose corn syrup labeling to the less offensive "corn sugar." Since the food industry's introduction of high fructose corn syrup into the food chain in the 1970's, the average amount consumed has gone from 19 pounds per year per person, to close to 60 pounds and rising.

Why then, after long-term consumption of pesticides, herbicides, fungicides, manufacturing chemicals, chemicals in household products, excitotoxins in our foods, dyes, solvents, and a myriad of chemical concoctions entering our bodies via the air we breathe, the water we drink, the personal care products we use, the food we eat is it a stretch of the imagination that having this go on day in, day out for years won't result in disease?

I don't care what the USFDA claims "acceptable levels" of these chemicals are. Why should *any* level be acceptable? I don't put things like "edible shellac" in my food when I cook, so why should it be okay for a Big Food conglomerate to lace our food with chemical replacements simply because it's cheaper than using nutritious ingredients, and tell us it's "acceptable?"

Some people have suggested to me that "everything in moderation" equates to safety. But to me, that's unacceptable! There is no such thing as "moderation." The idea that a little bit of chemicals every day is okay makes no sense because nearly everything we consume or touch has chemicals in it that are bio-accumulative. A perfect example is sodium lauryl sulfate which is in soap, dish and laundry detergent, shampoo, even toothpaste. Where's the moderation when people are using all of these products containing sodium lauryl sulfate not only every day, but sometimes all of them in one day, plus wearing this chemical in their clothing and sleeping with it in their bedding? Some people tell me our "bodies will take care of it." But while our bodies were designed to naturally detoxify, they haven't evolved to the point where they can handle over 80,000+ chemicals per year, or keep up with the constant onslaught of chemicals, and as a result these chemicals are accumulating in our bodies and we are getting sick as a result. Diseases that were once rare or non-existent 50 years ago, such as ALS, Multiple Sclerosis, Parkinson's and Alzheimer's are on the rise, with no sign of abatement.

The comment has been raised that nothing can be truly organic. This is true, because the grass organic cattle feed on and the vegetables an organic farmer grows all receive acid rain and are subject to the same air contaminants we are. Every breath we take is contaminated. But this doesn't mean we should simply shrug our shoulders or think that it's hopeless. We can try to eliminate as many toxins as possible from our lives. We can filter our water, eat organic food whose toxins are limited to non-existent. Will we ever be able to eliminate or prevent every single toxin from entering our body? No, but we can do everything possible to significantly reduce our toxic intake and lessen our toxic body burden.

FOOD SCIENCE

In the 1970's, a co-worker's husband was a "food scientist." I'd never heard of that term or job description before and couldn't imagine what a food scientist was, or did, or why anyone would need one. Who could predict that it was the beginning of the food science tidal wave to come?

This food scientist was responsible for the formula that creates coffee crystals and the new formula he was developing wasn't working. The coffee crystals weren't puffing up big enough, making the jars of crystallized coffee appear only half full. Eventually the problem was resolved and "food science" has "improved" upon the original formula so that the coffee crystals became larger, making it appear as though the container is just as full of coffee at 8 or 10 ounces as it had been at 16 ounces, making the consumer think they were getting the same amount of coffee, but it was just fluffier.

Food science is big business now, to the extent that most packaged, processed, and manufactured food is created in laboratories by food scientists and are chemical concoctions designed for taste, texture, and smell, making them more about illusion and artifice than nutrition.

Big Food isn't entirely to blame for our daily chemical consumption. If you think a "homemade" version of a commercially prepared food is better, think again. You can just as easily be served up a plate or bowl of "homemade" toxins from your friendly mom and pop establishment, or from your very own kitchen.

An ice cream store opened in a nearby town, touting "homemade" ice cream. One of my favorite flavors from this establishment was ginger ice cream. Having made my own organic ice cream, using organic cream, eggs, cane sugar, fresh fruit, raw cocoa, and nuts, I assumed the juice of fresh pressed, grated, or ground ginger root was used to flavor this "homemade" treat. But when I asked the owner how much ginger he used to flavor the ice cream, I was not prepared for his answer: a "food chemist" created the flavor in a lab using chemically-derived flavorings and manipulated until, when added to the ice cream, the taste was satisfactory. Unfortunately, this is how most commercial ice cream is flavored. As a result, the only ice cream I consume now is one I've made myself.

FOOD ADDITIVES

Processed foods make up everything in a supermarket that isn't raw. Typical supermarkets carry 50,000 or more items.

Any local supermarket, even a small one, offers aisle after aisle of pre-packaged "foods." Almost all of them have chickens cooking on a rotisserie, along with almost any food imaginable available in a can, jar, box or bag, waiting to be heated up and consumed. The food industry has made it so easy, people don't need to know how to cook anymore. They just need to be able to hit the buttons on their microwaves and dinner's ready. But is this what we should be eating?

Food product managers and marketers make pre-packaged foods look appealing and imply that they contain wholesome nutrition by using photographs of whole vegetables, or fruits, or a scenic farm on the packages. Some include photos of "chefs," but in reality, nothing could be further from the truth. The food scientists are the real chefs who "cook" and "flavor" everything in the lab. The food industry uses the cheapest ingredients possible substituting artificial chemical replacements and additives instead of whole, genuine foods pictured on the package.

These additives include synthetic vitamins, texturizers, emulsifiers, chemical dyes, chemical flavoring, and preservatives. And because they are not organic, they may include "acceptable" levels of pesticides and genetically modified ingredients.

Recently I was at the market on the checkout line when a nearby display case caught my eye. The cover of the "Blueberry Pancake and Waffle Mix" featured a stack of pancakes topped with maple syrup and fresh blueberries. But the ingredients didn't include real blueberries and the "blueberry flakes", or rather blueberry fakes as I like to call them, were made of "sugar (GMO), palm kernel oil (an artery clogging highly saturated hydrogenated oil); and blueberry powder," which was a concoction made of "cornstarch (GMO), maltodextrin (a form of corn sugar which is most likely GMO corn derived), blueberry flavor (chemical), and soy lecithin (a GMO emulsifier). (The descriptions in parentheses are my own.) In other words, every single ingredient in the package was processed or made in a lab.

Keep in mind when reading ingredients on food packages, that those listed first make up the largest percentage of the ingredients. "Enriched flour" usually is listed first, which consists of the poorest quality flour with zero nutritional value, not much better than floor sweepings with synthetic vitamins added to it. Unless the term "cane sugar" is used, it will be either high fructose corn syrup, or sugar derived from sugar beets, which are GMO crops. Most "sugar" in processed foods is high fructose corn syrup and no matter how safe they claim it to be, it is derived from GMO corn and I recommend avoiding it if you are suffering from LS.

ARTIFICIAL SWEETENERS

Unfortunately, sugar has become a bad word to many people. Yet the human species evolved consuming whole, natural, mostly unprocessed sugars that are found in whole fruits. And although processed sugar can raise the body's glycemic index, pure cane sugar, evaporated cane sugar or evaporated cane juice are derived solely from a cane sugar plant and have not been created in a lab. Although consuming large quantities of processed cane sugar is unhealthy, it's at least a food our bodies recognize, break down, utilize, store, or eliminate—as they were designed to do.

But artificial sweeteners including aspartame, aka NutraSweet, AminoSweet, Splenda, Sweet N Low, or Neotame are exactly what they say they are: artificial. How can that be good for us? Even if they are derived from a natural food source (corn or beets that are most likely GMO), they have been modified or altered in such a way that our bodies do not recognize them as food; thus we cannot process or utilize them properly the way we do with real food. When our bodies try to break down synthetic sweeteners, toxic metabolites are formed, something that doesn't happen with natural, whole plant sugar. Alas, the makers of artificial sweeteners claim that aspartame can be found in nature, which technically is true. But in nature, the components are combined synergistically with other nutrients. But that's not what happens with chemically created aspartame and that's why it creates toxic metabolites.

Unfortunately, as natural foods and ingredients are continually modified and "improved" scientifically, there are unintended side effects and consequences, which the food and chemical industries downplay. These side effects are denied and many doctors refuse to believe that patients' symptoms result from using artificial sweeteners. Yet there are a multitude of documented cases of the connection between the symptoms and the sweeteners, as well as people who have recovered from symptoms when they've eliminated artificial sweeteners from their diets.

Symptoms Induced by Use of Artificial Sweeteners

- Irritable Bowel Syndrome (IBD)
- Eye irritation (including itching, watery eyes, swollen eyelids)
- Headaches
- Swelling of the face, lips, throat, tongue
- Heart palpitations
- Joint pain
- Respiratory distress including coughing, tightness in the chest, shortness of breath, wheezing, sneezing, congestion
- Neurological disorders including anxiety, depression, dizziness, cognitive dysfunction
- Skin disorders including rash, hives, itching, oozing blisters

- Gastrointestinal distress including bloating, gas, severe and/or bloody diarrhea, stomach/intestinal pain, nausea and vomiting
- Brain tumors
- Cancer

Among artificial sweeteners, the excitotoxin Aspartame is linked to neurological disorders because it affects the protein synapses in the brain. Research including over 20 years of testing consistently shows the same results: cancerous tumors, especially in the brain. It took significant food industry and political maneuvering by lobbyists to get aspartame approved after the FDA had refused for 10 years based on testing that showed an alarming rate of tumor growth following regular consumption of the artificial sweetener. Aspartame is used in over 6,000 products, particularly diet or zero-calorie products. For instance, an average of one diet soda per day increases the risk of developing symptoms by 38%. Four or more diet sodas per day increases that risk by 78%. Even if soda is not consumed, but one eats a daily diet of zero-calorie foods, they increase their risk of developing any one of the symptoms listed above. It depends upon the individual how quickly they may develop symptoms. Some people report immediate reactions, while others may not have any indications for months or years, or none at all. Since 1983, when Aspartame came on the market, there has been an increase in the number of cases of Fibromyalgia and Lupus and six months later there was a 10% spike in brain tumors, a 30% increase in the need for kidney dialysis, and brain lymphoma increased by 60%. Today, over 80% of complaints to the FDA pertain to Aspartame.

HIGH FRUCTOSE CORN SYRUP (HFCS)

Introduced in the 1970's, high fructose corn syrup, or HFCS, was quickly embraced by the food industry as a cheap alternative to cane sugar, which explains that the use of "high fructose corn syrup keeps our foods affordable." As a result, in the 30 years since its introduction, the average person's consumption of HFCS has more than tripled. As of this decade, the overall U.S. per capita consumption of artificial sweeteners reached nearly 80 pounds, compared to 100 pounds per year for refined sugar.

In 2012, the Corn Refiners Association, or corn lobby, began a new public relations campaign to reposition HFCS as corn sugar, with frequent TV ads pressing the case that "corn sugar is just sugar. Your body can't tell the difference." Their website claimed that "high fructose corn syrup is simply corn sugar," and that it is *not* high in fructose. They'd even petitioned the FDA to change the name from high fructose corn syrup to corn sugar, claiming that the new name would more closely reflect the actual composition of the food additive. Instead, it appears that the Corn Refiners Association wished to disguise HFCS under the tidier name of corn sugar so consumers would believe they'd done away with harmful HFCS and that the "new" ingredient, corn sugar, was somehow less harmful. Why would they want to do this? Because high fructose corn syrup has been linked to a variety of serious health issues, including obesity, gout, and diabetes, and many consumers have become wary of HFCS, preferring *real* sugar instead. As of this writing, the FDA has refused the Corn Refiners Association petition to rename high fructose corn syrup as "corn sugar," but that may change at any time.

So what is the truth? Is HFCS, or corn sugar, the same as cane sugar and does our body really not know the difference? Do they really think our bodies are that stupid? Although all simple sugars are nearly identical as chemical formulae, each has its own distinct chemical properties.

High Fructose Corn Syrup is not a free molecular fructose such as the kind found in fruit. It is a *synthetically* manufactured treatment of hydrolyzed corn starch that converts glucose molecules to fructose. There are three types of high fructose corn syrups: HFCS-42, HFCS-55, and HFCS-90. The numbers reflect the percentage of synthesized fructose in the syrup. The first, HFCS-42, has the sweetness equivalent to table sugar and is found mostly in baked goods and processed foods. HFCS-55 is used as a sweetener in soft drinks, and the last, HFCS-90, which contains the highest fructose concentration, is only used to manufacture the lower fructose syrup HFCS-55.

The following chart is helpful:

Type of Sugar	Fructose/Glucose Ratio
Brown Sugar	1:1
Table Sugar	50:50
Maple Syrup	1:4
Molasses	23:21
Corn Syrup	0:35
HFCS-42	42:53
HFCS-55	55:41
HFCS-90	90:5

Every cell of the human body can metabolize glucose. But fructose goes straight to the liver for metabolization and interferes with the production of insulin. The livers of people consuming large quantities of high fructose resemble the livers of alcoholics, who frequently have fatty livers and cirrhosis. The conclusion is that this is an artificial sweetener to avoid.

People who consume high levels of high fructose corn syrup suffer from:

- Liver Disease
- Gout
- Obesity
- Diabetes

HFCS is found in a wide variety of products including bread, ketchup, apple sauce, and thousands of other processed foods, making it hard to avoid without careful scrutiny of packaged food labels.

Organic foods, on the other hand, often use juice from whole fruit as a sweetener, which is natural and not synthetic or synthetically derived. Still, it is the processed juice of the fruit and not the whole fruit, and is mostly fructose. Even though it may be organic, it is still a form of refined fructose.

WHAT'S IN THAT FRUIT JUICE?

If you need a sugar fix, it's best to opt for a piece of whole, raw fruit to satisfy the need for a sweet treat, rather than eating ice cream or other sweet packaged treats that probably contain a variety of artificial flavors and sweeteners.

Note too that almost all fruit juice, reconstituted from a juice concentrate or pure fruit juice, is a pasteurized concentration of fructose, glucose, and sucrose. While it is "natural," it contains a high concentration of sugar, with many calories, and it's devoid of nature's synergy. The high caloric value is due to the large quantity of fruit used to make one glass of juice. Most fruit juices are filtered and devoid of fiber, and the juices are concentrated. While a juice manufacturer may claim their product is "100% fruit juice," they are all reconstituted using water, and water is the first ingredient on the label, which means it's the major ingredient or the one with the largest percentage of the whole product. And the water used, filtered or not, most likely contains fluoride.

The only 100% real fruit juice is one that is fresh pressed or squeezed, is not filtered, and is not pasteurized. While manufacturers tout the amount of fruit in a single serving of their juice, most of the time it's flavored sugar water. And since the juice has been pasteurized, all of the beneficial bacteria have been destroyed, making it less useful to the consumer's overall health.

This same type of processing occurs with vegetable juices, which, like fruit juices, contain preservatives, some of which are carcinogenic, such as sodium benzoate.

It's important to carefully read the labels of fruit juices because many manufacturers add sugar in the form of high fructose corn syrup, as well as artificial sweeteners such as aspartame. The label on a well-known grape juice, which says it's "100% grape juice with added fiber," actually contains: Grape Juice from Concentrate (Filtered Water, Grape Juice Concentrate), Grape Juice, Maltodextrin (Dietary Fiber), Ascorbic Acid.

- Maltodextrin is a starch derived from corn, so it's technically "fiber," although it would make more sense if grape juice instead included fiber from the grape itself.

- Ascorbic Acid is artificial Vitamin C, and is used as a preservative, especially in highly acidic foods.

My absolute favorite, in terms of preposterous labeling, is another brand's "natural 100% apple juice with fresh pressed apples," which actually includes, according to the label, Apple Juice, Water, Apple Juice Concentrate. How does that add up to 100% apple juice and fresh pressed apples if it includes water and concentrate?

Only apple cider is 100% juice and fiber from fresh pressed apples, with no water added, no "concentrate," and no pasteurization.

As if all these labels aren't confusing enough, according to the USDA, six ounces of apple juice equals one fruit serving. Really? If you want one serving of fruit, the best source is the whole fruit. Then you'll be getting a lot more than just filtered water and liquid fructose/glucose/sucrose. Here's what you'll never find in a bottle of fruit juice, but you will get from eating an entire apple:

VITAMINS		
Nutrient	**Value**	**%DV**
Vitamin A	120 IU	2%
• Retinol	6.7 mcg	
• Beta Carotene	60.2 mcg	
• Beta Cryptoxanthin	24.5 mcg	
• Lutein + Zeaxanthin	64.7 mcg	
Vitamin C	10.3 mg	17%
Vitamin E	0.4 mg	2%
Vitamin K	4.9 mcg	6%
Thiamin	0.1 mg	3%
Riboflavin	0.1 mg	3%
Niacin	0.2 mg	1%
Vitamin B6	0.1 mg	5%
Folate	6.7 mcg	2%
Pantothenic Acid	0.1 mg	1%
Choline	7.6 mg	
Betaine	0.2 mg	

MINERALS		
Nutrient	**Value**	**%DV**
Calcium	13.4 mg	1%
Iron	0.3 mg	1%
Magnesium	11.2 mg	3%
Phosphorus	24.5 mg	2%
Potassium	239.0 mg	7%

MINERALS		
Nutrient	Value	%DV
Sodium	2.2 mg	0%
Zinc	0.1 mg	1%
Copper	0.1 mg	3%
Manganese	0.1 mg	4%
Fluoride	7.4 mcg	0%

AMINO ACIDS	
Nutrient	Value
Tryptophane	2.2 mg
Threonine	13.4 mg
Isoleucine	13.4 mg
Leucine	29.0 mg
Lysine	26.8 mg
Methionine	2.2 mg
Cystine	2.2 mg
Phenylalanine	13.4 mg
Tyrosine	2.2 mg
Valine	26.8 mg
Arginine	13.4 mg
Histidine	11.2 mg
Alanine	24.5 mg
Aspartic Acid	156.0 mg
Glutamic Acid	55.7 mg
Glycine	20.1 mg
Proline	13.4 mg
Serine	22.3 mg

OTHER		
Nutrient	Value	%DV
Protein	0.6 g	1%
Dietary Fiber	5.4 g	21%
Carbohydrates	30.8 g	10%
Phytosterols	26.8 mg	

Additionally, in whole fruits, there are whole-food synergistic values that fruit juices, artificial sweeteners, or even genetically engineered foods do not contain. What's actually missing in these processed products?

- Fruit skins – The skin is where fruit interacts with sunlight. Various pigments, colorations, absorb different wavelengths of light. These pigments include nutrient-rich carotenoids and flavonoids that help the body reduce the risk of cancer and provide protection against ultraviolet light. The skins also provide an important source of fiber.

- Fruit pulp – The pulpy part of fruits, especially the white pulp found in citrus fruits, is the primary source of flavonoids. The juicy part of the fruit contains not only fiber, but also natural Vitamin C. Vitamin C and flavonoids interact and have anti-viral, anti-allergic, anti-platelet, anti-inflammatory, anti-tumor, and antioxidant effects and properties.

- Fructooligosaccharides – Oligosaccharides are short chain carbohydrates that are derived exclusively from fruits and vegetables. Fructooligosaccharides are naturally occurring fructose sugar chains that constitute a prebiotic effect in the intestinal tract by enhancing growth and viability of beneficial probiotic bacteria such as lactobacilli.

Even orange juice isn't what you think it is. Florida's Valencia oranges are considered to be *the* oranges of choice by the orange juice industry, but those oranges are only in season from March through June. So how can we have "fresh" orange juice all year?

Well, some of that "juice" comes from oranges grown in the United States, as well as in other countries and imported. The orange juice industry stores the "juice" in million-gallon tanks through a process called "de-aeration." During this process, the juice is stripped of oxygen, which prevents oxidation, or turning rancid, and it can be stored for a year or longer. De-aeration also strips the juice of its flavonoids, which provide the fruit's natural flavor. What remains has been rendered tasteless and a lot less nutritious than what nature provided.

And when this tasteless, long-stored product must at last be turned into "fresh squeezed" orange juice, food science once again comes to the rescue with "flavor packs," which are chemically-altered products that have no relationship to what is found in an actual natural orange, and can contain high concentrations of ethyl butyrate, decanals, or terpene compounds, which are the chemically altered isolated flavors or fragrances that are now added to the tasteless sludge. Drink up!

If you actually want to drink real orange juice, the only way to get it is to buy some oranges and squeeze them yourself. You'll find that it looks and tastes nothing at all like industrialized OJ. Better yet, just eat the whole orange, preferably organic.

CHOCOLATE

Is nothing sacred anymore? One chocolate industry giant, so afraid of running out of cocoa, has vowed to overwhelm a major cocoa producing part of the world with genetically modified cocoa trees that will grow faster and produce more cocoa. In other crops that have been genetically modified, toxins that nature would keep in check have become more prominent, spurring new food allergies. Will this attempt to increase cocoa production take a natural antioxidant and delicious food and turn it into a less nutritious food allergen?

Alas, even chocolate has not been left untouched by food additives. Chocolate, especially bittersweet chocolate, is purported to contain naturally occurring antioxidants. But the cost of producing chocolate with rich raw cocoa butter puts a dent in a candy manufacturer's bottom line. So what's a poor multi-million dollar chocolate manufacturer to do? In 2006, the commercial chocolate industry made a pact to replace cocoa butter with PGPR.

What is PGPR? It stands for Polyglycerol Polyricinoleate and it's the chemical reaction (esterification) of condensed castor oil fatty acids with polyglycerol. It creates a water-in-oil emulsifier. And, aside from being a replacement for natural cocoa butter, PGPR is also used as a tin greaser by the food industry.

This can be tested readily by checking packages of chocolate candies and reading the ingredients. It won't matter what brand; PGPR is nearly always listed (along with high fructose corn syrup, artificial flavors and colors).

The following are ingredient lists from various kinds of chocolate:

Milk Chocolate Ingredients

- Sugar (unspecified form, could be beet sugar or corn sugar, both of which are GMO)
- Chocolate consisting of:
  - Cocoa butter (at least it's not PGPR)
  - Skim milk and milk fat (not organic, so probably from cows given rBGH and/or rBST)
  - Lactose
  - Soy lecithin (GMO)

- Salt
- Artificial Flavors (chemically derived)

Cornstarch – no doubt derived from GMO corn

Corn syrup - high in glucose and another form of GMO corn

Dextrin - derived from exposing starch to high heat or enzymes that polymerize it into a gummy substance; yet another form of GMO corn.

Artificial colors - Some colors are followed by "Lake," which refers to colorants derived from metal salts such as aluminum, calcium, barium, and others.

- **Blue 1** - Human allergen
- **Blue 1 Lake** - Linked to neurotoxicity (see Artificial Colors above)
- **Blue 2** – Neurotoxicity (brain cancer in animal studies)
- **Yellow 5 Lake** - (see Artificial Colors above)
- **Yellow 6** – Animal studies show tumor growth in adrenal glands and kidneys. Contaminated with carcinogens benzidine and 4-aminobiphenyl.
- **Yellow 6 Lake** - (see Artificial Colors above)
- **Gum Acacia** – A thickener often used to replace fats, but also used as glue on envelopes and stamps.

I won't buy or eat *anything* containing even one of those ingredients!

Peanut Butter Cups

Except for those with nut allergies, who doesn't love peanut butter cups? What combo could be better than chocolate and peanut butter? Chocolate is rich in antioxidants and peanut butter is high in nutrition and energy. They're a match made in heaven—or they were—until the food industry "massaged" out everything good. To read one manufacturer's description, peanut butter cups are "creamy" and "rich." That's certainly true, but ever wonder why?

They're "creamy" thanks to PGPR. And they're "rich" in sugar (no type specified, so it's most likely GMO beet sugar), Dextrose (high glucose sugar), TBHQ (tertiary butylhydroquinone is a form of butane that acts as a chemical preservative), and citric acid as a preservative. Oh, yum!

On the other hand, 100% certified organic peanut butter cups from small, independent companies such as Mama Ganache Artisan Chocolates will contain organic and fair trade cocoa, organic chocolate liquor, organic cane sugar, organic cocoa butter, organic whole milk, organic soy lecithin, organic vanilla, organic peanut butter, and sea salt. They're truly rich and creamy, and they melt in your mouth for the right reasons, not because of chemicals.

Beware of chocolates listed simply as "organic" and be sure to read the labels. Some do not contain 100% organic ingredients (non-organic soy lecithin is used, which is most likely GMO), and some brands, like Green & Blacks, have been purchased by Big Food.

To me, most chocolate always seemed to have a sharp or acidic taste and eating only the tiniest bit gave me a sour, acidic stomach. Now I know why—it's the chemicals. But it never happens with 100% organic chocolate.

Sadly, the entire commercial candy industry uses all of these artificial colors, artificial flavors, artificial sweeteners, chemical emulsifiers, chemical preservatives, and more, so my advice is: *Caveat emptor—let the buyer beware.*

MSG

"Plain and simple, MSG is a drug added to our foods that causes widespread toxicity."

Dr. George R. Schwartz

Some time ago, a prestigious TV chef devoted a segment to a non-scientific experiment involving MSG by taking a few dozen people to a restaurant without telling these "subjects" that they were participating in an experiment. They were divided into two groups, with one group given food prepared without MSG, while the other group ate meals containing MSG. After they'd eaten, the guests were asked if they felt any symptoms of MSG sensitivity, including headache, gas or bloating, dizziness, palpitations, or muscle tightness. A few people in each group complained of symptoms, with slightly more complaints from the MSG group. Then it was revealed to them that some of the diners who complained of MSG symptoms had not actually consumed any MSG. The conclusion drawn by the host and the chef was that MSG had been given a bad rap and that it isn't "the bad chemical it's made out to be."

But often the power of suggestion is enough to trigger a response. But what really made me take notice was the conclusion, something that stood out to me more than anything else. What I found shocking was that the host and the chef didn't refer to MSG as a flavor, a spice, or anything else that's natural. Instead, they called it a *"chemical,"* and one that's not bad for us. Viewers were being told by persuasive media in this instance that chemicals in our food are okay.

So what exactly is Monosodium Glutamate, or MSG? It's the third most popular flavor enhancer in the world, with salt and pepper taking the first two spots on the list. MSG is used in processed foods, fast foods, Chinese food, soy sauce, and most commercial soups. It's the staple of today's food industry.

In 1908, Dr. Kikunae Ikeda was able to isolate the flavor enhancer from Kombu seaweed, something Japanese households and chefs had used for thousands of years to flavor foods. What Dr. Ikeda discovered was that the flavor extract of the seaweed had *characteristics* of glutamic acid, and that the active substance was monosodium glutamate. A patent was secured and this seaweed-derived substance was manufactured by the ton and sold and used throughout Asia. It was a lot easier using MSG for flavor than tons of seaweed. Unfortunately, by isolating a single salt, the synergistic benefits of Kombu seaweed as a whole food are lost.

Meanwhile, in the United States, a milling company had a surplus of wastewater resulting from processing sugar beets and this wastewater contained substantial amounts of glutamic acid. And it thus became the goal of the beet producers to make MSG from this wastewater.

MSG as a flavor enhancer was ignored by the food industry until after World War II, when U.S. soldiers back from the Pacific described how much better Japanese rations tasted. That got the food industry's attention and they became interested in MSG.

Big Food companies, food service industries, meat packing and canning industries organized a symposium to taste test MSG and found that it suppressed undesirable flavors, made flavors and aromas more appealing, suppressed bitterness and sourness, and removed the "tinny" taste from canned foods. As a result, MSG began to be used widely in the food industry; in the last 30 years, its use in commercial foods has increased tenfold and continues to increase each year.

Seasonings such as herbs impart their own flavor when added to foods. MSG, on the other hand, intensifies the taste of the food to which it is added without altering the flavor.

MSG is claimed to be safe because glutamate occurs naturally in some foods. Keep in mind also that the flavor extract of the seaweed has *characteristics* similar to glutamic acid, but is not actually glutamic acid; yet another example of taking a nutritious whole food and synthesizing it. And the amount of MSG used in processing foods is far greater than anything found in nature and that's where the problems arise.

MSG sends taste messages directly from the tongue to the brain, and creates drug-induced nerve stimulation. MSG does not change the taste of food, but rather changes how the nervous system reacts to that food. The glutamate in MSG acts as a neurotransmitter that stimulates or excites brain cells, and in testing MSG, neurological stimulation has been observed for as long as half an hour. That's one reason you "can't eat just one" and it may also explain why so many of us have become food junkies.

MSG is classified as an excitotoxin meaning it stimulates or excites the nerve cells in our brain to the point of nerve cell death. Additionally, it also destroys the cells surrounding the affected nerve cells and may account for the headaches and dizziness that some people experience after consuming MSG.

When people have an adverse reaction after consuming MSG, they are said to be experiencing "MSG Syndrome." These reactions include:

- Acid reflux and heartburn occur because MSG weakens the stomach's sphincter, allowing stomach acids that are digesting food to escape back into the esophageal tube.
- Arthritis-like symptoms
- Asthma
- Cardiovascular effects are suspected from consuming MSG, although not fully understood or studied. Preliminary findings link heart murmur (mitral valve prolapse), and arrhythmia to the ingestion of MSG.
- Chest pain
- Depression
- Diarrhea
- Dizziness
- Headache (sporadic sharp pain in the temple)
- Migraine
- Mood swings
- Obesity
- Prostate problems
- Rage reactions
- Rash
- Schizophrenia
- Slurred speech
- In children, symptoms of headaches, vomiting, rash, hyperactivity, ADHD, shudder attacks, and seizures

I've been told by two different physicians that I had a "heart murmur" and for several years I experienced sudden and unexplained arrhythmia. When at work I would frequently dine at nearby restaurants for lunch, and at home frequently ate canned soups and other processed foods. Once I stopped frequenting restaurants and changed my eating habits, all my episodes of arrhythmia vanished and none of my current doctors have found any indication of a heart murmur.

HONEY

Instead of sugar, honey is often added to processed foods to make us think it's a healthier product. We all know that honey is supposed to be good for us. It's a complex carbohydrate made up of two sugars, levulose and dextrose, which our body converts to energy, and it contains enzymes that aid in breaking down and digesting starches. Honey also has antimicrobial and antioxidant properties.

But it's important to note that any honey, including raw honey, contains minute naturally occurring bacterial botulinum spores that no amount of processing can remove. This means that infants under the age of one year should not be given honey because their digestive systems are still too immature to produce enough acid to inhibit the toxin. It means babies can suffer serious or fatal food poisoning from the neurotoxic botulism bacteria in honey and must not eat it during that first year of life. Older children and adults produce sufficient acid to destroy these minute amounts of bacterial spores.

Raw honey that has not been processed is a whole food, and in its pure raw form appears as a waxy substance. It can be lightly heated and will melt to a pourable state. I had never consumed raw honey until recently and had for years used golden liquid honey in preparing certain dishes. After eating them, my husband always complained that it gave him indigestion, and I found honey by itself irritating to my mouth and throat, although it didn't upset my stomach in an occasional meal. Apparently there's a reason for our reactions. It turns out that, just as chocolate ingredients have been tampered with to increase profits, the same has been done with honey.

Even though honey sold in the U.S. is labeled as domestically produced, much of it comes from Asia and is simply packaged here. The USFDA is too understaffed to inspect every container unloaded in the shipyards or to check the millions of pounds of honey coming into the U.S. from abroad. This means it's anyone's guess whether the honey on your supermarket shelf is contaminated with:

- Lead from the buckets the honey is collected in
- Chloramphenicol – an antibiotic used to kill bacterial infestation in beehives, and is a known carcinogen and damages human DNA

And believe it or not, some "honey" has been made entirely without the help of real bees! Some honey adulteration tricks include:

- Mixing sugar water, malt sweeteners, corn or rice syrup, jaggery (a coarse, dark, unrefined cane sugar), barley malt sweetener, and other additives with a small amount of honey
- Using thickened, colored, artificial sweeteners made entirely of chemicals from the lab, as opposed to beehives

While there's no way to know whether the liquid honey we've consumed for years was genuine honey or not, one thing is fairly certain: most commercial honey is sold by large packers who didn't harvest the honey. All they did and still do is put their label on it.

By contrast, organic raw honey is certified organic, unpasteurized, unfiltered, and a completely different product because it's a natural whole food. It's creamy and has a mellow taste, and since we've switched, it doesn't irritate my throat or upset my husband's stomach. It tastes so good, once in awhile I'll eat a teaspoonful if I crave something sweet.

The raw honey manufacturer whose products we use has a website with history of their organic farm, along with photos, their mailing address, and their email address. Unlike the commercial producers, they are not a faceless conglomerate.

PESTICIDES

According to the Environmental Protection Agency, 30% of insecticides, 60% of herbicides, and 90% of fungicides used in food production are considered carcinogenic. Animal studies show pesticides to be carcinogenic, mutagenic, endocrine disruptors, neurotoxic, and reproductive disruptors. Pesticides have been linked to immune suppression, reduced male sperm, miscarriages, and diseases such as Parkinson's.

It's not easy and in some cases it's not even possible to remove pesticides from produce. Simply washing or peeling produce won't get rid of the pesticide residue because it is designed to be "rain proof" and stick to produce despite vigorous washing or scrubbing. Because pesticides have polluted "non-target" areas such as air, water, and soil, and has killed beneficial insects, to make pesticides "greener," industry has changed how pesticides work. Instead of being sprayed or dusted onto produce, pesticides are now designed to be absorbed internally by the plant, making it impossible to remove them.

In many cases, the "inert" ingredients (anything added to a pesticide that does not actively kill or control a pest) such as creosols in pesticides are more toxic than the active ingredients. For example, in the U.S. government's "Superfund" regulations, creosols are listed as "Hazardous Waste" and have been linked to skin and eye irritation, burns, inflammation, blindness, pneumonia, pancreatitis, central nervous system depression, and kidney failure. Inert ingredients, including creosols, are minimally tested, and in too many instances, they are not required to be listed on pesticide labels.

If that's not frightening enough, the biotech industry has taken pesticides to a new level by genetically engineering the plants to create their own pesticides! This has changed plants from food to pesticide factories. This is done by taking a naturally occurring soil bacteria, Bacillus thuringiensis (Bt), removing the gene that produces the toxin in the bacteria, and inserting it into the DNA of the plants so they will produce their own toxin. This toxin, called Bt Toxin, splits open the stomachs of insects that dare to take a bite out of the genetically modified plant.

It can't be a coincidence that people who never were allergic to certain foods are now having allergic reactions. It's very likely happening because every cell of these genetically modified plants produces Bt Toxin, making it 3,000-5,000 times more toxic than a spray, and at a toxic level not seen in nature. Plants containing Bt Toxin include non-organic corn, soybeans, sugar beets, yellow crookneck squash, zucchini, cotton, alfalfa, rapeseed from which canola oil is made, Hawaiian papaya, and even grass seed. Anything sold as a Roundup® Ready crop has this property of manufacturing its own pesticide. A hot area of research and development for the biotech industry and agri-business, the list of genetically modified plants grows almost daily.

The biotech industry claimed that Bt Toxin would not survive the hostile human digestive system. But they were wrong. A recent study out of Canada reveals that the Bt toxin is not only surviving in humans, it is now being passed on from one generation to the next as a genetic mutation.

As if all that wasn't scary enough, the Bt Toxin can also be inhaled. An entire Filipino village of 100 people developed symptoms of headache, dizziness, extreme stomach pain, vomiting, chest pains, fever, allergies, respiratory, intestinal, and skin reactions when an adjacent field of GMO corn was pollinating.

Since most fruits and vegetables are thin-skinned, they can readily absorb chemicals such as pesticides through their skin, as well as through their leaves, and any liquid chemical that reaches the ground can be absorbed by the roots as well. This means that even if a plant isn't genetically modified to produce its own poison, pesticides still are internalized by the plants and no amount of scrubbing will reduce them.

The Top Ten Contaminated Foods Grown or Produced in the USA

The following is the U.S. Food and Drug Administration's list of the top ten most contaminated foods growing and being produced in our country right now:

1. **Corn** – Topping the list as the number one contaminated food item is corn. Not only has corn been genetically modified (GMO) to become "disease resistant," it is also the crop most heavily sprayed with pesticides. Fifty percent of the pesticides used in the United States are used on corn fields. Corn is a staple in the

American diet and is in much of what we eat. To be safe, it's best to use organic corn if corn is an ingredient in a specific dish or food.

2. **Strawberries** - Considered one of the most contaminated of all fruits or vegetables on the market, in a study conducted by the Environmental Working Group, 70% of strawberries tested were contaminated with at least one pesticide. Thirty-six percent contained two or more pesticides.

3. **Bananas** - The pesticides that are used on bananas have been known to cause birth defects.

4. **Peaches** - Peaches have been found to have numerous violations of USFDA pesticide regulations. And pesticides are not limited to fresh peaches. Canned peaches are just as contaminated as fresh and can be even worse, depending on the chemicals and preservatives used in the canning process. Already underfunded and understaffed, the FDA frequently turns a blind eye or else misses violations for peach crops, including one crop that was contaminated at eighty times the allowed level. Things are likely to get worse; in 2011, the U.S. Senate gutted the USFDA's budget for food safety inspections.

5. **Rice** – Along with corn, rice is another staple of the American diet and is found in rice dishes and is used as a base in breads, cereals, snacks, rice milk, and in baby foods and formulas. The pesticides carbofuran, methyl parathion, and malathion are used to control rice crop damage from insects, while the herbicides molinate and thiobencarb are used to control weeds. Additionally, fertilizer nitrates, pesticide and herbicide residue runoff from

nearby conventional agri-farming via rivers, streams and tributaries also contributes to aquatic toxicity in the shallow surface water of the paddies that rice is grown in. Aside from these contaminants being absorbed by the rice, it results in significant mortality in aquatic organisms. And if that's not bad enough, rice is now another USFDA approved genetically modified crop.

6. **Oats and Grains** - Six to eleven servings of whole grains are recommended for daily consumption, so it would be smart to ensure that those servings are coming from pesticide-free, organically grown foods. Another example of Big Food's hubris is that at one point, it was discovered that one year's worth of a major cereal maker's products were found to be contaminated with illegal levels of pesticides. The company opted to let the contaminated product already on supermarket shelves remain but didn't release any additional products from their warehouses.

7. **Green Beans** – Because different states and different countries use different pesticide combinations, more than 60 pesticides are used to grow green beans. In an Environmental Working Group test, three separate pesticides were found in a sample of baby food green beans. It's been shown that green beans imported from Mexico tend to be the most contaminated.

8. **Leafy Greens** – Aside from contamination from heavy pesticide use, they are also frequently contaminated with e-coli from nearby conventional agri-farming residue runoff via rivers, streams and tributaries.

9. **Apples** - A widely distributed fruit, apples pervade the American diet. We eat them raw (an apple a day keeps the doctor away), we eat apple pies, applesauce, and we drink apple juice and cider. Unfortunately, apples contain 65% of the pesticides used on strawberries, the most contaminated fruit on the market. I once lived near a non-organic apple orchard and the pesticide sprayers would run all day, nearly every day of the week. Yet organic apples aren't much more expensive than their non-organic counterparts and they have a superior flavor than conventionally grown apples.

10. **Baby Food** - Last but certainly not least are those little jars of baby food. The Environmental Working Group conducted a test on baby food produced by some of the major baby food corporations and found 16 separate pesticides. Even if we don't want to bother making the change to organic for ourselves, we should at least try to do it for our children. Since babies spend the beginning of their lives eating only baby food, it should, at the very least, be pesticide free. It's also not difficult to prepare home-made baby food using a food processor. It's the best way to be sure of exactly what your baby is eating.

Eating the ten most contaminated vegetables and fruits will, on average, expose a person to nearly 20 pesticides per day, for an estimated 40 grams of toxins. If you're eating non-organic celery, for example, you may be consuming as many as 67 different pesticide residues along with it. Fruits and vegetables with soft skins are most susceptible to pesticide contamination because their thin skins absorb more pesticides. Consuming non-organic versions will introduce 47 to 67 different pesticide residues into your body per serving.

While the United States Food and Drug Administration has its list of the top ten most contaminated foods, the Environmental Working Group has its own "Dirty Dozen and Clean Fifteen." You can download the list from the Environmental Working Group's website (www.ewg.org) and carry it with you while you shop. The list is designed to help you save money by showing you which non-organic fruits and vegetables are the least contaminated by pesticides and safer to eat, as well as the ones that should be avoided and substituted with the organic version. It's worth taking the time to find out what's safe and what isn't.

The Environmental Protection Agency, the Food & Drug Administration, and the U.S. Department of Agriculture set tolerance levels for pesticides, claiming that their consumption in small amounts isn't harmful. That's like saying small amounts of rat poison every day won't harm you in the long run. Although there are no long-term studies pinpointing specific pesticides as being linked to specific diseases, clinical studies show that children with higher percentages of pesticides in their blood and urine are 20% more likely to have ADHD, nervous system disorders, and weak immune systems.

According to the Department of Preventive Medicine at Mount Sinai School of Medicine, studies show that it takes only two weeks for people who switch to an organic diet to reduce 95% of the pesticides in their bodies. That sounds like a quick and easy way to reduce toxic overload.

PESTICIDE NEUTRALIZING SYSTEMS

People have asked about home food cleansing systems to neutralize pesticides and kill microbes and viruses.

In reviewing the available units, those that claim to neutralize pesticides and reduce microbes couldn't back up those claims with test results. Their test results state that of the 23 pesticides (they didn't specify which ones) tested, only *"50% were sufficiently reduced,"* and the other half were reduced by 80%. Not neutralized, or even eradicated 100%. It may be possible to "sufficiently reduce" pesticides by 80% simply by scrubbing them in plain water—unless they're in genetically modified pesticide producing produce. The only sure way to protect yourself is to buy organic food.

As for killing the microbes and viruses, that's a good thing...maybe. But that presents the problem of killing off the good microbes that we need along with the pathogenic kind.

Yes, there are a lot of people who swear by this type of pesticide neutralizing product, but have they really investigated what's in the water they wash the produce in? These neutralizing products don't say anything about removing chlorine or fluoride. What about trihalomethanes? Or lead? Or volatile organic compounds? Lindane? Alachlor? Atrazine? Benzene? Trichloroethylene? Methyl Tertiary Butyl Ether? How about pharmaceuticals that water treatment facilities are recycling back to us via our faucets? There are a lot more dangerous things in our water supply to be concerned about than removing all of the microbes on our produce. Ultimately it's your decision.

GENETICALLY MODIFIED FOOD (GMO)

Genetic modification of organisms (GMO), or the genetic engineering of food, is a growing and potentially health hazardous factor in our lives. Because there is so much information regarding the health risks in consuming bio-engineered food, I have devoted a great deal of discussion on the topic.

According to consumer advocate Jeffrey Smith of the Institute for Responsible Technology, *"After GMO's were introduced in 1996, the percentage of Americans with three or more chronic illnesses jumped from 7% to 13% in just 9 years, food allergies skyrocketed, and disorders such as autism, reproductive, digestive, and others are on the rise."*

As Jeffrey Smith's quote above indicates, many believe that genetically modified foods are dangerous for a variety of reasons. And with that in mind, here is a question to consider: What do cocoa trees, cotton, corn, sugar beets, canola oil, Hawaiian papaya, alfalfa, wheat, rice, soy, a salmon that grows twice the size in half the time, or grass seed all have in common? They have all been genetically modified, and there is no end in sight as to what food staple the bio-tech industry will tamper with next. It seems that they won't be happy until they have modified every single plant that nature has created, as if they know better than nature itself.

Some people think genetically altered food isn't "so bad." But to me, only someone who has not delved into the topic would believe this. Every living thing on this planet has evolved over 4 billion years and during that time, nature has fine-tuned plants, trees, animals, and humans so that with each new generation, the organism enhances traits that allow it to maximize its potential. Nature has perfected the balancing act between good and bad traits in each organism so that with each new generation, the modified organism is better than the previous ones. Nature performs this modification through mating (cross breeding) or pollination and has perfected the process through natural selection, or the survival of the fittest. This means that only the strongest survive to create the next generation, thereby passing along the characteristics and traits that have helped it survive.

For years, breeders have been mating/cross-breeding/cross-pollinating similar plant and animal species to get specific traits or outcomes. This is how new breeds of dogs are created, such as when a cocker spaniel and a poodle are bred to produce a new breed, the Cockapoo, for example. And although it's a new breed, it's still a dog. But sometimes cross breeding doesn't always bring out desired results and some breeds have developed physical problems such as hip dysplasia as the result.

I grow amaryllis, and one year cross-pollinated two Hippeastrum amaryllis. One was all red with a black throat, while the other was mostly white with deep red veining and a green throat. The seeds produced by each of these plants resulted in six separate bulbs and the seeds from the all-red amaryllis produced flowers that were mostly red, while two had a white-star pattern in the center; but not a single one was identical. The bulbs from the seeds of the white amaryllis ranged from solid white with a blush of pink to salmon with white edges; again, no two were alike.

Emboldened, I cross-pollinated two different amaryllis species; an hippeastrum amaryllis, which has wide petals, with pollen from a cybister amaryllis, which has very narrow petals. Then I reversed the procedure, pollinating the cybister amaryllis with pollen from the hippeastrum variety. Both pollinated plants developed seed pods, but late into their development there were unintended results. The hippeastrum seed pod inexplicably yellowed, withered, and died while the cybister amaryllis produced a full-term seed pod that produced only half the usual number of seeds. Soon after planting and germination, half of the original seeds died and a few only lasted a month or two. Out of 50 original seeds, only 17 survived and are flourishing, but I can't predict how the resulting flowers will look. However they turn out, they will be a new organism, but they will still be amaryllis.

Will they be viable? Will they be disease resistant and able to grow as well as their parents did? Will they flower? Have I unintentionally created a failure that won't be able to reproduce? Will the bulbs thrive or die after a few years? Those questions won't be answered for at least 5 years when the bulbs are mature enough to flower. Until then I'll have to wait, watch, and observe in the "laboratory" of my own home before giving any away.

Unfortunately, this is something the bio-tech industry fails to do. Because their new "creations" are deemed "similar" to the original organism, they do not conduct testing of new "creations" for longer than 30 days before the genetically engineered crops are approved for release into the environment. This is a significantly insufficient length of time to determine undesirable traits, which may not surface until the next generation or even the second or third generations. This is a serious concern because it means that nobody really knows how those genetically modified crops will affect animals, humans, or other crops they pollinate. Will the animals or humans who consume GMO foods on a regular basis develop illnesses or die? Will their reproductive cycles be affected? Wouldn't it be wiser to wait and see, before putting these crops into circulation?

Because the bio-tech industry considers all of its information to be patented scientific and intellectual property, their test results are not made public. As a result, research data hasn't been made available even to independent scientists who request it. And it's worrisome that scientists who are not affiliated with the bio-tech industry have performed their own animal testing with less than satisfactory results. For example, cows fed GMO corn experience spontaneous abortions and are rendered sterile, and baby pigs from a mother fed a GMO diet have been born without genitals, meaning they would not be able to reproduce—if they were able to survive. One rat study done by Monsanto, made public via a lawsuit, showed a significant increase in three types of blood immune cells: basophils, which indicates an allergic reaction, lymphocytes and total white blood cell counts, which the body produces in response to infection, toxicity, and diseases, including cancer.

Animal studies show significant changes to the intestines and major organs, including the liver, kidneys, pancreas and genitals of mice, rats, pigs and salmon fed a GMO diet versus those fed a non-GMO diet. In the GMO-fed group, there were alterations to the intestinal tract that affected their ability to digest proteins.

How might a diet consisting of mostly GMO food affect us? Quite possibly it could alter our ability to digest proteins, which in turn means that our body will be less able to produce amino acids. Amino acids are the building blocks for proper cell growth and function.

Despite what the bio-tech industry would have us all believe, truly natural, non-GMO whole foods contain beneficial, synergistic components that genetically modified foods can't provide, simply because the bio-tech industry can't wait billions of years to fine-tune the genome in the way that nature has.

Even in a family, no one knows, unless they are identical twins, how individual children will look or what physical characteristics they will display. No one can predict if a child will have brown eyes, blue eyes, red hair, black hair, or even what gender it will be. Why is that? It's because all the science in the world still does not fully understand how genes express themselves. There are a multitude of forces in play at the time of conception and afterward. Studies show that outside forces also affect the outcome of an organism, including the amount of chemicals like pesticides or heavy metals present at conception and throughout fetal development.

In nature there are specific divisions and there is an order to reproduction. Dogs breed with other dogs, cats with cats. A flower doesn't cross pollinate with a tree, a beet doesn't cross pollinate with an ear of corn, and a mammal doesn't mate with a fish. This is true because the DNA of one is not compatible with the DNA of the other. Nature knows that to combine two totally different species would create a freak of nature with less than desirable effects. Even Dr. Frankenstein put together his "creation" by using human parts instead of components of other species.

But now, along comes the bio-tech/bio-science industry, and instead of following the natural order of things, Big Bio-Science takes a bit of this DNA from one species, a bit from another, entirely different species, and creates a hybrid organism that has never previously existed in nature, and one that did not evolve naturally. And on top of this, they don't take a wait and see approach to find out if it's safe, since they claim that the GMO hybrid is food that is "similar" to the original.

Enter the USFDA, which accepts this claim, and deems the new item Generally Regarded As Safe, or GRAS. This designation means that the item does not need to be tested for safety and as a result, the item is quickly approved for release into the environment. Unfortunately, once this new creation is released into the environment, it can never be recalled. If undesirable and unexpected characteristics or problems develop, it nevertheless will contaminate everything around it that is "similar," changing all of those organisms as well, and not necessarily for the better.

Before I began researching genetically modified foods, I thought the modified corn, soy, or beets were simply the best characteristics of one breed crossed with the best of a different variety of the same breed, such as an all-yellow corn cross pollinated with a yellow-and-white corn. But that's not the case.

Without knowing the long-term repercussions, it doesn't make sense to inject the DNA of one organism, such as bacteria, into another organism, such as corn, and expect the outcome necessarily to be beneficial or positive. For example, the inserted gene can become truncated, fragmented, mixed with other genes, inverted, or multiplied, creating unintended characteristics. Native genes can be mutated, deleted, permanently turned on or off, and hundreds can change how they work.

Yet the bio-tech industry tries to make us believe that only they can feed the world, and that nature-compatible farming, which has fed us through the entire history of humanity, is not the answer. And yet, experiments have proven that to be untrue. Genetically modifying crops by inserting foreign DNA into the plants, and manipulating their own DNA, has had negative results. Crops that were naturally able to fend off certain diseases are no longer capable of doing so. These crops have been modified to withstand being blasted with Roundup®, which contains the chemical glyphosate. Glyphosate binds the nutrients in the soil, preventing plants from taking nutrients from the soil that it needs to be healthy. The result is that crops become sick, prone to disease they naturally would have been able to fend off, may suffer sudden death syndrome (SDS), and have lower yields.

The bio-tech industry claims there is no need for testing the safety of GM foods on humans. As long as the introduced protein is determined safe, food from genetically modified crops are determined to be "substantially equivalent" and "not expected" to pose any health risks.

But "substantially equivalent" does not mean that it is equivalent. "Not expected to pose health risks?" Are they serious? Even species created in nature that have evolved over billions of years can pose health risks. They can be poisonous if we eat them, such as specific poisonous mushrooms categorized as amanitas, false morels, and a category known as little brown mushrooms (LBMs), or cause us problems if we come into contact with them, such as Poison Ivy.

Genetically modified organisms are now being released into the wild on a regular basis, with no regulation or long-term studies. They are combining their artificially modified genes with the DNA of plants that have evolved over billions of years. What if the bio-tech industry is wrong about their safety?

The bio-tech industry is fighting to prevent "clean" products from being labeled as "non-GMO," and has poured millions of dollars to fight state initiatives to demand labeling of GMO ingredients. One argument they raise against labeling GMO ingredients is that it would be expensive to change labels and would make the products cost prohibitive.

This is a ridiculous scare tactic because manufacturers repeatedly change the labels of their products every time they alter the ingredients list, add a new flavor, change the recipe, or when the FDA demands a change. For instance, package labeling changed when listing trans fats was required by the FDA, and in late 2013, the FDA mandated that no products could contain trans fats, which means that companies not only had to switch to using non-hydrogenated oils, but their packaging had to change as well. This would be a huge undertaking for the food industry, and yet none of the products involved would be unaffordably priced.

Now the Grocery Manufacturers Association, which is a front for the bio-tech industry and Big Food, is pushing for a federal law that would prevent states from passing GMO labeling initiatives.

But consumers need information about potential health risks of genetically modified food in order to be able to make their own choices.

The long-term effects of GMO foods on humans are still unknown and scientists conducting independent research have been thwarted by the bio-tech industry through loss of research grants, thus removing the scientists who are doing the research, and ensuring that their study results never see the light of day.

If the bio-tech industry truly has nothing to hide, then what are they afraid of? In 2012 Monsanto spent millions in pro-GMO advertising to defeat California's Proposition 37, which would have required the labeling of GMO ingredients in products sold in California. Other states that have proposed similar legislation have backed down after threats of lawsuits by Monsanto. By objecting so strenuously to labeling, by refusing any type of short-term or long-term safety testing, the biotech industry raises more questions than they answer.

If you still believe that genetically modified, genetically engineered food is harmless, ponder this: Two of the biggest players in bio-engineering are Monsanto, Inc. and Dow. No matter what they call themselves they are, plain and simple, chemical companies.

Monsanto and Dow both produced the chemicals needed to make Agent Orange, the defoliant used during the Vietnam War to prevent enemy soldiers from hiding in the heavy jungle foliage. It derived its name because it was shipped in orange-striped 55-gallon barrels, and is an herbicidal mixture of the toxic chemicals 2,4,5-T (2,4,5-Trichlorophenoxyacetic acid) and 2,4-D (2,4-dichlorophenoxyacetic acid).

These chemicals not only physically harmed the Vietnamese, causing spontaneous abortions and grotesque birth defects that mostly affected males, but also American soldiers—Vietnam veterans who came into contact with Agent Orange—it continues to affect their offspring three generations later because the chemicals (2,4-D and 2,4,5-T) used in Agent Orange are not only environmentally persistent, they are also bio-accumulative and persistent in humans. They literally mutate human DNA and are being passed on from generation to generation.

Monsanto also developed DDT, touted as safe for decades until its ill-effects proved otherwise; along with Dioxin, called the most toxic synthetic man-made chemical on the planet, and PCB's (Polychlorinated Biphenyls) which, according to the U.S. EPA, have an adverse impact on the immune, reproductive, nervous, and endocrine systems, as well as being a recognized carcinogen. PCBs not only remain in the environment for years, they also accumulate in the human body after exposure.

As if introducing these toxic chemicals into the food chain and environment wasn't enough, Monsanto has now introduced genetically modified hormones recombinant bovine growth hormone (rBGH) and recombinant bovine somatotropin (rBST) into milk production which is passed on to anyone drinking the resulting milk.

To top it all off, the same company has created Roundup® Ready genetically modified crops that are ending up on our plates. This means it's not just fresh produce we have to be wary of because genetically modified corn, sugar beets, soy, and canola oil end up in most processed foods, as well as in a variety of "healthy" products including vitamins.

To protect yourself from these genetically modified foods, read package labels carefully, even though it's unlikely to find a list of ingredients that spells out genetically modified ingredients. Keep in mind that if the ingredients are not organic and contain any form of corn, beets, soy, or canola oil, they are genetically modified. Corn flakes, corn chips, soy milk, texturized soy, soy protein, products containing corn oil, and canola oil are also genetically modified, and any sugar that is not specified as pure cane sugar or evaporated cane juice is derived from beets, or from corn in the form of corn syrup, corn solids, high fructose corn syrup, maltodextrin, or else it is beet sugar, which has been genetically engineered.

The extent to which these genetically modified ingredients can be found in most processed foods should not be taken lightly. When Monsanto formally requested FDA approval for their genetically modified stearidonic acid (SDA) soybean oil, the company projected the intended use for this soybean oil *"...as an ingredient in baked goods and baking mixes, breakfast cereals and grains, cheeses, dairy products, fats and oils, fish products, frozen dairy desserts and mixes, grain products and pastas, gravies and sauces, meat products, milk products, nuts and nut products, poultry products, processed fruit juices, processed vegetable products, puddings and fillings, snack foods, soft candy, soups and soup mixes."*

The other problem with genetically modified plants is that they are built to withstand the herbicide Roundup®. The main component or active ingredient of Roundup® is a chemical called glyphosate.

Glyphosate binds with the nutrients in the soil, suppressing the growth of unwanted plants or weeds, and prevents them from taking in nutrients from the soil, thereby starving the undesirable plants. Sounds great in theory, but what happens to the plants we want to grow when they can't get nutrients from the soil around them because glyphosate prevents it?

While genetically modified crops have been engineered to withstand Roundup®, nutritionally-deprived soil also affects the crops. The vital minerals a healthy plant needs to resist soil-borne diseases are significantly reduced. Glyphosate also destroys beneficial soil organisms that live around a plant's roots and naturally enable the plant to absorb nutrients while suppressing disease-causing organisms. Without these beneficial organisms, and because they're getting less nutrition, the plants become weak and more prone to disease and insects. Photosynthesis is disrupted, reducing water efficiency, and damaging root systems, causing plants to release sugars that change soil pH in harmful ways.

Aside from weakening the plants, glyphosate, by binding with nutrients such as minerals in soil, deprives crops from absorbing and using those vital nutrients. A side-by-side analysis of organic, non-GMO grown produce and Roundup® Ready crops shows that for the organic crops, the uptake of iron, manganese, and zinc was 100%. But using only ½ ounce of glyphosate per acre (1/40th of the recommended dosage), the genetically modified Roundup® Ready crops absorbed only 50% of the available iron, manganese is below 20%, and zinc is roughly 90%. The dispersion of these minerals into the plant in organic non-GMO crops is also 100%. However, in the genetically modified Roundup® Ready crops, iron levels were approximately 10%, manganese barely 2%, and zinc about 15%—certainly not sufficient to keep us healthy.

Other micronutrients are reduced as well in genetically modified Roundup Ready crops. In a study of alfalfa treated just once with Roundup® showed the following reductions:

Nitrogen	-13%	Boron	-18%
Phosphorous	-15%	Copper	-20%
Potassium	-46%	Iron	-49%

Calcium	-17%	Manganese	-31%
Magnesium	-26%	Zinc	-18%
Sulfur	-52%		

The human body requires daily replenishment of these vital micronutrients in order to function optimally. You'd be wrong to think that by eating non-organic potatoes, crook-neck yellow squash, zucchini, papaya, corn, or soy you are eating healthy and getting your day's ration of essential vitamins and minerals. A 1991 study showed that as much as a staggering 76% loss in nutritional value was found in foods, compared to those same food nutritional studies conducted in 1940.

The analyzed liver of a stillborn calf revealed *no detectible levels of manganese.* This is important because Roundup® Ready crops are the food fed to non-organically raised livestock that eventually end up on our plate. By adding manganese to herd feed, disease rates plummeted from 20% to less that 0.5%. This means that the comment that "you've been eating this food all your life and it didn't make you sick" is based upon fiction, not fact.

Glyphosate accumulates and can remain in soil for a very long time. One study showed that it took 22 years for glyphosate to degrade by 50%. But nobody knows what happens when we ingest glyphosate grown crops. In a recent German study, every urine sample collected from people who lived in and around the city of Berlin tested positive for glyphosate. Does glyphosate inhibit our ability to absorb and use the micronutrients we eat? Are we, like the Roundup® Ready crops, becoming weak and disease-prone? There are no studies yet to determine the answers to these questions.

But Don Huber, Ph.D., is an eminent plant pathologist and retired Army colonel who advised the U.S. government on biological threats to our food supply for over 30 years. Monsanto, Inc. hired Dr. Huber to study their genetically modified organisms and when he raised concerns about a pathogen, he was fired and Monsanto immediately discredited his work, suggesting that he was incompetent.

Distressed by his discovery, Dr. Huber wrote an open letter to the U.S. Secretary of Agriculture in 2011, requesting that there be a halt to the deregulation of genetically modified organisms, and alfalfa in particular. According to Dr. Huber, a virus-size fungal pathogen may have proliferated as a result of using glyphosate, which creates soil conditions favorable for allowing that pathogen to thrive.

Dr. Huber believes that because of this organism's proliferation in genetically modified Roundup® Ready plants, soybeans are now suffering sudden death syndrome, corn is exhibiting Goss' wilt, along with at least 40 other plant diseases. He also describes escalating infertility and spontaneous abortions in the U.S. cattle, dairy, swine, and horse populations, with 20% infertility in dairy heifers and up to 45% spontaneous abortions in cattle. The connection with these problems is that cattle are fed alfalfa hay or silage, which is ground up corn, stalks and all. When 2,000 heifers were used in a feeding study, half were fed non-GMO alfalfa and the other half fed GMO corn silage subjected to glyphosate. As a result, nearly half the 1,000 cows fed GMO silage had spontaneous abortions, while none of the heifers fed non-GMO alfalfa aborted. Independent animal studies also show an alarming abnormal proliferation of cells in the intestines, liver, and pancreas.

Alas, Dr. Huber's warning has fallen on deaf ears, and the bio-tech industry has received approval to introduce into the environment just about any genetically modified organism it can dream up. In addition, genetically modified alfalfa has been deregulated. Because it is pollinated by wind, it will contaminate any non-GMO alfalfa nearby. This poses a serious threat to organic cattle farms that depend on non-GMO hay to feed their livestock in winter.

Genetic engineering is even reaching our lawns through an exclusive marketing agreement between Scott's, which makes lawn care products, and Monsanto. Scott's has the exclusive right to sell Roundup®, and recently Scott's applied for permission to exclusively market Monsanto's genetically modified grass seed that will withstand being sprayed with Roundup®. And because grass is also pollinated by wind, it will contaminate all the other grass around it. This becomes a problem for organic farms because organic cattle and dairy farmers depend on unadulterated, GMO-free grass to pasture their animals that produce GMO-free milk, cheese, or are slaughtered for meat that we consume.

It may also pose a health risk to humans. An entire village became ill when a neighboring GMO corn field pollinated, so how might GMO grass pollination impact human health? How might it affect people living next to GMO lawns, or children playing on GMO grass, especially after it has been treated with Roundup®? Scott's and Monsanto claim it is safe, but no independent studies have been conducted.

While Monsanto takes most of the heat, other chemical companies also play a part in spreading GMO crops and chemicals. Because many weeds have mutated to the point they are impervious to Roundup® alone, Dow AgroSciences, a division of Dow Chemical has announced another, even more toxic multi-herbicide called Enlist®, which will include a combination of glyphosate, glufosinate (a neurotoxin that causes birth defects), and 2,4-D choline (an Agent-Orange ingredient derivative). While nearly 100% of soy grown in the U.S. is already GMO, now it has also been re-engineered to withstand this deadly combination of chemicals. Using even more toxic combinations of chemicals will only create more mutated weeds, and potentially more health risks that are already associated with pesticides and herbicides.

Just think, the same companies that brought us dangerous chemical agents such as DDT, Agent Orange, Dioxin, PCBs, and rBGH/rBST milk are now releasing Agent Orange's cousin and Roundup® Ready crops for our consumption.

Now, if you still really want to believe that if this wasn't safe, the USFDA wouldn't allow it, then ponder this: genetically modified white potatoes were created for mass production for use as fresh potatoes in our supermarket produce aisle, as French fries in every fast food chain, as frozen potatoes, potato chips, and every other conceivable potato product, even potato starch. And because these potatoes were able to generate their own pesticide, the potato "seeds," or starter potatoes, came with a label identifying them as a "pesticide!"

And as a "pesticide," they fell under the jurisdiction of the EPA, which ruled them to be food, and therefore the EPA contended that it was up to the FDA to determine whether they were safe. However, since they were labeled as a pesticide, the FDA ruled that it was up to the EPA to determine whether they were safe. Thus, these little pesticide factories fell between the cracks and no long-term safety testing occurred. This means that all of us might have taken part in that experiment—without knowing or consenting to it. But because fast food chains, to their credit, did not embrace the potatoes, the "pesticide potato" line was discontinued.

But there isn't one single crop that the bio-tech industry isn't tinkering with and then targeted for mass production. Just like genetically modified corn, soon more vegetables will most likely be genetically engineered.

In late 2013, approval for a genetically modified apple came before the USFDA. The GMO Arctic Apple (a combination of the Golden and Granny Smith apples) has been genetically engineered to not turn brown when sliced and exposed to air. The genetic engineering process uses a type II gene from E. Coli Tn5 and is grown on a medium containing Kanamycin, which is an antibiotic.

Every cell of the Arctic Apple tree, including the fruit, will show resistance to Kanamycin. Why is this alarming? It's worrisome because the antibiotic, Kanamycin, is commonly used in human medicine to treat a wide variety of infections. Do we really want a fruit that if we eat it will render an antibiotic useless just so we can have an apple that won't turn brown after you slice or bite into it? What happens to insects that pollinate the blossoms, or wildlife that eat the fruit? How will it affect the surrounding soil? What's to stop pollinating insects from transferring the gene to non-GMO apple trees? There is no testing or proof that these genetically modified apples are harmless to humans, wildlife, or the environment. Approval of this pointless apple is still pending. If approved, it will be with scant review from the FDA, the very agency that was created to protect us.

Forty of fifty years ago, the FDA used to conduct its own testing before issuing approval for any new product. Today, the agency does none of its own testing and typically it depends upon studies provided by the petitioner. Government scientists review the material, and then it is rubber-stamped by the FDA and approvals granted.

According to the April 7, 2011 Federal Register, the USDA requires a bio-tech petitioner to submit environmental reports that the Animal and Plant Health Inspection Service (APHIS) uses to base its preliminary assessment. From there, in a joint agreement between the petitioner and APHIS, an outside contractor is hired to prepare "independent" environmental analyses before any genetically engineered plant or animal is deregulated and released into the environment. Sounds promising, doesn't it? Except that the hiring of the "independent" contractor, the "independent" environment impact study, analysis and document preparation is totally funded by...the petitioner, which is major conflict of interest!

If the Department of Agriculture was really serious about the long-term impact of genetically modified organisms on every aspect of the environment, including on humans, a growing number of independent studies are available using credible science to determine that impact. These independent studies are not funded by parties that have a vested interest in a favorable outcome, but the bio-tech industry claims to be "unaware" of such studies, or else claims that the studies are "flawed" if they dispute industry's dogma. It appears that if the bio-tech industry didn't fund the study, then it must be either non-existent or else science fiction. Alas, the FDA appears to be equally as dumb and blind.

Chemical companies are tampering with what's already perfect in nature in order to sell more chemicals. Do we really want to believe their press that this stuff can't hurt us? Is there really any federal agency protecting us? If you believe that, then I've got a bridge to sell you.

Most of us have no interest in becoming hosts to an internal pesticide factory, and I personally do not want to wait and see the effects on myself or future generations. What nature provided has served us well for 170,000 years, and while we still have a choice, organic food is the only safe way to eat.

LABELING

Don't let words like "natural," "hand made," "homemade," or even "organic" trick you. Read every label and ask questions. The FDA uses three categories for labeling organic products:

- **Natural:** This term is meaningless, especially when it comes to processed foods and advertising. A manufacturer may make a product using genetically modified canola oil, genetically modified corn, and MSG flavoring, and yet it would still be considered "natural" under FDA guidelines. Some very prominent *all natural* breakfast cereals consist of nearly 100% GMO and synthetic ingredients. Meats and poultry are also sometimes labeled as natural when in fact they are factory farmed. *Natural* or *all natural* are labels to be shunned because nothing backs up the claim: no testing, no rules, and no guidelines. These terms are simply marketing ploys to entice the public to buy products that most likely are anything but *natural.*

- **100% Organic:** This means a food item is made with 100% organic ingredients. These products will display the green and white USDA certified organic label. Some manufacturers of 100% organic foods have their products tested and certified by the Non-GMO Project, an independent non-profit organization committed to on-site inspections, testing, verification, and assurance that companies whose products contain their seal are certified GMO-free. Only those that make the grade are certified and can show the label stating that they are "Non-GMO Project tested/certified GMO-free." Note that some companies claim to be "enrolled" in the Non-GMO Project but their products have not been tested or certified. However, the USDA Organic label does not guarantee safety or purity. It's still necessary to examine every package with care. It is also helpful to investigate who owns the organic brands you use, because many large food companies, including Kellogg's, General Mills, Pepsi, Heinz, and many others have taken over organic companies (*See* "Who Owns Organic" at www.cornucopia.org/who-owns-organic/).

- **Organic:** This term means a product is made with *at least* 95% organic ingredients. Big Food has managed to weaken this guideline so that 5% non-organic ingredients may be included, even some of which may be synthetic.

- **Made with Organic Ingredients:** This designation means that the product is made with a minimum of 70% organic ingredients, and with restrictions on the remaining 30%, with GMOs strictly prohibited. Note that food products with less than 70% organic ingredients are permitted to list the organic ingredients on the side panel of the package, but they cannot make any front of the package claims about being organic.

The USDA's regulations for growing and preparing organic foods further stipulate that:

- The use of irradiation is prohibited
- Sewage sludge is prohibited from being used as fertilizer in organic farming because contaminants in the sludge may be absorbed by crops
- Genetically modified organisms cannot be used in the production and processing of food

- Antibiotics and synthetic hormones are prohibited from being used in meats and poultry
- 100% organic feed for all organic livestock is required
- Synthetic pesticides are not allowed.

It's interesting to learn that synthetic pesticides evolved from chemicals including mustard gas and nerve poison, both developed for chemical warfare during World Wars I and II. Eager to unload these stockpiled toxins without having to pay to dispose of them, the chemical companies who had developed them began to tout such toxic matter as a way to control insects, fungi, bacteria, weeds, and other pests. By their nature, pesticides are inherently toxic and were designed to kill living organisms, including humans. They are known to pose significant health risks to humans, including:

- Birth defects
- Nervous system damage
- Hormonal and endocrine disruption
- Respiratory disorders
- Skin and eye irritation
- Various cancers
- Immune system suppression
- Testicular cancer and low sperm count in men, and birth defects (hypospadias) in male babies

Pesticide exposure is especially harmful to children and the toxins are passed from mother to fetus. Early chemical exposure is linked to the sharp rise in children's health problems, including autism, asthma, brain cancer, and other cancers.

- More than 1 million children in the U.S. aged 5 and under consume at least 15 pesticides every day from the fruits and vegetables used in baby foods they're fed.

- Nearly 600,000 of the million children eat at least one dose per day of organophosphate insecticides that the federal government considers unsafe.

- Over 10% of these million children take in doses of pesticides that are greater than 10 times the level considered "safe" by government standards.

Even if products are labeled organic, it doesn't mean you can skip reading their labels. That's because members of The National Organic Standards Board (NOSB) used to be represented by organic farmers. Now the membership is dominated by representatives from Big Food that only have an organic product line because they acquired organic brands. As a result, the rules that govern organic products were changed in 2006, making them less strict. In addition, approved organic ingredients were typically reviewed every five years and either re-approved or disapproved based upon the most current studies. In 2013, that ruling was overturned and no review has taken place. Now *organic* simply means that 95% of the ingredients must be organic. The other 5% do not have to be.

Unfortunately, with more and more small organic companies being purchased by Big Food, and the influence Big Food has over the FDA, the list of the 5% synthetic ingredients approved for the organic label by the FDA is growing, making it necessary to read *all* labels, regardless if a product is listed as organic.

For example, some of the previously unapproved synthetic ingredients that are now allowed under the organic label include:

- MSG which is typically listed as yeast extract
- Preservatives sodium benzoate and polysorbate 80
- Ingredients treated with sulfuric acid
- Ingredients extracted with hexane
- Non-nutritive sweeteners such as aspartame

At least this watering down of the "organic" label stopped at permitting sewage sludge to be used as fertilizer, which is often the case for non-organically grown products.

It is best to choose products that are 100% organic, state they are GMO-free, and include the FDA organic symbol. There are still a handful of independent companies dedicated to uphold the 100% organic tradition, and do not include GMO's or synthetic ingredients. Here are a few:

- Amy's
- Lundberg Family Farms
- Nature's Path
- Rising Moon
- Woodstock Farms

To find a current downloadable shopper's guide of companies who most likely do not use synthetic or GMO ingredients, go to www.CenterForFoodSafety.org.

Whenever you see the term *natural*, chances are it's anything but natural, and not what you expect. For example, when you purchase 100% organic bread, it is made with whole grains such as whole wheat and the list of ingredients is very small. You won't find "enriched flour" anywhere on the label, and this is because the flour in 100% organic bread has not had all the nutrition milled out of it, nor does it need synthetic nutrients added as a result.

When it comes to corporate processed foods, I envision the product looking like a blob of colorless paste that "food scientists" alter with additives that will make it look, smell, and taste appealing—like the real bread used to and still does if it's organic. But processed bread includes additives including artificial color, artificial flavor, artificial texturizers, and the usual very long list of chemical ingredients that do not occur in nature but are created in the lab.

IRRADIATED AND MICROWAVED FOOD

Irradiation

When food irradiation first was being discussed, it sounded like a great idea. If you irradiated food, then all bacteria would be destroyed, meaning it would be possible to irradiate a piece of chicken, then vacuum seal it, and it would last on a shelf indefinitely without refrigeration. Now, not only could you store poultry in a bag on a shelf in the pantry instead of the fridge or freezer, you also could do this with any perishable product, from meat, to fruits, to vegetables, and just about anything else.

It sounded like a great invention, but like most innovations that seemed like great scientific leaps forward, sometimes they can be a detriment to human health. Why?

- Because irradiated food is dead. Not only have all bacteria, fungi, or parasites been rendered dead, so have all of the beneficial, living micro-organisms and micronutrients our bodies need, including probiotics, amino acids, and enzymes. Here's why we need them: Probiotics are beneficial bacteria that aid in the breakdown and digestion of food. Approximately 25 pounds of these beneficial bacteria are found internally and externally, and help keep pathogenic (bad) bacteria in check.

- Amino acids are the building blocks for all proteins and are essential in building muscle, connective tissues, bones, and other structures. They also provide the nitrogen essential for growth and maintenance of all our living tissues and structures and have specific functions in human physiology and biochemistry.

- Enzymes are complex proteins that cause the chemical reactions necessary for life. Enzymes enable digestion and are secreted by the pancreas and gastrointestinal tract. Together with microbes, enzymes break down protein, carbohydrates, and fats. When we eat raw foods, the enzymes in the food begin to break down the food even before our digestive system starts working on it. This pre-digestion means our bodies don't have to do all of the work. But enzymes are fragile, and at temperatures above 118°F become inactive. This means that when food is heated at high temperatures during processing, the enzymes are killed and no longer able to perform their vital functions and the human body must carry the load. This overburdens the digestive organs and increases the likelihood of diseases such as pancreatitis and diabetes.

Irradiated food has been rendered nutritionally dead, and although it looks and tastes like the original food it has no nutritional value. This means that a steady diet of irradiated food will deprive the body of the essential nutrients it needs for health and survival.

Some manufacturers go the extra step and state on their packages that their product has not been irradiated. Luckily we like to label nearly everything in the USA, and irradiated food has its own symbol. Avoid eating anything labeled with this symbol, shown here, because it has been irradiated and is therefore without nutritional value and potentially dangerous to your health.

Microwave Ovens

Many people believe that microwaving food briefly will heat the food but leave its nutritional value intact. But this is a fallacy because microwaving changes the composition of the food. In fact, foods that are microwaved have been shown to:

- Lose valuable nutrients (up to 97%)
- Have chemical structural changes

Microwaving food also creates radiolytic compounds not found in nature.

And no matter how long you microwave food, whether for 1 minute or 1 hour, it's still microwaved and therefore damaged. There's also a reason microwaving is often referred to as "nuking" food.

Like most people, I used to think that microwaving food worked by making the molecules in the food vibrate, which created friction, which in turn created heat. This sounded harmless enough.

But the reality is that the atoms, molecules, and cells in food are forced by electromagnetic radiation to reverse polarity anywhere from 1 to 100 billion times per second. This tears apart the structures of the molecules making them deformed so that they no longer hold any nutritional quality.

These structural changes have been shown to lead to degenerative health. Just as grilling meat creates carcinogens, these "nuked" compounds increase the chances of colon cancer.

In an experiment conducted by the Swiss Federal Institute of Technology, in conjunction with the University Institute for Biochemistry, eight volunteers from the Swiss Macrobiotic Institute at Kientel, Switzerland, were fed eight whole and microwaved foods over a period of 2-5 days, as follows:

1. Raw organic milk
2. The same milk conventionally pasteurized
3. The same raw milk microwaved
4. Pasteurized non-organic milk
5. Raw organic vegetables
6. The same organic raw vegetables cooked conventionally
7. The same organic raw vegetables microwaved
8. The same organic vegetables frozen, then defrosted in a microwave

The eight volunteers each received only one food form, meaning that, five volunteers ate food prepared conventionally, while three ate foods prepared via the microwave. Blood samples were taken immediately before and after each food type was eaten, and significant changes were detected in the volunteers who had eaten microwaved food. Those changes included:

- A decrease in hemoglobin needed for oxygenation of the blood
- A reversal in HDL/LDL cholesterol ratios, (lowered "good" HDL, increased "bad" LDL)
- An increase of white blood cells, which signals illness in the body.

Today, many foods are processed for microwaving, including frozen foods in plastic bags or on plastic food trays, and snack foods in bags, including popcorn. And, as if microwaving food isn't destructive enough, there are the added detriments of the long list of chemical ingredients used in the product, along with the dangers of all the plastic and packaging. Let's use a very popular snack, popcorn, as an example of the dangers of microwaved food.

Since the corn used in most commercial pre-packaged microwavable popcorn is not organic, it's most likely GMO. And, aside from being high in fat and sodium additives, the flavorings in microwave popcorn are made of chemicals, whether it's butter, cheese, nacho, or some other flavor. These chemicals, especially the artificial butter, have been associated with a debilitating and eventually terminal disease, *bronchiolitis obliterans*, also known as "popcorn lung." This dreaded condition is caused by inhaling the vapors from a bag of freshly-popped microwave popcorn, and these inhaled chemicals are proven to irreversibly destroy the small airways in the lung(s). The only cure is drastic: a single or double lung transplant. As of 2010, three consumers have been stricken with "popcorn lung." The law firm handling these cases has devoted a website to this debilitating and potentially fatal disease, and the *New York University Review of Law & Social Change* has chronicled these case studies.

The chemicals and lung-destroying vapors aside, the coatings on the inside of the microwave bags have a grease-repelling coating that contains chemicals that can metabolize into an even more dangerous form called perfluorooctanoic acid, or PFOA, and just 10 bags of microwave popcorn per year is estimated to account for 20% of the PFOA levels measured in the average American. PFOA has been linked to:

- Birth defects

- Cancer
- Immune disorders and toxicity
- Impaired liver function
- Dangerous changes in lipid levels

Microwaving causes fluorotelomer coatings to give off gases people inhale and which is also absorbed by the food. So by using microwaved popcorn, the consumer is both breathing in and eating a dangerous substance that has been linked to a variety of health problems.

PFOA is found on fast food wrappers and even on disposable plastic plates. These coatings are also used in non-stick cookware and utensils.

Additional container coating chemicals that can leach into microwaved food include:

- Polyethylene Terephthalate (PET or PETE) – A synthetic polymer linked to liver damage
- Benzene – A known carcinogen, neurotoxin, immunotoxin, hematological toxin
- Toluene – A neurotoxin
- Xylene – Exposure includes neurotoxicity, organ toxicity, eye and skin irritant, musculo-skeletal abnormalities, and pulmonary edema

After learning about these dangerous coatings and chemicals used in non-stick cookware and utensils, I replaced all non-stick bake pans with glass or stainless steel ones and now all my cooking utensils are stainless steel. I also use high-heat silicon spatulas, and instead of non-stick cookie sheets, I use stainless steel pans covered with untreated parchment paper.

I admit that I consumed many bags of microwave popcorn over the years, and fresh organic popcorn, made the old-fashioned way in a stainless steel stovetop popcorn popper, as opposed to microwave popped corn, is a great snack that is low in calories, high in fiber, and non-toxic.

But it's important to note that popcorn should only be made in a stainless steel pot or pan. Aluminum is to be avoided, and pans made of aluminum with aluminum covers also pose a threat because aluminum leaches into the food being cooked in it when it's exposed to high heat. Studies have shown high levels of aluminum accumulation in the brains of people with Alzheimer's Disease.

Unfortunately, air poppers are not safe, either, because although they do not contain the chemicals, the plastics with which they are made, when subjected to high heat, also leach chemicals into the food, including:

- Bisphenol-A
- Dioxin

To avoid trouble, I now use only organic, non-GMO popcorn that I pop in a stainless steel, stove-top popcorn popper using only two ingredients besides the popcorn: Himalayan pink salt and organic virgin coconut oil.

When I cook I use stainless steel, glass, or CorningWare pots, pans, and bowls. I also use them to re-heat food on the stove and somehow it doesn't seem inconvenient, especially knowing all the toxins I'm avoiding. I eat most of my food raw, steamed, or baked, and use a stainless steel pot filled with boiling filtered well water and a stainless steel strainer to steam organic corn on the cob, rather than poisoning myself, not only by microwaving ears of corn, but also covering them with plastic wrap! I know better now, and I advise everyone to follow suit. Remember that the most nutritional food is living food, and is best in its rawest form, when it's full of beneficial micro-organisms. This is why living food decays quickly—because it's alive. If it has an artificially extended "shelf life," it actually has no life left in it. Dr. Randy Wysong explains "shelf *life*" as *"a misnomer—it refers to dead food that has no life because it has been processed, packaged, and all but embalmed."*

FACTORY FARMING

- In April 2011, over 27 tons of turkey products were recalled due to salmonella contamination that sickened people in 10 different states.

- In August 2011, a major meat packer recalled 36 million pounds (that's 18,000 tons) of factory-farmed turkey products due to salmonella contamination that sickened over 100 people in 32 states.

- In September 2011, the same company recalled 92 tons of ground turkey that tested positive for salmonella.

- In 2011, the U.S. Department of Agriculture Food Safety and Inspection Service had pending 11 Salmonella, 5 E.coli, and 3 Listeria open cases.

- Before 2011 ended, there were nearly 100 pending cases where chicken, turkey, and beef products were recalled for E.coli, Salmonella, and Listeria contamination, mislabeling, spoilage, adulter-ation, under processing, and miscellaneous other health risks.

POULTRY

Factory farm chicken eggs come from chickens that are inoculated at birth and routinely fed antibiotics to keep disease at a minimum. Their feed consists of the cheapest available and to keep parasites down, arsenic is routinely added to their feed; and their eggs, instead of being laid in nests, simply roll down a chute to a conveyor belt. These unnatural, inhumane conditions contribute to 36% higher cholesterol levels in factory-farmed eggs, along with diseases including salmonella, compared to eggs from organically raised free-range chickens.

One of the largest egg recalls in U.S. history took place in 2010. At that time, salmonella sickened and killed people who ate affected eggs. Over a half million eggs were recalled with the outbreak linked to a particular factory egg farm in Iowa.

In case anyone thinks these recalled, salmonella-tainted eggs were destroyed, guess again. Instead the eggs were pasteurized and used in food products that contain powdered eggs or liquid pasteurized eggs, as well as in pet food, all of which appeared on supermarket shelves. And the factory farm responsible for these contaminated eggs received only a slap on the wrist from the FDA, without being shut down even briefly to improve conditions and rectify the handling issues that led to the salmonella. As a result, nothing has changed.

Aside from the poor conditions for egg-laying hens, chickens themselves have been tampered with by food scientists working for food giants. Here's a comparison of chickens raised the old fashioned way and the new, reengineered kind:

The life cycle of a humanely raised, free-range chicken is fairly long at 10-15 years. A chicken raised this way will mature in 3-6 months, and a hen can lay one egg per day and up to 300 eggs per year while in their egg-laying prime of up to 5 years of age. Most egg layers are not meat birds, although some large breed chickens can weigh between 6-8 pounds and be raised for egg laying and then used for meat when they've surpassed their egg-laying prime.

On the other hand, reengineered, corporate agribusiness chickens raised as meat birds have been redesigned to have larger breasts and therefore more meat. On corporate chicken farms, chickens mature in 48 days rather than 3-6 months, and then their short lives end. According to the IRS publication Poultry Industry, "Market Segment Specialization Program," Training 3123-013 (03/2002), typical meat chickens known as "broilers," are, at the age of 21 days placed in "grow-out facilities where they are fed, watered, and medicated" in order to maximize their weight to feed ratio. They are fed artificial growth diets without being allowed to forage for food. As a result, their organs and bones cannot support their weight and these birds cannot walk.

Chickens that are designated as layers are bred to be egg producing machines. They are bred to be small, weighing only about 3 pounds, and most would fit the average person's palm. These laying hens are kept in laying houses and are stacked in cages holding between 2 and 10 hens each. These cages are crammed one on top of the other into barns with no windows or natural light. The hens are packed in the cages so tightly that they are unable to spread their wings. Their beaks are cut so they can't peck at and wound each other and their wings are clipped, even though they have no opportunity to fly. These laying houses are fully automated to provide constant feed and water to each cage. As previously described, their eggs roll down onto a conveyor belt for collection and once these egg-laying chickens are no longer productive, they end up as "animal digest" or "chicken meal" in pet foods because they are so small and without enough usable meat for any other purpose.

Why is chicken and egg farming so inhumane? Perhaps The National Chicken Council provides an explanation. Here it is, in their own words: *"We are not producing chicken, we are producing food. We're producing more chickens, using less land, at a very affordable price. Somebody explain to me what's wrong with that?"* As one chicken grower for a major chicken-producing corporation says, *"Smells like money to me."*

Turkeys are raised exactly the same way, except they are not used in egg production. Farmers who raise poultry for corporations provide facilities, utilities, and labor, but the chickens and turkeys are owned by the corporations, which provide the poultry, feed, veterinary, technical, and catch and haul services.

Compare this with local farmers. The chickens roam everywhere, even laying their eggs in the goat barn feed hay. The eggs range in size from small to large depending upon the breed of chicken, the yolks are bright orange, the shells are much harder, and they taste better than store-bought eggs. They taste like the eggs I remember from childhood. Factory farm produced eggs pale by comparison.

Chicken and turkey from an organic farm is also better, with tender meat that's juicy, tasty, and not fatty. They are also normal sized birds, not the grotesque sized factory farmed poultry.

But even organic poultry is threatened. In 2013 the USFDA came out with new guidelines for raising organic poultry and eggs.

The FDA, in its convoluted wisdom, has deemed that it isn't factory farming that causes salmonella-tainted eggs. No, it's free-roaming chickens' exposure to wild birds! It has been proposed that organic egg producers raise their hens just like factory farms where the birds have no access to the outdoors, or are permitted screened porches. If the farms insist on free-ranging their chickens, then cannons must be set off to scare away wild birds. No doubt these guidelines will not reduce the incidences of salmonella-contaminated factory farmed eggs, but may increase the chances of less healthy organic egg production because the chickens will not be allowed to forage the way they evolved to do, and will have limited access to direct sunlight.

MEAT

- In July 2011, over 114 tons of ground beef were recalled for possible E.coli contamination.

- In October 2011, over 188 tons of beef products were recalled due to E.coli contamination.

E.coli is another bacteria that threatens our food chain and is now prevalent in cows and humans, thanks to the agri-business methods of fattening up beef cattle as quickly as possible. Because cattle are grass eaters, also known as ruminants, pasture-fed cattle are much leaner and their bodies use the grass they eat in a healthy way. As a result, they don't become fat the way that agri-business raised cattle do.

Agri-business-raised beef is farmed much in the same way as poultry in that these cattle are not allowed to roam in a pasture to mature naturally. Instead, they are kept in barns and fed at concentrated feeding stations known as "CAFO's," where they eat a diet of corn to fatten them up quickly, and that corn is quite often genetically modified. But cows did not evolve eating corn, and as ruminants designed to eat grass, their bodies are unable to absorb the nutrients from corn, which means their bodies turn the corn into fat.

There is a serious public health downside to this type of cattle feed, aside from producing fat cows, in that the cattle that are corn-fed produce E.coli in their stomachs, which does not occur if they are allowed to eat grass, and this deadly bacteria is excreted in the cattle's manure. In these giant agri-business farms, the cattle can't move around because they are crammed into pens, standing knee deep in their own manure and their fur is caked with it. When cows are slaughtered to become food some of the E.coli contaminates the meat that ends up in the supermarkets of the nation.

Yet if cattle are taken off the corn diet and fed only grass, as they were designed to eat, within only 5 days they will shed 80% of the E.coli bacteria in their intestines. This obviously is a very simple solution that would guarantee that the beef in your supermarket would be free of E.coli contamination. But is that what the agri-business beef industry does? Take a guess. Think about it the next time you consider buying "cheap" hamburger meat. You might want to opt for organic ground beef or bison or some other grass-fed, organic meat.

Why?

Pink Slime

There's the whole "pink slime" situation, for starters. Back in 2002, an FDA microbiologist coined the term "pink slime" for the "filler" used in nearly 100% of all non-organic and non-bison hamburger meat. It's all the waste trimmings a butcher would normally throw out, including the outer fat. But some of that waste contains bits of flesh, so the agri-business meat industry puts that waste into a centrifuge, which separates the fat from the tissue, and what is left is "pink slime," which formerly was sold to the pet food industry, but now is used by the meat-packing industry as filler for hamburger meat, which saves the producers anywhere from 3 to 5 cents per pound.

And because it's from the outer carcass of the cow, it's most likely loaded with E.coli, so it's soaked with ammonium hydroxide in an attempt to kill off the bacteria. But FDA testing confirms that the E.coli bacteria still exists, and as a result, we have major recalls of hamburger meat as a result of E.coli outbreaks.

So, the next time you buy non-organic, non-bison hamburger meat or stop for a burger at a fast-food chain, you'll not only be getting a good dose of ammonium hydroxide and some E.coli bacteria, but you'll also be eating pink slime. In other words, you'll be eating what used to be considered dog food. Bon appetite!

Aside from E.coli contamination of meats, there have been E.coli outbreaks in produce crops including lettuce and spinach. And how does the E.coli end up in our produce? In some cases it comes from runoff water dumped by cattle factory farms into the waterways that irrigate produce farms. The other source of E.coli is non-organic farming, which allows the use of "sewage sludge" to be used in growing crops. Sewage sludge is made of non-organic agri-business, E.coli packed manure that's spread out on the fields where non-organic crops are grown, thereby contaminating the produce with E.coli. It means even eating a non-organic salad can have a serious downside and E.coli can be fatal.

Antibiotics in Factory Farming

It's surprising that any of us ever needs antibiotics, considering how much of it is in the meats we eat. According to the FDA, in 2009, the reported and non-independently reported use of approved antimicrobial drugs used in food-producing animals shows:

TABLE 1-Antibiotics		
Destination	Antimicrobial Class	Annual Totals (kg[1])
Domestic	Aminoglycosides	339,678
	Cephalosporins	41,328
	Ionophores	3,740,627
	Lincosamides	115,837
	Macrolides	861,985
	Penicillins	610,514
	Sulfas	517,873
	Tetracyclines	4,611,892
	NIR[2]	2,227,366
Export	Tetracyclines	515,819
	NIRE[3]	1,115,728

[1]kg = kilogram of active ingredient. Antimicrobials which were reported in International Units (IU) (i.e., Penicillins and Polypeptides) were converted to kg.

[2]NIR - Not Independently Reported. Antimicrobial classes for which there were less than three distinct sponsors actively marketing products domestically were not independently reported. These classes include: Aminocoumarins, Amphenicols, Diaminopyrimidines, Fluroquinolones, Glycolipids, Pleuromutilins, Polypeptides, Quinoxalines, and Streptogramins.

[3]NIRE – Not Independently Reported Export. Antimicrobial classes for which there were less than three distinct sponsors exporting products were not independently reported. These classes include: Aminocoumarins, Aminoglycosides, Amphenicols, Cephalosporins, Diaminopyrimidines, Fluorquinolones, Glycolipids, Ionophores, Lincosamides, Macrolides, Penicillins, Pleuromutilins, Polypeptides, Quinoxalines, Streptogramins, and Sulfas.

TABLE 2-Antibiotics Antimicrobial Drugs and Drug Classes Approved for Use in Food-Producing Animals	
Aminocoumarins: Novobiocin	**Macrolides:** Carbomycin

TABLE 2-Antibiotics
Antimicrobial Drugs and Drug Classes Approved for Use in Food-Producing Animals

Aminoglycosides:
Apramycin
Dihydostreptomycin
Efrotomyci
Gentamicin
Hygromycin B
Neomycin
Spectinomycin
Streptomycin

Amphenicols:
Florfenicol

Cephalosporins:
Ceftiofur
Cephapirin

Diaminopyrimidines:
Ormetoprim

Fluoroquinolones:
Danofloxacin
Enrofloxacin

Glycolipids:
Bambermycin

Ionophores:
Laidlomycin
Lasalocid
Monensin
Narasin
Salinomycin
Semduramicin

Lincosamides:
Lincomycin
Pirlimcycin

Erythromycin
Oleandomycin
Tilmicosin
Tulathromycin
Tylosin

Penicillins:
Amoxicillin
Ampicillin
Cloxacillin
Hetacillin
Penicillin

Pleuromutilins:
Tiamulin

Polypeptides:
Bacitracin
Polymixin B

Quinoxalines:
Carbadox

Streptogramins:
Virginiamycin

Sulfas:
Sulfachlorpyridazine
Sulfadimethoxine
Sulfamerazine
Sulfamethazine
Sulfaquinoxaline
Sulfathiazole

Tetracyclines:
Chlortetracycline
Oxytetracycline
Tetracycline

Organically raised animals do not need the pharmacy of drugs that factory farm animals are routinely given to keep them from getting sick. This is because organically raised animals are naturally healthy and as a result, organic meat contains less fat and none of the growth hormones or antibiotics that non-organic meat is laced with.

PROCESSED MEATS

In addition to factory farmed meat full of antibiotics and growth hormones, as well as ammonium hydroxide filler, processed meats are loaded with processing additives.

The first category to consider is dyed or color-enhanced ground beef. Have you ever noticed that a package of ground beef is a healthy deep pink on the outside but looks dark grey on the inside? That's because ground beef, unless freshly ground that minute, is actually somewhat grey in color. But because we equate pink flesh with health, meat producers spray dyes on the exterior surface of the ground beef to give it that bright pink, healthy looking color.

This is not commonly known, and when a neighbor complained to me 15 years ago that the supermarket in a nearby town dyed their meat, I couldn't believe it. But when I saw the unnatural bright red ground beef in the meat section of that store, I knew it was true. Never before had I seen ground beef with such a bright red color. But not all supermarkets do this so it's worth asking questions. And it's worth the extra time to have the meat ground while you wait and ask to watch as it is ground.

The second, and far worse category of processed meats are deli meats, bacon, ham, salami, corned beef, and the mystery meats found in hot dogs, bologna sausage, commonly known as baloney and sausage. The World Cancer Research Fund, in a review of over 7,000 clinical studies that examined the connection between diet and cancer, found an undeniably strong relationship between a diet heavy in processed meats and bladder and bowel cancers.

These meats are "cured" so they last a long time in the fridge without spoiling. Decades ago, meats were "cured" with salt or were smoked, and the curing process took months to years. Now meat processors do not have the luxury of curing meats slowly so they speed up the curing process by using chemicals that are added as preservatives, coloring, and flavoring. These chemicals include, but are not limited to:

- Sodium Nitrate and Sodium Nitrite, which are preservatives that help processed meats retain their color, even after cooking. They also retard the growth of botulism toxins, which can be fatal if eaten. The danger of these two sodium preservatives results when they react with chemicals in the stomach, including stomach acid, because they then convert to nitrosamines that are associated with an increased risk of certain cancers.

- Sodium Benzoate was FDA approved in early 2013 to be used as a preservative to control the growth of Listeria and other pathogenic bacteria in "ready-to-eat" meat and poultry products. Sodium benzoate is a carcinogen and has also been linked to DNA damage.

- Sodium Propionate used as a preservative to control the unwanted growth of bacteria in processed meat and poultry products was approved by the FDA in March 2013. Sodium propionate has been linked to gastrointestinal upset and respiratory problems.

- Benzoic Acid is another preservative given FDA approval for use in ready-to-eat meat and poultry products to suppress pathogenic bacterial growth. In documents submitted to the FDA by Kraft Foods Global Inc., the corporation claims that these three chemicals "do not conceal damage or inferiority, or make products appear better or of greater value than they are." Benzoic acid is believed to promote asthma and hyperactivity, especially in children. In addition, Kraft admits that it adds Lem-O-Fos to its meat and poultry products to "enhance antimicrobial activity." Studies have shown that when benzoic acid is combined with citric acid it forms neurotoxic benzene.

According to the documentation, all three of these newly approved preservatives in ready-to-eat meat and poultry products will provide greater anti-microbial stability, better handling and shipping, improved visual characteristics of the products, and speed up the FDA food safety approval process.

- Polycyclic aromatic hydrocarbons (PAHs) – Many processed meats are smoked, either as a flavor enhancer or as a curing process. Grilling food can cause Polycyclic Aromatic Hydrocarbons to form when dripping fat burns and creates excessive smoke, and these hydrocarbons are carcinogenic.

- MSG – Monosodium Glutamate is an excitotoxin that literally excites cells to cellular death, especially brain cells. MSG is often disguised using different names, including *autolyzed yeast extract*, *hydrolyzed vegetable protein*, and the blanket terms, *spices* and/or *seasoning*.

- High Fructose Corn Syrup (HFCS) – High fructose corn syrup is an artificial sweetener derived by changing the molecular structure of corn starch by using high heat.

- Artificial colors – These consist of synthetic chemicals that do not occur in nature. Depending upon which dyes are used, they have been linked to hyperactivity in children and linked to cancers of the brain, bladder, testes, adrenal gland, kidney, and thyroid, as well as liver damage.

- Artificial flavor – Artificial flavors, by their name designation alone, provide sufficient warning about exactly what they are: artificial. They are simply a mixture of chemicals that mimic a natural flavor. These chemicals have taste and smell activation components.

- Caramel color - One of the most widely used artificial colorings is "caramel color," which can be found in nearly every commercially produced food product. It is derived by heating carbohydrates, like sugars, with acids, alkalis, and especially ammonium compounds. When produced with ammonium, caramel coloring contains two types of contaminants that are linked to cancer. And don't be misled: caramel color has absolutely nothing to do with the caramelization of cane sugar, which means the sugar turns brown when it's heated.

- Natural flavor – In the food processing world, natural flavor has nothing to do with nature. It can be dozens, or even hundreds of chemicals known as esters that are interacting to create specific tastes and smells; chemicals such as Octyl Acetate (orange flavor), Isoamyl Acetate (banana flavor).

The World Cancer Research Fund found in a 2007 analysis that eating 1.8 ounces of processed meat daily increased the likelihood of cancer by 20%. Other studies link processed meats to the increased likelihood of the following types of cancers: colon (50%), bladder (59%), stomach (38%), and pancreatic (67%). Processed meats are also linked to diabetes, lowered lung function, and an increased risk of chronic obstructive pulmonary disease (COPD).

MEAT GLUE

And if all of this weren't bad enough, an Australian investigative reporter revealed that the commercial food processing industry uses something called "meat glue" to hold pieces of protein together. That's right, meat *glue,* otherwise known as transglutaminase. If you ever wondered how that deli meat, which you readily recognize as bits and pieces of meat put together in a "loaf," stays together, or how a hot dog holds together without a casing, along with that imitation crab meat, fish sticks, or even Chicken McNuggets, the answer most likely is meat glue. If you go to a restaurant and order steak, look for seams, joints, or the grain of the meat going in different directions. If any of those characteristics are visible, you'll know that the delicious steak is nothing more than pieces of lesser meats glued together to form a bigger one.

Meat glue is also used to:

- Improve the texture of emulsified meats like sausages and hot dogs, especially if they do not come in casings
- Improve the texture of deli meats, also called PSE meat (pale, soft, and exudative meat)
- Make non-fat milk products seem "rich and creamy" without the fat
- Make noodles firmer

Meat glue is derived from two sources: the coagulant proteins in animal blood, and from the cultivation of bacteria. In powder form, it is considered toxic if inhaled and factory/lab handlers must wear masks.

The whole point of meat glue is to take inferior cuts of meat which formerly would have been considered waste, and turn them into something that looks appealing. But it's just another food industry trick to turn waste that used to be deemed unfit for humans, into money.

One microbiologist claims that meat glued products are hundreds of times higher in bacterial contamination than conventional meat. In 2010, the European Union banned glued meat products, but alas, and as usual, the United States has not issued such a ban. The Centers for Disease Control concluded that glued together meat products are prone to food poisoning because the different pieces of protein cook at different rates, meaning the bacteria in the meat parts are not thoroughly killed by cooking. In addition, these pieces of meat come from different sources, which mean that if a food contaminated illness becomes an epidemic, it will be even harder for the CDC to track down the source.

After learning all this about how processed meats are made, I thought I'd never eat another hot dog, and I rarely do. But there's nothing that can beat the taste of a hot dog on a bun with mustard. Luckily I found an organic replacement for hot dogs along with everything else in my home. While I wouldn't recommend making hot dogs a regular food staple, an occasional one can be a treat. Look for organic *uncured* hot dogs that are 100% muscle meat with no "mystery" in them whatsoever. Organic and uncured, means they don't have fillers, preservatives, or synthetic ingredients. Look for them in the freezer section of your food store or refer to the "Resources" section in this book for where to order them online.

I also found organic whole wheat hot dog and hamburger buns, which are big and heavy and made with no artificial or unnecessary ingredients. I was in hot dog heaven and so were our friends when they tasted my organic hamburgers and hot dogs on organic whole wheat buns, with organic mustard and ketchup. "What did you do to the hamburger meat to make it so moist and beefy tasting?" they asked. Or, "I bet this is very lean beef," they supposed. Or, "Where did you get this great ketchup?" But all I did was feed them 100% organic food with no additives, fillers, artificial color, texture enhancers, no MSG, and no meat glue.

Our local food co-op also carries wonderful uncured maple ham from a nearby farm. When I brought hors d'oeuvres to a party made from this ham, I was constantly asked where I got it because the other guests hadn't "tasted ham like that in years!"

We've all been seduced into believing that the "artificial" and "imitation" slop we've been consuming these last 20 or so years is actually food. But once we try "real food," our taste buds immediately know the difference. I've now successfully replaced all of the meats and poultry in my freezer with organic versions raised by local organic farmers or ordered from organic websites. Nothing is "cured," and now I don't have to be cured either.

FISH

We've been urged to eat more fish because it contains precious Omega-3's that do everything from reducing inflammation to protecting our heart. Alas, even fish are now subject to the same unsustainable, disease-breeding farming practices that the beef, poultry, and pork industrial producers use.

Most people hearing about farmed fish envision a safe environment where the fish live healthy lives free of contaminants, but nothing could be further from the truth. In reality, major fish producers maintain hundreds of thousands of "net cages" in the ocean, each of which can contain nearly 750,000 fish. In these crowded conditions, unable to eat food their bodies thrive on, and which they evolved eating, the fish are fed a diet intended to speed up and increase their growth. These overcrowded, unnatural conditions pollute the environment, encourage disease, and require the use of antibiotics to keep the fish "healthy."

These industrial fish farms harm the aquatic environment, are bad for human health, and certainly aren't good for the fish. The following are some of the downsides to farming fish:

- **Sea Lice** – These are parasites that attach to fish and feed off them. This happens to wild fish too, but occurs in huge numbers of fish living in crowded, farmed conditions. Fish living in captivity provide unnatural breeding grounds for various infestations that also contaminate the surrounding waters and infect other nearby marine life. Sea lice attaching to immature fish whose scales are not yet fully developed are much more likely to kill off the young fish. To control sea lice, industrial fish farmers add a pesticide, Emamectin Benzoate, to the fish feed. This chemical kills the Sea Lice that feed on treated fish, but now sea lice are becoming resistant to this pesticide and alternatives such as deltamethrin are being tested. But no matter which chemical is used, anyone who eats the farmed fish treated with pesticides is eating it right along with the fish on their dinner plate.

- **Infectious Hematopoietic Necrosis (IHN)** – IHN is a highly infectious virus found in industrially-farmed fish such as salmon and rainbow trout. While IHN can also infect wild fish, it is especially virulent for crowded farmed fish. Infected fish develop symptoms of swollen bellies, bulging eyes, darkened skin, abnormal behavior, and anemia, and they eventually hemorrhage from the mouth, behind the head, and on the pectoral fins, weakening until they float "belly up." There is no treatment for these fish, who suffer a slow death.

- **Furunculosis** – This is another highly infectious bacterial disease that causes large boils on the fish's skin. While it can occur in the wild, it is especially prevalent in factory farms growing Atlantic salmon, Atlantic cod, turbot, American eel, carp, catfish, minnow, northern pike, and smallmouth bass, among others. In 2005, furunculosis wiped out 1.8 million salmon spawn at a single factory farm hatchery on Vancouver Island in British Columbia, Canada. The disease also is found in salmon farms throughout Scotland, Norway, Canada, Washington State, and the Broughton Archipelago in British Columbia.

- **Bacterial Kidney Disease** – This chronic bacterial infection afflicts salmon, trout, chars, and freshwater white fishes, killing off significant numbers. Treatment consists of inoculated vaccines, and antibiotics either through medicated baths, or through feed. Not only do these treatments end up in the environment, they end up at your dinner table.

These are only a handful of examples of the many aquatic diseases that afflict factory farmed fish. Other pesticides and antibiotics fed to fish growing in factory fish farms include:

- Ivermectin
- Oxytetracycline
- Florfenicol
- Romet 30
- Sulfadimethoxine
- Ormetoprim
- Sulfadiazine
- Trimethoprim
- Tricaine methanesulfonate
- Formaldehyde

Another problem with eating factory farmed fish is the high incidence of PCB's and other contaminants found in those environments and their harmful impact on human health. In the same way that factory-farmed animals are fed ingredients unfit for human consumption factory fish are similarly handled.

What's more, only two companies control the entire factory-fish feed market, and here's what's listed on the feed label from one of them:

- **Byproducts** – Farmed fish can be fed factory-farmed poultry by-products, including feathers, necks, and intestines.

- **Genetically Modified Organisms (GMOs)** – Some farmed fish may be fed genetically modified corn, soy and canola.

- **Other** – Wild fish would never eat the items in the following list, but farmed fish living in pens have no other choice but to eat poultry meal, whole wheat, soybean meal, corn gluten meal, and feather meal.

As a result of eating soy, canola, and maize, factory farmed fish have an imbalance and higher propensity of Omega-6 fatty acids, which increase inflammation if they dominate a diet. The ratio of Omega-3 essential fatty acids should be higher than that of Omega-6 fatty acids in a healthy diet, which keeps them in proper balance, both for humans and for animals, including fish. But farmed fish do not eat a healthy diet for the same reason cows are fed corn and growth hormones: it's cheaper than the species' natural choice food, and the high Omega-6 diet and chemicals are given to grow and fatten up the fish much faster, which means they can be sold sooner and end up on all of our dinner plates.

Because of the high level of contaminants for factory farmed salmon, which in the wild is one of the most nutritious fish available, in North America we are warned not to eat factory-farmed salmon more than once every 2 ½ months due to the high concentrations of PCB's and other contaminants found in the fish. There are no such restrictions on wild salmon, which should be a regular part of any healthy diet as they are rich in Omega-3's and are in the proper balance with Omega-6's. Wild is far safer than factory farmed fish, and a comparison between wild salmon and farmed salmon shows higher levels of vitamins in the wild salmon, but increased levels of dangerous contaminants in the farmed fish:

Salmon Nutritional Content		
100 Gram Serving (3.5 oz)	**Farmed Salmon**	**Wild Salmon**
Vitamin A	40 IU	154 IU
Vitamin D	60 IU	533 IU
Fat Content	13%	2.5%
PCB's	27 parts/billion	5 parts/billion

Other hazards found in factory farmed fish include:

- **Colorants** – Like our processed foods that contain artificial colors, our fish do too! Factory farmed fish, fed unnatural diets, aren't all that healthy so they become pale, the same as sick humans. Unlike wild salmon, which normally dine on krill that give wild salmon their naturally pink hue, salmon bred in factory farms are fed an unnatural diet of soy, canola, wheat, and corn, making them as grayish-white as their diet. But who'd want to eat a pasty-looking piece of salmon? Nobody, until food chemists step in with their magic "Salmo Fan," a paint-strip-like device showing the shades of salmon pink, from light to very dark that factory salmon farms use to pick the color they want for their unnaturally grayish-white salmon. Then they feed the fish *synthetic* forms of the naturally-occurring astaxanthin found in krill that gives them and the salmon who eat them their color. This means that, through industry smoke and mirrors, a sickly looking, factory-farmed salmon is turned into a healthy looking, freshly caught wild sockeye salmon. Alas, it's a far cry from wild salmon on every level.

- **Fungicides** – Fungicides are used to treat fish eggs, fish, and shellfish with external fungal and parasitic infections.

- **Antibiotics** – Because of the high density of fish in factory farm "net cages," bacterial infections can be rampant and swift. To stave off infection, "preventive" antibiotics are routinely used, adding to the ever-growing problem of antibiotic resistant microbes.

- **Disinfectants** – Because bacterial infections are so prevalent in farmed fish, disinfectants are used as security measures to control bacterial infections on nets, boats, boots, raingear, diving equipment, containers, platforms and decking to prevent the spread of bacterial infections from one fish farm site to another. Some of these disinfectants are known endocrine disruptors and can end up on or in the fish we eat.

Even though disinfectants are used throughout the fishing industry to sanitize boats and fishing gear after a fishing expedition, wild-caught fish do not live in a disinfected environment, and because they are usually quickly cleaned and frozen at sea as soon as they are caught, they do not ingest or absorb these chemicals.

- **Metals** – Copper-based paints are used on fish farm cages and nets to prevent marine-life buildup. The reason for concern is the amount of copper that can be absorbed by the fish, producing toxic effects for humans who need only trace amounts of copper in their diet. Currently there is no monitoring of copper levels in farmed fish.

- **Sodium tripolyphosphate (STPP)** - Some unscrupulous fisheries use STPP as a chemical preservative when freezing and packaging fish. It gives shrimp/prawns a soapy texture, turns seafood (especially scallops) lighter in color, making it tasteless, bitter, watery, or metallic. STPP is listed on the EPA's Federal Insecticide, Fungicide and Rodenticide Act as a registered pesticide. Contact with skin can produce acute irritation, and it is a suspected neuro-toxin.

DO ORGANIC FISH EXIST?

The more accurate question is: Can fish be organically certified? Fish in the wild are considered "organic" by doing what nature intended. But to label fish organic is ludicrous because no fish in the wild is going to follow guidelines set by humans; they're just going to eat what they always eat. Some factory fish farms want to label their fish as organic, but beware. Do not buy fish that's been "certified as organic" unless you see the seal of approval of independent organizations such as The Living Oceans Society, The Coastal Alliance for Aquaculture Reform (CARR), and The Marine Stewardship Council.

GMO FISH

As if factory-farmed fish isn't a bad enough idea, the bio-tech industry is busy modifying the fish population, too. Recently the FDA gave preliminary approval to genetically engineered Atlantic salmon that would grow much larger, fatter, and faster than any normal salmon does in its natural lifetime by modifying its genetic structure to include genes from Alaskan Chinook salmon and an eel-like creature called ocean pout, and then pumping the genetically-manipulated fish full of growth hormones. There was public outcry and demonstrations against the proposed "Frankenfish," but negative public response has been ignored and this new type of "salmon" is expected to be sold to fish markets in the near future as fresh salmon. Currently there is no intention to label this fish as genetically modified. Should the FDA give GMO salmon the green light (with industry insiders entrenched in our government, it's only a matter of time), and with the biotech industry fighting to avoid having to label their GMO "Frankenfood," one of these laboratory-created "Frankenfish" monsters may soon be on ice at your local supermarket.

FISH FRAUD

Selling fish can be a fishy business in more ways than one. When Randy Hartnell, Founder and CEO of Vital Choice, toured New York City's famed Fulton Fish Market in 2004, he was distressed to find cheap, farmed Atlantic salmon being marketed as the superior, sought-after, more expensive wild Pacific Chinook salmon. An investigation was conducted by The New York Times and an expose written. In 2011, The Boston Globe and the conservation group Oceana both launched their own investigations. So what, if anything has changed? According to Craig Weatherby of Vital Choice, as of December 2012, fish fraud remains business as usual.

Unfortunately, this isn't surprising, and it turns out that nearly 50% to 70% of all fish sold in supermarkets and restaurants are not as labeled or marketed. The suppliers substitute cheaper, less desirable, and more readily available fish in place of many of the most popular, more expensive varieties. Some examples of typical fish fraud include:

Sold As	Actual Species
Red Snapper	Ocean Perch Crimson Snapper Colorado Snapper Tilapia
Albacore Tuna	Escolar (excess oil causes gastrointestinal upset)
Grouper	Tilefish (high in mercury)
Wild Pacific King Salmon (chinook)	Farmed Atlantic Salmon

Other premium fish which have cheaper fish substituted in their place include:

- Albacore tuna
- Cod
- Haddock

- Catfish
- Grey Sole
- Halibut
- Lemon Sole
- Sockeye Salmon
- Yellow fin Tuna

So what's a seafood lover to do? There is a small but growing practice of raising fish in controlled, enclosed environments that provide filtered water and reduce the risk of contaminants and disease. These practices remove the risk of harming humans and other marine life, as well as providing farmed fish with a better, healthier environment in which to spawn and grow.

To find out where to get these fish, consult a copy of *Seafood Watch*, a downloadable, printable pocket-sized booklet that lists fish that are sustainably caught and low in contaminants, along with those fish to avoid because of poor fishing practices and contaminants. *Seafood Watch* is available from The Monterey Bay Aquarium website. It's helpful when dining out, but in many instances, restaurants have no idea where the fish came from that they serve, or whether they are farmed fish or wild.

MILK

Milk is the liquid of life and mother's milk is the foundation of human nutrition for newborns. We are born with no immune defenses, having spent 9 months in a safe environment sharing our mother's immunity. Babies who are breast fed receive colostrum, which is a mother's first milk, and it provides those newborns with the enzymes, peptides, vitamins, minerals, proteins, carbohydrates, fats, immunoglobulins, growth hormones, and antibodies that will jumpstart a baby's immune system. These bioactive components decline by 50%-70% for the second nursing, by another 30%-50% for the third nursing, and are no longer present by the fourth nursing.

According to research, without this first milk, mammals have a greater lifelong chance of contracting infections.

In the Twentieth century, the way we got our milk changed drastically in the U.S. For people not on farms, a local milkman delivered fresh milk in glass bottles from local farms. By the 1960s, milk was sold in wax lined cardboard cartons at local supermarkets and grocery stores. In the last few decades, milk producers began lining the cartons with a plastic coating containing the toxin BPA, and the milk has been pasteurized.

In 1994, rBGH (recombinant bovine growth hormone) was introduced to the dairy industry and by the 21st century, the dairy industry transformed from a large number of independent local dairy farms providing fresh milk to local stores and customers, to a consolidated industry made up of a handful of national companies that distribute pasteurized/homogenized milk to the entire country.

Dairy cows raised on industrial factory farms are injected with growth hormone rBGH to increase their milk production. As a result, these animals develop mastitis, which is an infection of the udder routinely treated by high levels of antibiotic that are passed into the milk. The infection causes a secretion of pus, which means that the milk now contains that unpleasant additive, as well as an insulin-like growth factor, IgF-1, which has been linked to breast and other cancers in humans. This is what's found in the milk on our supermarket and grocery store shelves, and it's bad enough that adults consume it, but much worse, it's fed to our infants and children. This pus-filled milk is also found in the supermarket cheese aisle, in non-organic yogurt, and in processed foods containing milk/cheese ingredients such as frozen pizza.

It is estimated that 32% of all dairy cows are injected with the hormone rBST (recombinant bovine somatotropin), which is made by isolating a gene from the growth hormone that lactating cows produce. That isolate is inserted into E.coli bacteria and grown in vats, and cows injected with this drug produce approximately 25% more milk. Forcing cows to continually produce milk in large quantities increases the risk of mastitis and contributes to their early death by putting additional stress on their bodies. In fact, cows injected with rBGH or rBST usually are slaughtered within three years compared to the 20-year life span of organically fed, pasture raised dairy cows. The hormone-injected cows live such short lives because their udder infections spread throughout the cows' systems, and unfortunately, those infected animals end up in our supermarket meat cases and in pet food. Furthermore, most large commercial pet food companies use meat from "4D" animals (diseased, disabled, dying, dead) and deemed unfit for human consumption.

The glut of milk from hormone-laced factory-farmed cows helps keep milk prices low, but those low prices, coupled with rising feed cost and dairy association fees, have forced many small dairy farmers out of business because they can't compete with the big milk producers at those low prices.

Many dairies had begun to label their milk as rBGH- and/or rBST-free and as a result, Monsanto, the huge multinational bio-engineering chemical company which makes rBGH and rBST, brought suit against Oakhurst Dairy of Maine, claiming that Oakhurst, by labeling their milk "hormone-free" implied that milk from hormone-laced cows was inferior and that the labels were "misleading, unfair, and deceptive." The companies eventually settled and Oakhurst agreed to add labels that read, *"Our Farmers' Pledge: No Artificial Growth Hormone Used."* Oakhurst also was instructed to note on their label that "The FDA claims there is no significant difference in milk from cows treated with growth hormones." Some dairies add that *"Currently there are no tests that can confirm if non-organic milk contains growth hormones or antibiotics."*

But organically raised cows cannot be given rBGH or Posilac (also known as rBST) and still produce organic milk according to the legal definition of *organic.* It's been possible to test hormone levels in milk since 1995 using patented technology developed at Cornell University that makes it possible to determine the difference between milk from organically raised cows and those injected with growth hormones but the test has never been approved by the FDA because of successful political maneuvering by Monsanto.

In 2007, Monsanto filed a complaint with the USFDA requesting organic dairy producers be banned from claiming on labels that their milk is from cows not given growth hormones. Most milk producers will stand by the claim that there is no difference between non-organic pasteurized milk and pasteurized organic milk, and to a great extent, they are correct. And while organic milk has fewer pesticide residues, is free of growth hormones and antibiotics, and has few somatic cells, pasteurization renders both organic and non-organic milk nearly identical in that any live nutrients found in them are killed by the process, making the milk a dead food. Ultra-pasteurization is the deliberate second high heating of milk, ensuring that it is an ultra dead food.

Proponents of pasteurized milk cite key nutrients in milk, such as calcium and Vitamin D, but pasteurization alters the structure of milk proteins and destroys enzymes, beneficial bacteria, and greatly reduces vitamins such as B-complex vitamins, as well as Vitamins C and D. During pasteurization, most of the beneficial calcium becomes insoluble, meaning the body cannot readily break it down, absorb it, or use it. This is why synthetic vitamins and calcium are added back into pasteurized milk.

Contrast pasteurized, processed milk with raw, unpasteurized milk and the differences are startling. Along with keeping all nutrients intact and bio-available so the body may absorb and use them, there are many additional beneficial nutrients in raw milk. Raw milk from cows raised organically without antibiotics or growth hormones that are truly free-range pastured contains vital nutrients pasteurization eliminates, including:

- **Phosphatase** – an enzyme that aids in the absorption of calcium.

- **Lipase** – an enzyme that helps absorb fats.

- **Butterfat** – a nutrient that helps the body absorb and use vitamins and minerals in the milk and contains vitamin A and acids with strong anti-carcinogenic properties.

- **Unoxidized cholesterol** - healthy cholesterol that the body uses in cell production and repair.

- **CLA** - Conjugated Linoleic Acid, which has a variety of benefits including weight stabilization and anti-carcinogenic properties.

- **Omega-3/Omega-6 Ratios** – high omega-3 and low omega-6, which are the beneficial ratios between these essential fatty acids.

Aside from these differences, there is another important factor to consider in choosing raw milk rather than pasteurized milk and that is homogenization. When milk is homogenized, it is mechanically processed using a technique that breaks apart the fat globules in the milk so that the cream no longer rises to the top but becomes evenly mixed with the other components. This mechanical process creates its own high heat, thus pasteurizing the milk a second time (or a third time if the milk has been ultra-pasteurized before homogenization), killing off any live nutrients that may have survived initial pasteurization. This type of processing changes the milk and the restructuring and fragmenting of the fat globules have been linked to the increasing number of people with milk allergies.

Milk-related allergies and diseases can also be triggered by the type of dairy cows that produce the milk. There are two classifications of milk from cows A1 and A2. In nearly all commercial milk production, dairy cattle are Holsteins or a mixture of breeds, which are considered new compared to the traditional dairy breeds. These "new" breeds produce milk that contains A1 beta-casein, which is considered a mutation because in the past, milk-producing mammals, from humans to sheep, goats, camels, oxen, and the "original" dairy cow breeds such as Jersey and Guernsey cows, have produced milk with type A2 beta-casein protein.

The problem with A1 beta-casein protein is that it releases a peptide that A2 beta-casein does not. This peptide, which is a fragment of protein, has opiate-like characteristics, and once it passes through the stomach and into the bloodstream, it causes an auto-immune response in whoever drinks it. Diseases linked to using A1 beta-casein milk include:

- Type I diabetes

- Heart disease
- Atherosclerosis
- Lactose intolerance (which may actually be an A1 intolerance)
- Delayed neurological psychomotor development in children
- Worsened Autism symptoms (requires further study)

The reason lactose intolerance may instead be A1 intolerance is because supposedly lactose-intolerant people are often able to consume goat milk and Jersey cow milk without digestive issues and the milk from these sources contains A2 type beta-casein. There is some speculation on whether pasteurization and/or homogenization enhance the mutant A1 protein, but this has not yet been determined.

Most people know nothing about A1 and A2 beta-casein proteins in milk and the link between A1 milk and auto-immune responses. And the commercial dairy industry works hard to keep it that way as it produces predominantly A1-type, or mutated milk, which is also pasteurized and homogenized. Naturally, the dairy industry is concerned about the impact this information about the two types of milk could have on the sales of the A1-type milk it produces.

Outside the US, other countries are being proactive and quietly replacing A1-type dairy cows with A2-type. Unfortunately this is not the case in the United States, where the efforts of dairy industry lobbyists protect the industry's status quo, with little regard for the health of American citizens and as a result, there is no incentive to change the type of milk being processed and produced.

These facts also explain why raw dairies are being targeted by the U.S. Department of Agriculture. It has less to do with the safety of raw milk or "protecting" the public and much more to do with protecting the milk profits of Big Dairy. In fact, ninety percent of the world drinks raw milk, and milk in the U.S. wasn't pasteurized until the 1930's, and doing so puts the U.S. in the minority. If raw milk is so dangerous and so bad for humans, then how is it that 90% of humanity has managed to survive on raw milk? In the 1920's, Dr. J. R. Crewe, founder of the Mayo Clinic, used "The Milk Cure" in the successful treatment of numerous diseases, including chronic conditions, tuberculosis, diseases of the nervous system, cardiovascular and renal conditions, hypertension, and gastritis. He considered raw milk so beneficial and important to human health that he referred to it as "white blood."

Every time I hear someone say that raw milk contains "dangerous bacteria," it makes me want to slap my forehead in frustration. That same false accusation is mentioned repeatedly by "experts" on television, and in newspaper stories describing federal agents raiding raw milk farms and forcing them to destroy their product, and not even the Amish have been spared. This means that raw milk dairy farms are under siege, even when there are no complaints filed against them. This siege defies logic because the human race has survived and evolved for thousands of years on raw milk, millennia long before pasteurization was invented, and long before the FDA was formed to "protect" us.

Pasteurization was important and necessary in the early 1900's when not much was known about germs and sterilization, and milk was coming from unscrupulous New England "distillery" dairy farms, which fed their penned in, poorly raised dairy cows a form of low-grade, cast-off distillery grain slop. The animals refused to eat the deficient food and were forced into submission via starvation and dehydration. Actually, those conditions don't seem so different from the way factory-farm animals are raised and fed today.

The "distillery" dairy cows were diseased and so was their milk, and many people living in the Boston area were sickened and died from consuming the pathogen-laden milk. Pasteurization of milk began soon after and the practice eventually spread across the United States, even though there had been no problems of people becoming sick from drinking raw milk in other parts of the country.

Today, raw milk production in the United States is conducted under scrupulous hygienic guidelines and methodology and the cows are humanely raised, without growth hormones, are grass fed in pastures and alfalfa fed, with zero to miniscule amounts of grain feed and no corn silage. If a cow requires an antibiotic, it is separated from the herd and not returned to milk production until *after* the antibiotic is no longer detectable in the animal's urine. And yet, the mention of raw milk elicits a negative response from many who have been brainwashed to believe old wives tales and media hype.

But human breast milk is raw and considered the most nutritious milk of all for humans. What makes it any less "safe" than raw milk from organic cows or goats using sterilized equipment?

Organic raw milk contains not only good bacteria that aids in healthy digestion (probiotics), it contains the healthy bacteria that protects against disease-causing bacteria. Mark McAfee, founder and CEO of Organic Pastures Dairy, the largest raw dairy in the United States, performed pathogen testing on raw milk and pasteurized milk. He contaminated both milks with the pathogens for E.coli, Listeria, and Salmonella. In the raw milk, none of the pathogenic bacteria survived because the "good" bacteria in the raw milk destroyed them. But in the pasteurized milk, the pathogens survived and actually flourished because all natural defense mechanisms had been destroyed via pasteurization and homogenization.

Pasteurization kills the beneficial bacteria and enzymes that keep the pathogenic ones in check.

When buying raw organic milk, it's not a bad idea to investigate how that milk is processed, the type of cows (A1 or A2) used to produce it, and the type of sterilization methods used in milking the cows and bottling the milk. It has been my experience that most farmers are proud to give a tour of their farm, show how the animals are raised, and answer questions. But you don't always have to inspect a farm. Many farms have websites with photos and contact information. Because some of the dairy farms providing raw milk to the food co-op I frequent are far from where I live, I contacted the farms via email to ask what type of dairy cows they raise, if they are pastured, and how the milk is processed. As a result, photos of the cows, along with histories of the farms and their dairy practices are now posted for everyone's benefit on the glass door of the co-op's raw milk refrigerator.

A great alternative to raw cow milk is raw goat milk from an organic farmer. I became a raw goat milk fan one weekend after visiting a local organic Farmer's Market. One vendor was offering samples of goat milk. Overcoming my initial reluctance I took the sample of goat milk and was hooked after one taste. Here are some facts about raw goat milk:

- It tastes like milk, only better than pasteurized and homogenized whole milk, with a flavor that's richer, fuller, and sweeter.
- It looks white, like ordinary milk, and it's creamy.
- It smells like milk.
- It can last as long as 8-10 days in the refrigerator.

- Raw goat milk can be frozen using freezer-safe canning jars or vacuum sealed. Goat milk can be frozen for up to 3 months, but after 3 months, the delicate enzymes are destroyed, preventing the thawed raw goat milk from regaining the proper consistency between liquid and fat components.

- Frozen raw goat milk is defrosted by thawing in the refrigerator for several hours and shaking the container periodically to help recombine the milk fat and watery components.

On almost all counts, goat milk is nutritionally equal to or better than cow milk, except for being lower in folic acid. Proper processing of goat milk and goat cheese requires that male and female goats be kept separate at all times. The reason is that male goats produce a pheromone that sticks to anything the animal touches. The scent of the pheromone also is quite penetrating, and if the male goats are not kept separated from the females and not kept away from the milking area, the goat milk and cheese may have a strong "goaty" taste.

Goat milk does not contain agglutinin, and as a result, the fat globules in goats' milk, do not cluster together, making them easier to digest. Goat milk has more essential fatty acids than cow milk, along with a higher proportion of short- and medium-chain fatty acids that are easier to digest. Goat milk contains predominantly A2 beta-casein protein, which is more like that found in human milk.

Raw Milk vs. Pasteurized (Retail) Milk & Infant Formula					
Component	Breast Milk	Raw Goat Milk	Raw Cow Milk	Retail Cow Milk	Infant Formula
B Lymphocytes	X	X	X	—	—
Macrophages	X	X	X	—	—
Neutrophils	X	X	X	—	—

Raw Milk vs. Pasteurized (Retail) Milk & Infant Formula					
Component	Breast Milk	Raw Goat Milk	Raw Cow Milk	Retail Cow Milk	Infant Formula
T-Lymphocytes	X	X	X	—	—
lgA/lgG Secretory Antibodies	X	X	X	—	—
B-12 Binding Protein	X	X	X	—	—
Bifidus Factor	X	X	X	—	—
Fatty Acids	X	X	X	X	X
Fibronectin	X	X	X	—	—
Gamma-Interferon	X	X	X	—	—
Lactoferrin	X	X	X	—	—
Lysozyme	X	X	X	—	—
Mucins and Oligosaccharides	X	X	X	X	—
Hormones and Growth Factors	X	X	X	X	—

Raw Goat Milk vs Raw Cow Milk: Nutrient Values		
Component	Goat Milk	Cow Milk
Weight (grams)	244.0	244.0
Water (grams)	212.0	214.7
Carbohydrate (grams)	10.9	11.4
Calories (grams)	168.0	150.0
Fat (grams)	10.1	8.2
Saturated Fatty Acids	6.5	5.1
Monounsaturated Fatty Acids (grams)	2.7	0
Polyunsaturated Fatty Acids	0.4	0.3
Cholesterol (mg)	28.0	33.0
Vitamin A (IU)	451.0	307.0
Vitamin B-1 (mg)	0.12	0.09
Vitamin B-2 (mg)	0.34	0.40

Raw Goat Milk vs Raw Cow Milk: Nutrient Values		
Component	Goat Milk	Cow Milk
Vitamin B-6 (mg)	0.11	0.10
Vitamin B-12 (mg)	0.16	0.87
Vitamin C (mg)	3.0	2.0
Calcium (mg)	326.0	290.0
Copper (mg)	0.112	0
Folic Acid (mcg)	0.7	12.0
Iron (mg)	0.12	0.12
Magnesium (mg)	34.0	33.0
Manganese (mg)	0.044	0
Nicotinic Acid (mg)	0.7	0.20
Pantothenic Acid (mg)	0.76	0.77
Phosphorus (mg)	270.0	227.0
Potassium (mg)	499.0	368.0
Sodium (mg)	122.0	119.0
Zinc (mg)	0.73	0.93

Federal law prohibits the interstate sale of raw milk, and the regulation of raw milk sales and distribution varies from state to state in the United States. Some states allow raw milk to be sold directly from the farm but not from retailers or in restaurants, while other states allow sales from both farm and retailer, and some states prohibit the sale of raw milk entirely. To find out if your state or neighboring state supports the sale of raw milk, visit: www.realmilk.com/state-updates/

I've stopped using industrial pasteurized/homogenized milk, including commercial organic brands, for more than 3 years and instead from two local certified organic farms buy only fresh raw registered Jersey cow milk and cream, and raw goat milk that my family drinks and I also use in foods I prepare. I find that organic raw milk tastes better, fuller, richer, and sweeter than industrial pasteurized milk, even when that pasteurized milk is "organic."

MILK SUBSTITUTES

Many people turn to milk substitutes for philosophical or medical reasons. These milk substitutes tend to be watery and therefore need to be enhanced in some way for them to mimic the fullness and creaminess of real raw milk.

Carrageenan is the most often used thickener in milk substitutes, as well as in many other processed foods, and is portrayed as "natural" because it is derived from seaweed. Carrageenan is actually a gel extracted from red seaweed, but it is processed using caustic solvents and it coats the intestinal tract and stomach with an oil-like film that unfortunately impedes proper digestion. Carrageenan has been associated with stomach discomfort and there is research suggesting that this food additive is carcinogenic.

Carrageen is a multi-purpose substance; in addition to being an additive to milk substitutes, it's also used as an ingredient in plane de-icing.

INFANT FORMULA

As the Raw Milk versus Pasteurized and Infant Formula chart indicates, commercial infant formula can't hold a candle to breast milk or raw milk. Every time I hear the warning that infants should not drink raw milk, it makes me wonder if raw breast milk is going to be banned next. Never having had children, analyzing infant formula never crossed my mind. But after looking at the comparison chart and seeing no nutritive values, I decided to examine baby formula. I was in for a shock! The list of ingredients on containers of the most well-established and trusted names in baby foods and formula was appalling. It seemed obvious to me why babies have colic, diarrhea, gas, and require special formulas, including "sensitive" formulas. Even soy varieties and those touted to be "organic" made me wonder how babies thrive at all, and made me think that it's no surprise that younger and younger children are being stricken with Lichen Sclerosis, asthma, and other chronic illnesses.

Examining the formulas, there didn't seem to be much variation and all appear to be equally deficient. Some manufacturers claim that their formulas most closely resemble breast milk, but breast milk doesn't include any of *these* ingredients:

- **Corn syrup** – Consists of genetically modified sugar

- **Corn syrup solids** – Same as Corn Syrup

- **Dextrose** – A "cleaner" name for glucose made from corn that is most likely genetically modified

- **Fructose** – A sugar derived from corn that is most likely genetically modified

- **Corn Maltodextrin** – An anti-caking agent most likely made from genetically modified corn

- **Soy Lecithin** – An emulsifier derived from genetically modified soybeans

- **Canola Oil** – Made from genetically modified crops

- **Mono- and Diglycerides** – Emulsifiers derived from reduced fat

- **Vegetable Oil** – Made of palm olein, coconut, soy, sunflower, some of which are most likely genetically modified
- **Soy Protein Isolate** - An isolated protein, and genetically modified
- **Mortierella Alpina Oil*** - Synthetic genetically modified oil
- **Crypthecodinium Cohni Oil**** - Synthetic genetically modified oil
- **Natural Flavor** – Synthetic chemical flavor
- **Vitamin A Palmitate** – Synthetic vitamin isolate
- **Vitamin D_3** – Synthetic vitamin isolate
- **Vitamin E Acetate** – Synthetic vitamin isolate
- **Vitamin K_1** – Synthetic vitamin isolate
- **Thiamin Hydrochloride** – Synthetic vitamin isolate
- **Riboflavin** – Synthetic vitamin isolate
- **Hydrochloride** - Synthetic vitamin isolate
- **Vitamin B_{12}** - Synthetic vitamin isolate
- **Niacinamide** - Synthetic vitamin isolate
- **Folic Acid** - Synthetic vitamin isolate
- **Calcium Pantothenate** - Synthetic vitamin isolate
- **Biotin** - Synthetic vitamin isolate
- **Ascorbic Acid** - Synthetic vitamin isolate
- **Choline Chloride** - Synthetic vitamin isolate
- **Inositol** - Synthetic vitamin isolate

- **Potassium Phosphate** - Synthetic vitamin isolate

- **Magnesium Chloride** - Synthetic vitamin isolate

- **Ferrous Sulfate** - Synthetic vitamin isolate

- **Zinc Sulfate** - Synthetic vitamin isolate

- **Cupric Sulfate** - Synthetic vitamin isolate

- **Potassium Iodide** - Synthetic vitamin isolate

- **Sodium Selenite** - Synthetic vitamin isolate

- **Sodium Chloride** - Synthetic vitamin isolate

- **Potassium Chloride** - Synthetic vitamin isolate

- **Potassium Citrate** - Synthetic vitamin isolate

- **L-Methionine** - Synthetic vitamin isolate

- **Taurine** - Synthetic vitamin isolate

- **L-Carnitine** - Synthetic vitamin isolate

* A source of Arachidonic Acid (ARA)
** A source of Docosahexaenoic Acid (DHA)
(Synthetic vitamins are discussed in Chapter 9.)

The Mortierella Alpina and Crypthecodinium Cohni oils are manufactured by Martek Biosciences Corporation. According to the processing documentation submitted to the FDA, the "nutritional" oils are derived from soil fungus and algae that have been genetically modified by Monsanto Corp., grown in a medium comprised of dextrose, which is genetically modified corn glucose, along with yeast extract, and/or hydrolyzed soy (most likely genetically modified) protein. The oil is extracted using hexane, a neurotoxic chemical solvent. (For information on products containing these synthetic oils and sold in other countries, visit Martek Bioscience's *Life's DHA* website: www.lifesdha.com/Products-Containing-lifesDHA-/Partner-Products/tabid/683/Default.aspx

Are organic formulas any better? While they may not contain synthetic ARA/DHA oil, they are also loaded with sugar in the form of brown rice syrup, as well as numerous oils and synthetic vitamin isolates.

Packaging is another concern with infant formula. Cans of formula are most likely lined with hormone-disrupting Bisphenol-A (BPA), which can leach into the formula.

We in the United States are warned against and afraid to feed our babies raw milk, the complete natural food nature provided for infants to thrive and survive for over 170,000 years, yet we are encouraged to use infant formulas that are a laboratory-created concoction of sugar, synthetic isolated vitamins and genetically modified synthetic oil. There is something very wrong with this picture!

WHAT ELSE COULD BE HIDING IN MILK PRODUCTS?

Commercial dairy industry lobbyists have petitioned the Food and Drug Administration to *"amend the standard of identity for milk"* for the purpose of defining what is a *"safe and suitable"* sweetener, including *"non-nutritive"* sweeteners. What are those "safe, suitable, non-nutritive" sweeteners? Sucralose and Aspartame. The dairy industry is requesting that milk products containing sucralose or aspartame NOT be labeled as such because "reduced calorie" milk would not appeal to children, and that by not labeling sucralose or aspartame, "consumers are not misled regarding the characteristics of the milk they are purchasing." In other words, the milk industry doesn't want the consumer to know that they might be purchasing modified milk products containing ingredients that might cause brain tumors.

If the FDA approves this petition, products that could possibly contain unlabeled aspartame or sucralose include:

- Flavored milk
- Sour Cream
- Eggnog
- Yogurt including low- and non-fat
- Ice cream and ice milk
- Goat milk ice cream and ice milk
- Frozen desserts containing milk or cream
- Condensed milk
- Evaporated milk
- Non-fat dry milk
- Dry cream
- Light cream
- Light whipping cream
- Heavy cream

We've already learned the dangers of aspartame, yet unlabeled, sweetly poisoned milk products would, according to the petition, "particularly benefit school children" and is aimed at "improving the nutrition and health profile of food served in the nation's schools." What will the dairy industry dream up next to turn a naturally nutritious food into an unhealthy one?

WATER

We are liquid beings and our cells are 70% water. We can survive quite awhile without food, but we will die within days without water. We need water to hydrate our cells and to flush out toxins.

But increasingly our water is polluted from chemicals in the air, which is the most obvious form of pollution. Acid rain occurs when rainwater combines with chemicals released into the atmosphere during the manufacturing process and through automobile emissions, air-borne pesticides, and so on. Acid rain pollutes our lakes, rivers, and even our soil. When massive flooding of farms and homes occur, the flood waters carry chemicals with them, including lawn fertilizers, herbicides, pesticides, animal manures, gasoline, oils, chemicals from building materials, and the chemicals in household goods and personal products. The list of water-borne toxins is huge, but we rarely hear about the chronic illnesses and shortened life-spans people suffer after dealing with aftermath toxic cleanup, aside from lawsuits generated by 9/11. Many first responders in the 9/11 tragedy, as well as cleanup crews for the Exxon Valdez and the BP oil spills, have suffered chronic illnesses, cancers, and untimely death.

Our water is polluted in other ways as well, and comes to us from municipal water supplies with chemicals such as fluoride, synthetic and organic chemical waste products, antibiotics, hormones and other pharmaceuticals, including heavy metals and chlorination by-products. Tap water can contain biological parasites such as Cryptosporidium and Giardia, which are chlorine-resistant and cause flu-like symptoms or more serious illnesses.

In the U.S., we use over 80,000 chemicals every day and industry scientists develop and synthesize over 1,000 new ones every year. These often end up in our drinking water, meaning that pure clean water is almost non-existent.

Nature has always had the means of purifying water through leaching as water filters through the earth's layers of large, small, and micro soils. Some micro-organisms seem to thrive on some contaminants, making them useful bio-cleaners for water, while others cannot. But Nature is having an increasingly tough time keeping up with the pace of industrial pollution. The following is a description of how our water is "purified," along with alternatives.

CHLORINATION

Careful review of over 10,000 Environmental Protection Agency documents by the Center for Study of Responsive Law found that: *"U.S. drinking water contains more than 2,100 toxic chemicals that can cause cancer."*

Although there is technology available to better purify municipal drinking water, it is deemed too costly to undertake. One technology is reverse osmosis, which sounds great except that in addition to removing contaminants from water; it also removes minerals necessary for human health. Without adding those minerals back into the water supply, the human body will extract them from teeth, bones, and organs. Returning vital minerals to the water supply would require time, money, and careful management; things which are impractical for most municipalities.

Another water purification technology is similar to how nature handles it, and that is by filtering water through granular carbon filters and carbon block filters that remove pathogens, organic and inorganic matter, as well as sediment, metals, and cysts. This is very effective and is the most common type of filtration system especially in homes.

Unfortunately, these technologies are not used by municipalities, which rely on the fastest and least expensive techniques to clean up the public water supply. In most of the U.S., municipal water is force filtered through sand beds that remove visible particles. Then chlorine is added to the water, which basically is like adding bleach to the water to kill off most of the bacteria. But there are no mechanisms for removing synthetic chemicals, pharmaceuticals, pesticides, herbicides, and everything else that gets dumped down the drain.

And chlorine is indiscriminant when it comes to killing bacteria, dangerous or beneficial. It's important to note that bathing with chlorinated water destroys the beneficial bacteria on our skin, and it harms our skin and hair in another way by destroying their natural oils, which can cause skin conditions including:

- Dandruff
- Dry, brittle hair
- Eczema
- Psoriasis

In addition to what it does to the skin and hair, note that the vapors in a hot, steamy shower include chlorine and other contaminants, which we inhale faster and in greater quantities than from bathing in a tub of water, or even from drinking it. These inhaled chlorine-chemical vapors cause lung irritation and can trigger asthma attacks.

Chlorine in drinking water is bad enough, but also dangerous are the toxic disinfection byproducts (DBP's) generated when chlorine reacts with organic matter such as plants and algae.

So what can you do to protect yourself and your family? Here are some suggestions:

WATER FILTRATION SYSTEMS

According to Sun Systems, a good water filtration system is **certified** to remove the following:

- **Alachlor** – A chemical used in crop herbicides, and found in groundwater. Long-term exposure causes cancer as well as damage to liver, kidney, and spleen.

- **Atrazine** – A chemical used in crop herbicides and a groundwater contaminant. It is an endocrine disruptor and a carcinogen.

- **Benzene** – Used as an industrial solvent in the production of drugs, plastics, synthetic rubber, dyes, and in making other chemicals. It is also found in the exhaust of motor vehicles and industrial emissions, and is a known carcinogen that damages bone marrow and the immune system.

- **Chlorine** – Adversely affects the immune system and damages the circulatory, cardiac and respiratory systems.

- **Cysts** – Organic pathogenic bacteria and parasites.

- **Lead** – A neurotoxin, lead causes nerve damage and is harmful to the kidneys and reproductive organs.

- **Lindane** – A chemical used by the agricultural and pharmaceutical industries, lindane is a neurotoxin that affects the nervous system, liver, and the kidneys, and is a known carcinogen.

- **Methyl Tertiary Butyl Ether (MTBE)** – MTBE is made by blending chemicals such as isobutylene and methanol, and it is used as an additive in gasoline. It sticks to particles in ground water and is linked to brain tumors, and cancers of the blood, liver, and kidneys when inhaled from or consumed in tap water.

- **Trichloroethylene (TCE)** – TCE is used as a solvent and sticks to particles found in ground water. It causes neuro-toxicity, immuno-toxicity, and organ toxicity.

- **Trihalomethanes (THMs)** - THMs are byproducts that are created in the water via chemical reaction when chlorine comes into contact with organic matter during water disinfection. THMs remain in the water after the disinfection process has ended and include chloroform, bromodichloromethane, dibromo-chloromethan, and bromoform.

- **Volatile Organic Compounds (VOCs)** – VOCs are emitted gases from solids or liquids. They can be found in paints, cleaning supplies, pesticides, building materials, glues and adhesives. Health problems caused by exposure to VOCs include respiratory difficulties, neuro-toxicity, allergic reactions and cancer.

An on-line water filtration system comparison study by Sun Systems was very useful and we opted to install an Aquasana under-counter filter at the kitchen sink. We use this filtered water for drinking and cooking and it was relatively easy to install. Aquasana also sells filtering shower heads, and whole house filters.

FLUORIDE

According to the Centers for Disease Control and Prevention, *"Water fluoridation is the deliberate addition of the natural trace element of fluorine..."*

While fluorine does occur in nature and is listed on The Periodic Table of Elements, nature keeps it under lock and key in the form of a crystal and it does not appear in nature as a "free" element.

But what is added to our municipalities' water supplies does not appear on The Periodic Table of Elements and is not the naturally occurring fluorine, but rather a man-made, synthetic mixture of chemicals. In fact, *fluoride* is merely a blanket term used for a combination of three toxic ingredients: Sodium Fluoride, Sodium Fluorosilicate, and Fluorosilicic Acid. These chemicals actually are components of waste material that is purposely added to the water supply in many states or municipalities allegedly to prevent cavities, but it may actually be harmful to the public health.

Where does fluoride originate? For nearly a century, the fertilizer, cement, and armaments industries released two extremely poisonous gases into the atmosphere: Hydrogen Fluoride and Silicon Tetrafluoride. These two toxic ingredients are the main components that make up fluorosilicic acid, the most often used chemical in "fluoride."

Hydrogen Fluoride is a chemical compound containing fluorine that takes the form of a colorless gas, a fume-emitting liquid, or a solid that dissolves in water. As a gas, it is used in the production of aluminum, making electrical components, and in etching glass. It is also used to separate uranium isotopes, in manufacturing refrigerants, as a catalyst in high-octane gasoline by the petroleum industry, in stainless steel "pickling," as well as in the production of pharmaceuticals, plastics, and fluorescent light bulbs.

According to the Hydrogen Fluoride Material Safety Sheet, it is described as a "corrosive and toxic product, very hazardous to human health and the environment." Health problems from exposure to hydrogen fluoride include:

- Severe respiratory damage, including pulmonary edema
- Risk of permanent eye lesions, corneal damage, and blindness
- Skin burns
- Convulsions
- Arrhythmias and death from cardiac or respiratory failure
- Binding with calcium in the body, resulting in low levels of calcium (hypocalcemia)
- Damage to lungs, liver, and kidneys (animal studies)

The chronic effects of exposure to hydrogen fluoride include:

- Dental fluorosis, defined as mottling or pitting of teeth
- Skeletal fluorosis, defined as pathological bone formation
- Irritation and congestion of the nose, throat, and bronchi
- Abnormally increased bone density
- Damage to the liver, kidneys and lungs
- Pulmonary effects, renal injury, thyroid injury, anemia, hypersensitivity, and dermatological reactions.

Reproductive and developmental effects include:

- Fluoride ingested by pregnant women crosses the placenta, thereby exposing fetuses even before birth
- Menstrual irregularities
- Children born to mothers with high levels of fluorides when pregnant will have dental fluorosis.
- Impaired reproduction and malformation of fetal bones and teeth (according to animal studies). Degenerative testicular changes (found in animal studies)

Silicon Tetrafluoride toxicological properties:

- Are corrosive and irritating to all living tissues
- Are corrosive and irritating to the upper and lower respiratory tracts, skin, and eyes resembling those from exposure to acid
- Cause acid burns and skin lesions
- Cause chemical pneumonitis and pulmonary edema (fluid accumulation in the lungs) in the lower respiratory tract and deep in the lungs
- Cause residual pulmonary malfunction
- Cause eye lesions and possible vision loss
- Fluorosis resulting in an abnormal calcification pattern of the skeletal system.

The use of these chemicals, hydrogen fluoride and silicon tetrafluoride that make up the fluoride in municipal water supplies began in the 1940's during WWII when the U.S. was building as many munitions as possible, along with the production of fertilizer, cement, and aluminum.

Decades later, under pressure from environmentalists, industry eventually was forced to capture these greenhouse gases by using a water spray. When hydrogen fluoride and silicon tetrafluoride gases are dissolved in water, they become hydrofluoric acid, also known as fluorosilicic acid. With it comes all of the heavy-metal manufacturing by-products, including aluminum, arsenic, barium, cadmium, chromium, lead, and mercury.

This toxic slurry, according to the EPA, is considered a hazardous waste product that must be handled with the correct HAZMAT gear and disposed of properly. This is serious stuff that the U.S. Environmental Protection Agency regards as hazardous and is deemed an ecological disaster if it is released into the environment.

The Occupational Safety and Health Administration (OSHA) requires operators handling this slurry to wear a respirator, face mask, neoprene gloves that are a foot long, encapsulating suits, and acid-proof boots. If that doesn't raise a red flag about the toxicity of "fluoride," then perhaps this statement in the CDC's Morbidity and Mortality Weekly Report of 1995 might: *"The water supply industry has a high incidence of unintentional injuries compared with other industries in the United States."*

To dispose of highly toxic chemical waste such as fluorosilicic acid requires specially lined tanks, with special berms built around the tanks. It costs a great deal of money to dispose of the acid, which requires extraordinary handling and storage to prevent fatal injury, and/or leakage that will contaminate the air or ground water. It cannot be dumped just anywhere...or can it?

Thus began the great hoax of fluoridating our drinking water. Take a toxic waste product that would be considered an environmental disaster if it were to end up in our rivers, lakes, or streams, but truck it around the country and dump it into our community water supply, and it miraculously becomes "beneficial." What a brilliant scheme! Convince the dental community and the public that toxic waste is a dental preventative and rake in the money from public water authorities dumb enough to pay to have poison unloaded into their drinking water!

While natural *fluorine* does have cavity-preventing properties if *directly* applied to teeth by a professional, a growing mountain of evidence shows that drinking *fluoride* has no effect whatsoever on cavities. In fact, countries that have never fluoridated their water have the same level of dental health as we do, and in many instances, far better dental health.

The logic behind fluoridating water is flawed. Would you pour gallons of cough syrup into community drinking water to prevent a cough? What if not everyone is prone to coughing? Would you force them to drink the cough syrup too? How would you regulate how much cough syrup each person would consume? Should every single person have cough syrup in their glass of water, cup of tea or coffee? Should they have to rinse their produce in it? Cook with it? Wash their clothes in it? Bathe in it? Put it in their baby formula?

No? And yet, this is exactly what pouring toxic fluorosilicic acid into community drinking water amounts to, logical or not. Does someone who drinks vast amounts of water each day consume more fluoride than another person? And if so, how does that fluoride affect them? Even if a small amount were deemed harmless, anything can become toxic if you ingest enough of it. In the 15th century, Paracelsus, a physician and considered the father of toxicology, wrote: *"All substances are poisons: there is none which is not a poison. The right dose differentiates a poison and a remedy."*

This is what has been happening for over 50 years: we have all been force-fed fluoride, whether we needed it or not, regardless of age, weight, gender, and without our consent. Keep in mind that this form of fluoride is *not* naturally occurring fluorine. Rather, it is man-made toxic waste that is being deliberately put into our water supply. This waste does not exist in nature, and contains other manufacturing contaminants such as heavy metals.

Fluoride is so hazardous that the U.S. is on constant alert against this form of chemical warfare lest it be used by terrorists to contaminate our water supply. And yet, the U.S. government sees fit to add it to its own citizens' drinking water. It defies logic! Gradually, however, the American public is beginning to awaken from their drug-induced slumber and understand the consequences. If fluorosis is what happens to teeth and bones exposed to high levels of fluoride, it stands to reason that other organs will be affected. Here are just some of the health problems fluoride causes:

- **Dental Fluorosis** - Approximately 1/3 of all children in the United States suffer from Fluorosis, which is a tooth-wasting disorder that results from ingesting too much fluoride. Dental fluoridosis causes white spots and brown mottling of teeth, the erosion of tooth enamel, and in the worst cases, causes the enamel to flake off. Fluorosis is a visible sign of fluoride toxicity.

- **Skeletal Fluorosis** - Since bones and teeth have similar molecular structure, fluorosis of the bone creates bone wasting and brittle bones. The material data safety sheet for silicon tetrafluoride describes it as an "abnormal calcification pattern of the skeletal system." Osteoporosis may not be so much a lack of calcium as it is a result of continued ingestion of fluoride. Studies show that women living in areas where the water contains naturally-occurring fluorine and is not artificially fluoridated have a lower incidence of osteoporosis and bone fracture.

- **Osteosarcoma** – Fatal bone cancer

- **Arthritis Chronic fatigue syndrome**

- **Gastrointestinal problems**

- **Hypothyroidism** - Lowered thyroid function due to fluoride's ability to mimic TSH, the thyroid stimulating hormone.

- **Endocrine disruption** – Disruption of important proteins that are key building blocks for hormones

- **Neurotoxicity** - Impaired mental development and reduced IQ in children, and dementia in adults

- **Apoptosis** – Cell death

- **Ataxia** – Muscular disorders

- **Immunotoxicity** – Disrupts the immune system and inhibits antibody formation

- **Reproductive toxicity** – Damages sperm and increases sterility

- **Bio-accumulation** – Causes the kidneys to excrete only 50% of the fluoride taken in, with the remainder accumulating in bones, the pineal gland, and other organ tissue.

But that's not all. The beginning of this section listed three toxins that make up the blanket term "fluoride." Fluorosilicic Acid (the combination of hydrogen fluoride and silicon tetrafluoride) is the poison most often added to our water, but there are two other waste-product chemicals also used in "fluoridation," and those are Sodium Fluoride and Sodium Fluorosilicate.

Sodium Fluoride is a pesticide/fungicide used in wood preservatives, especially in pressure-treated lumber. We're told not to burn this type of lumber because it will release dangerous toxins into the atmosphere. And yet, our government has given the green light to corporations to dispose of this pesticide/fungicide in our drinking water.

Technicians applying sodium fluoride to products must wear chemical resistant gloves, elongated, chemical resistant sleeves, and a face shield, and there is a dire warning that, *"Equipment for brush-on applications is limited to only brushes that have handles that are several feet in length."* In other words, don't get near it, but it's ok to drink it.

Symptoms of exposure to sodium fluoride via inhalation, ingestion, or contact with eyes or skin are:

- Irritation to skin or eyes
- Headache
- Salivation, nausea
- Burning or cramping abdominal pain
- Intense vomiting or diarrhea
- Muscle weakness
- Tremors or convulsions
- Spasms of the extremities
- Respiratory arrest
- Heart arrhythmias leading to cardiac arrest

Although sodium fluoride is not the most common compound to be used in water fluoridation, it is often referred to as the "safest" because industry studies submitted to the government to evaluate the risk to human health by using pharmaceutical grade sodium fluoride rather than the toxic waste product being used in community water supplies.

Sodium Fluorosilicate is the second most commonly used fluoridation compound, also known as sodium silicofluoride. It is an "inert" ingredient in pesticides, and inert ingredients can make up to 99% of pesticide formulations. Just because a substance is "inert" does not mean it is safe. According to the Material Safety Data Sheet, sodium fluorosilicate is listed as a hazardous product for human health and the aquatic environment. The exposure effects range from mild to severe, and include:

- Irritation of the mucous membranes of the nose, irritation of the throat, eyes, and skin.
- Risk of cardiac and nervous disorders
- Cardiac arrhythmia
- Skeletal fluorosis
- Severe burns and gastrointestinal perforation
- Nausea with bloody vomiting and diarrhea
- Convulsions
- Coma
- Cardiopulmonary arrest
- Animal studies have shown toxicity of the liver, bladder, lungs and spleen

Sodium fluorosilicate is not only a product of pesticide manufacturing; it may also be used in powdered laundry detergents. This means that besides drinking it, it also ends up as residue on and in our food when we wash it or cook with it, and permeates our "clean" clothing, bedding, and other laundered linens.

Fluoride in Food

We are exposed to fluorides in numerous and insidious other ways as well. Any liquid we drink made from water, even if it's organic, may contain fluoride. And any food you eat, whether it comes out of a bottle, bag, box, or is fresh, probably has been exposed to fluoridated water during processing.

Fluoride is in everything from baby formula and baby food, to that fresh produce in your salad or the dressing you add to it. Quite possibly any cup of coffee or tea, or glass of fruit juice or soda is a cup of fluoride. Fluoride levels in processed food will surprise you. It's in cereal, crackers, and even bread because these products all have been processed using water that may well have been fluoridated.

Another form of the chemical is sulfuryl fluoride, which is used as a fumigant for non-organic fresh produce after it has been harvested, and for stored and processed non-organic food.

Fluoride in Pharmaceuticals

Water is a main component of most liquid pharmaceuticals, including cough syrup, nasal spray, eye drops, SSRI antidepressants, and some antibiotics, and it is used as a base for cream medications. We might hope that the water used in pharmaceuticals is free of fluoride, but there is no evidence that this is the case so we may assume that fluoride is an unintentional ingredient in these pharmaceutical products as well.

But Fluoride is also purposely added to pharmaceuticals. In Chapter 2, which describes Toxic

Topicals, Clobetasol is described as *a synthetic fluorinated* corticosteroid. Do you still wonder why it burns your skin, or why it is advised to use it sparingly? Once again, it's not because it is so potent or so effective. It's used sparingly because it is so toxic.

And don't forget that it's in one of the most legal addictive drugs: cigarettes. Fluoride is inhaled with every puff of a cigarette, and is present in cigarette smoke.

Fluoride Exposure from All Sources

In 2011, the U.S. Department of Health & Human Services lowered the recommended fluoride levels in community drinking water to 0.7 mg/L from the previous range of 0.7 mg/L to 1.2 mg/L. This occurred after a review of the EPA's drinking water standards by the National Academy of Sciences' National Research Council, which recommended that the level be lowered. Although the review was published in 2006, it took 5 years for the change to be implemented.

The review took into account fluoride levels from naturally occurring sources and from pollution and pointed out that at the higher, pre-2011 guidelines (0.7 mg/L – 1.2 mg/L), consumption of that much fluoride over a lifetime increased the odds of bone fracture. When fluoride intake from all sources is totaled including from food, beverages, toothpaste, mouthwash, and medications, the total consumption of fluoride may add up to more than 7 mg/L per day, well over 500% of government guidelines.

Is *Your* Water Fluoridated

To find out if your water is fluoridated, the Centers for Disease Control and Prevention have a "My Water's Fluoride" page that contains a map of the United States. There you are able to search by state, city or town, right down to every water authority servicing your area. The website is: http://apps.nccd.cdc.gov/MWF/Index.asp.

In 2011, the Centers for Disease Control decreased the "acceptable" levels of fluoride for infants, as if any level should be acceptable. But what about the rest of us? When will our government put a stop to this absurd and outrageous practice? My guess is never, since this "dental health" hoax has continued for over 50 years, and it's such a great way for the chemical industry to avoid paying megabucks to dispose of their toxic waste—and make money at the same time!

More and more communities are refusing to add fluoride to their water. With dwindling demand for a product that is more harmful to health than good, what's a fluoride manufacturer to do? They simply find new ways to sneak it into consumer products. Recently my husband bought a package of dental floss and when he got home discovered that the floss was coated with fluoride! Needless to say, he returned it. Where will fluoride show up next? Some toothbrush bristles are being coated with fluoride and it proves we can't ever let down our guard.

But there are organizations joining together to fight on our behalf to rid our water supply of fluoride, but it's not our government. Here are some of the groups willing to fight for our health and safety: The Environmental Working Group (EWG), the Fluoride Action Network (FAN), some dentists, and ordinary citizens just like you. These organizations are fighting to stop the water poisoning, one state, one community at a time.

BOTTLED WATER

Evian is "naïve" spelled backwards. Bottled water is one of the greatest, most lucrative, most deceptive marketing campaigns ever launched. Independent tests have shown that the majority of bottled water isn't any better than what comes right out of your faucet. Not only is it expensive, but in many ways it's worse than your own tap water. Here's why:

First, it comes in plastic bottles which have contributed to massive pollution of landfills and oceans. A plastic island, the size of all of the Gulf states combined, floats off the coast of California. The Container Recycling Institute estimates that over 67 million plastic water bottles are discarded every day in the U.S. alone.

Second, the Sierra Club estimates that it takes 1.5 million barrels of oil every year to produce those plastic water bottles we discard every day. Even worse, processing plastic bottles releases toxic compounds into the environment, including carcinogens such as benzene, as well as ethylbenzene, ethylene oxide, and nickel.

Finally, plastics contain endocrine disrupting chemicals such as bisphenol-A (BPA), nalgene, and polycarbonate that can leach into the bottled water and cause a variety of health problems.

Rather than coming from pristine mountain streams, studies reveal that as much as 40% of bottled water comes right out of municipal water supplies, which, as previously discussed, are treated with chlorine and fluoride. And on top of this, the bottled water industry has no regulatory agency overseeing the purity of its water.

In 2010, independent laboratory testing initiated by the Environmental Working Group found 38 contaminants, including DBP's (disinfection by-products), nitrate, caffeine, arsenic, Tylenol, industrial chemicals, and bacteria in ten brands of bottled water.

But as previously mentioned, our greatest consumption of all of these chemicals is not necessarily from drinking water, or even from soaking in a tub of it. Rather, it comes from our daily showers, where we inhale 25 times more of these chemicals than from any other form of ingestion. We can inhale up to 20 times more chlorine in a shower than from drinking a glass of chlorinated tap water. A quick shower can increase by 700% our blood levels of Trihalomethanes (THMs), the common chemical byproducts from disinfected water that include, but are not limited to chloroform, bromodichloromethane, dibromochloromethan, and bromoform.

The human body needs clean water in order to purify itself. If we do not filter out these contaminants before using our water, it means our already overburdened bodies are forced to become the filter.

Water Bottles

After researching the possible causes of my LS, not only do I filter my home's well water, I bring my own water with me everywhere I go. Glass is my number one choice of carrying container, and I save the glass bottles that various food items come in and re-use them not only for storage of my homemade food, but also as water bottles. But because glass breaks, my second choice is stainless steel water bottles.

To find a stainless steel water bottle that is not lined with Bisphenol-A (BPA), several websites list comparisons, including Go Green Travel Green and the Safe Water Bottle Review. There are also individual websites, such as Klean Kanteen or Life Without Plastic, devoted to BPA-free stainless steel water bottles. Still, whenever possible, I simply refill my glass jars or bottles.

AIR

Even the air we breathe is full of chemicals, including pesticides from the spraying of farm crops, toxins from manufacturing plants, some of which are hundreds of miles away, pollutants from automobile emissions, to name the most obvious sources. However, you may be contaminating the air you breathe right in your own home, and then breathing in as many as 133 chemicals from that contamination.

How is that possible? The easiest way to find out is by using your nose. That's because if you can smell it, then a chemical is giving off gases. And even if your nose can't detect an odor, chemicals may be everywhere, surrounding you in your own home. These chemicals are found in air fresheners, scented candles, perfumes and building products. Here are the reasons to avoid as many as possible:

Air Fresheners

These unnecessary products are nothing more than liquid or solid chemicals in a bottle and they are extremely toxic because they can contain over 80 different chemicals. Television ads abound for air fresheners that you plug into your wall or spray into the air; some automatically emit a spray of chemicals and others are activated by a motion sensor. And now a new one can "detect odors" on its own, and then unleash a spray of chemicals without human intervention.

Some television ads show actors spraying air freshener on every piece of upholstered furniture, draperies, or directly into the air to remove unpleasant odors. What is so infuriating about these commercials is that they are encouraging the use of 80 or more chemicals that can trigger asthma, anaphylaxis, eye irritation, swelling of face, and pulmonary inflammation. These adverse reactions occur not only in humans, but can also spur deadly reactions in pets. Here are some of the culprits found in air fresheners:

- Sensitizers
- Broncho constrictors
- Respiratory irritants
- Skin Irritants

The chemicals found in air fresheners are categorized as "fragrance," and as previously discussed, are not required to be labeled. Here are just a few of the chemicals found in air fresheners:

1. **Denatured Alcohol** – Also known as methylated spirits, this is actually ethanol mixed with a poisonous additive that makes the alcohol extremely dangerous to drink with very ill effects. Denatured alcohol can contain acetone, methyl ethyl ketone, methyl isobutyl ketone, or denatonium benzoate, all of which are toxic chemicals.

2. **Acetaldehyde** – Part of the formaldehyde family. When inhaled, acetaldehyde can constrict airways and cause suffocation. It is an ingredient in fragrance and a known carcinogen. Acetaldehyde is also linked to immunotoxicity and is a known skin, eye, and lung irritant.

3. **Alpha-pinene** – This oil constituent has been linked to numerous allergic reactions. Although alpha-pinene is commonly used by the fragrance industry, it has not been assessed for safety by the cosmetics industry panel.

4. **Benzaldehyde** – A member of the formaldehyde family, it is a known asthma trigger, is carcinogenic, and a skin irritant.

5. **Trimethyl Pentanyl Diisobutyrate** – A plasticizer most often used in nail polish, it is a skin irritant.

6. **Limonene** – Part of the terpene (turpentine) family, limonene is a volatile organic compound (VOC) used most often in building materials. It is linked to allergies and immuno-toxicity, and it irritates the skin, eyes, and lungs.

7. **Butylated Hydroxytoluene (BHT)** – This toluene-based chemical is used as a food additive as well as a fragrance ingredient. It has been linked to cancer, developmental and reproductive disorders, immuno-toxicity, and is a powerful allergen.

8. **Benzyl Acetate** – This chemical compound produces respiratory irritation. Continued exposure to this compound at 50 parts per million will cause kidney damage. It is also suspected of having carcinogenic properties.

9. **Benzothiazole** – A fume associated with asphalt, this additive has not been assessed for safety by the cosmetics industry panel.

10. **Hexadecane** – As part of the hexane family it is used in solvents and is petrochemical based. This chemical has not been assessed for safety by the cosmetics industry panel.

11. **Butylphenyl Methylpropional** – Also called Lilial, this chemical is used as a fragrance ingredient and is found in hair coloring, conditioner, moisturizer, styling gels and lotions. It is viewed as persistent and bio-

accumulative, and has been linked to organ system toxicity and immunotoxicity, and is associated with allergies and contact dermatitis. This toxic chemical is banned in Europe.

12. **Cyclamen Aldehyde** – Used as a fragrance ingredient, this is another member of the formaldehyde family.

13. **Geraniol** – While it is a naturally-occurring scent ingredient found in essential oils such as rose and citronella, it is banned in Europe and is restricted in the U.S. It is closely associated with immuno-toxicity and severe allergic reactions.

14. **Methylpyrrolidone Ethyl Acetate** – It is an ingredient that dissolves chemicals and when inhaled, is toxic to the brain and nervous system. Aside from use in air fresheners, it is also used as a paint stripper.

15. **Fragrance** – Already discussed in Chapter 2: Toxic Topicals, fragrance is a blanket term for a multitude of chemicals a manufacturer deems proprietary and is therefore not forced to specify.

There are many other chemicals included in these products aside from the ones listed above, but I hope these will be sufficient to prevent someone from using any type of air freshener or cleaning agent in their home.

None of this is new. In the early days of TV, in the 1940s or 1950s, there was a black and white commercial that showed a well-dressed mother spraying a new miracle mist in every closet, pantry, and even into the air. This fine mist was designed to control every pest imaginable, from moths in your clothing, to ants in your food pantry, and would kill any insect in your home. It was described as "perfectly safe." And what was this miracle spray? Nothing less than DDT! And we all know how that turned out.

Scented Candles

In the past, not only did I purchase scented candles, but I received them as gifts. Once when our power went out, I lit many of these candles and recall feeling nauseated by what I thought was the mixture of scents. I now know it was from the release of gases from all those toxic chemicals.

Scented candles can be used as a form of aromatherapy mood enhancers, but there are better choices available that use beeswax and organic, GMO-free soy with pure essential oils for scent. However, even essential oils can be toxic to sensitive individuals, and we must remember that just because it grows in nature doesn't mean inhaling it is safe. To avoid problems of toxicity, I've replaced scented candles with battery-operated lanterns or lamps. Not only is the air cleaner, but they can't set the house on fire, either.

Perfume

Perfume, sad to say, is just another term for *fragrance*, which is covered in Chapter 2: Toxic Topicals. Some people have severe, life-threatening reactions to the chemicals used in different perfumes, including anaphylactic shock. It doesn't matter how exclusive or expensive the brands, perfumers are not required to list the chemicals in their perfumes because it is deemed proprietary. But perfumes are just chemicals in a bottle and ones you apply directly to your skin.

And now our most vulnerable, non-consenting segment of the population is being subjected to potentially harmful chemicals in a bottle. In 2013, high end fashion house Dolce & Gabbana released a baby perfume and cologne that supposedly "accentuates that natural baby smell." Johnson's Bulgari and Burberry also have fragrance lines specifically targeting preschoolers, and no doubt more brands will follow this toxic trend that may trigger asthma, allergies, or even anaphylaxis in defenseless children.

If you, or a family member, want to smell good, I recommend investing in pure organic essential oils. These essential oils have strong scents, so you need only a drop or two. But keep in mind, even though they are organic essential oils, it doesn't mean you can't still have a reaction to them. Always apply a tiny test drop to see how your skin reacts to a particular essential oil. Producers of essential oils advise that they be diluted with a few drops of organic extra virgin olive oil before applying them to your skin. A 3:1 ratio of 3 drops organic extra virgin olive oil to 1 drop of essential oil is recommended.

Building Products

Vinyl flooring contains phthalates, and phthalates are found in plywood that was used in older homes for subflooring, as well as in cabinetry. Phthalates are dangerous because they give off formaldehyde gas.

Some hardwood floor finishes can emit toxins into the air, and synthetic fiber carpeting gives off the flame retardant polybrominated diphenyl ethers (PBDE), and upholstery dirt repellants (including older Scotch Guard) contain the flame retardant polytetrafluoroethylene (PTFE).

All of these chemicals are now found in the blood and urine of nearly 100% of the U.S. population. Today, some contractors are building "green" homes using products that are free of these chemicals, but most of us do not live in these types of safer homes. So what can we do about it, if we aren't able to move to a new, "green" home? There are several ways to cope.

AIR PURIFICATION

Is there anything we can do to help cleanse the air in our own home? Use a HEPA filtration system? Buy room air purifiers? It's certainly possible to invest in some very good air filtration systems, and if you live in a rural environment that might have reduced air pollution, the best way to get clean, fresh scented air is to simply open some windows. However, millions of people live in busy metropolitan areas where the outside air may not be healthy to breathe. Even people living in a natural setting can be exposed to toxins, including the fumes from a neighbor's dryer sheets wafting in through open windows that can cause illness.

Once again, look to nature, which surrounds us with air fresheners and purifiers in the form of trees and plants. Anything that is green and leafy, especially ferns, has the ability to clean the air in your home. Plants were designed to thrive on toxins such as carbon dioxide, which we exhale, and to emit clean oxygen. It is said that the air in a house filled with green leafy plants will be 95% purified. Plants are much better than filtration systems because they run on sunlight, which is free, along with water. Houseplants are undemanding, yet quite rewarding in so many ways. And outside your home, if you've got more trees in your yard than lawn so much the better.

AUTOMOBILE EMISSIONS

Automobiles are toxic externally and internally for many reasons.

- **External Emissions** - Automobile exhaust contains a multitude of toxins, including heavy metals such as cadmium, particles of which may collect along roadsides. These particles are light and can easily float on air currents up to 150 feet away with just the slightest breeze. People walking or biking along roadsides busy with automobiles, logging trucks, trucks with smokestacks emitting black clouds of smoke are inhaling these toxic emissions. It's unfortunate that even healthy outdoor activities expose us to heavy metals.

- **Internal Emissions** – Nearly everything in our cars is plastic, from the dashboard to the synthetic leather (pleather) seats. That "new car" smell everyone is so fond of is actually the gases being emitted by all those new plastics.

HEAVY METALS POISONING

Heavy metals are a serious health threat. But how do they enter the body? Heavy metals are everywhere, sent out as exhaust from manufacturing plants and from automobile emissions; wherever they come from, we breathe them in. We take them in through the chemicals in fluoridated water and in the foods we eat. Heavy metals are also used in home and personal care products, meaning that we also consume them and absorb them through our skin.

Types of heavy metals include cadmium (automobile emissions), mercury (vaccines as well as dental amalgams), lead (used in plumbing, the manufacture of crystal glassware, enamel, and computer monitors, and as a stabilizer in the manufacture of plastics), and aluminum (deodorant, baking powder, cookware, vaccines). In other words, there's no escaping heavy metals in our daily lives.

Mercury

Mercury is a prominent heavy metal and we hear a lot about mercury in fish. But there's a source of mercury that's much closer to home. In fact, I've got a lot of it myself. And that common source of mercury is the fillings in our teeth. Silver fillings, also known as amalgam fillings, contain up to 50% mercury. Even crowns contain mercury, and I've seen photographs showing mercury vapors emitted in the mouth. Chewing food can also emit mercury vapors, which are then absorbed into the body. Brain damage, neurological problems, and effects on the kidneys have been associated with mercury from amalgam fillings. It's advised by some health practitioners to have mercury fillings removed and replaced with non-toxic materials by certified biological dentists. This is not covered by dental insurance, but many swear by the improvement in overall health from having this mercury removed.

Removal of mercury fillings cannot be handled by an ordinary dentist because without proper handling, even more mercury will be released into the body than if the fillings had been left in place. It requires special damming that only a qualified, certified biological dentist has been trained to do.

Since learning this startling and frightening fact about mercury in dental fillings, I've considered having this expensive work done, but I've had these fillings for most of my life. And yet, if I'd believed they were the cause of my bout of LS, I'd have had the fillings replaced. But when we consider that children the age of 2 and younger are being diagnosed with LS, mercury in dental fillings cannot be a factor for them. Also, one LS sufferer explained to me that she'd undergone the removal and replacement of her mercury fillings but she still had LS. And while I still have all of my fillings, I no longer have LS. While it's best to avoid mercury dental fillings, it doesn't seem likely that it's a major factor in contracting LS.

Many dentists have stopped using mercury fillings and it is wise to confer with your dentist about what's in the fillings being used. Alternative restorative dental materials include:

- Resin composite
- Glass ionomer
- Resin ionomer
- Porcelain
- Gold alloys

To find a certified biological dentist, visit the website of the International Academy of Biological Dentistry & Medicine (www.iabdm.org/cms/). The website lists participating dentists by U.S. state, as well as in other countries.

Aluminum

Aluminum is another heavy metal that is quite prominent but often overlooked. As early as 1980, a study of the brains of Alzheimer's victims showed unusually high levels of aluminum. It was then that my husband insisted we eliminate every aluminum pot, pan, and utensil we owned, but that was not the end of aluminum poisoning in our household.

That's because various forms of aluminum (aluminum sulfate, aluminum chloride, aluminum oxide) are used in the production of baking powder and other food manufacturing ingredients (cake mixes, frozen dough, pancake mixes, foods in aluminum cans), deodorant, plant fertilizer, soaps, pharmaceutical drugs (vaccines, over-the-counter medications, buffered aspirins, diarrhea and hemorrhoidal medications), in water disinfection, cosmetics, dyes, insecticide, paint, synthetic rubber, lubricants, wood preservatives, aluminum metals, and in aluminum foil. It's even used as an additive to the leather used on baseballs to harden and toughen their hides. In fact, one way or another we come into contact with aluminum every single day.

Signs of aluminum toxicity include:

- Disturbed sleep
- Nervousness
- Memory loss
- Headaches
- Impaired intellect
- Emotional instability
- Muscle aches
- Speech problems
- Anemia
- Digestive problems
- Lowered liver function
- Impaired kidney function
- Colic

The human body cannot readily break down and eliminate heavy metals such as aluminum so they end up being stored in our tissues, and in our brains.

STILL NOT CONVINCED?

As already discussed, there are numerous toxins that may contribute to LS, but it's not possible to identify just one thing as the cause because it may not be *the* thing.

Why is it that although we accept the dangers of smoking, we ignore the serious problems caused by long-term exposure to pesticides, herbicides, fungicides, manufacturing chemicals, chemicals in household products, excitotoxins in our foods, along with dyes, solvents, and a myriad of chemical concoctions entering our bodies via the air we breathe, the water we drink, the food we eat, and the personal and home maintenance products we use? Is it a stretch of the imagination that this toxic overload won't result in disease?

Is it because most of the toxins in our lives are, for the most part, invisible, odorless, tasteless, and undetectable that we think we're safe? Is it because we're told they are at "acceptable levels" by the government?

It is impossible to list every single food item containing some sort of preservative, food additive, artificial colorant, artificial flavoring, texturizer, emulsifier, etc., or to list every single product containing toxins. My goal here is to raise the reader's awareness of how prevalent and insidious toxins are in our everyday lives, how they are affecting us, and empower the reader to make healthier choices so they can begin to heal their bodies. With children being born with nearly 300+ chemicals already in their bodies, is it any wonder they are developing illnesses such as Lichen Sclerosis at astonishingly younger and younger ages?

HOW DOES ALL OF THIS RELATE TO LICHEN SCLEROSIS?

Lichen Sclerosis has been detected in humans for longer than 124 years, and for most of those years it was considered a rare, menopausal woman's disease. No longer is that true, however. Today it is the silent plague affecting all age groups, races, genders, and countries around the globe. In 124 years, no "cause" has been named, and no "cure" has been developed. How did LS expand from a rare, menopausal woman's disease to affecting every segment of the human race? What do we all have in common?

The effects of toxins such as heavy metals are devastating to the human body. Individually or combined, they affect every organ, including the brain, as well as every tissue, hormone, and cell. Disease does not spring up out of nowhere and toxins are the culprits for many, if not all of our modern-day illnesses that either didn't exist previously or were extremely rare fifty years ago.

Symptoms of toxic overload on the human body manifest as "diseases" and often those symptoms overlap. This means that many chemicals affect the human body in the same way and because we are subjected to so many chemicals, it's nearly impossible to pinpoint exactly which toxins or chemicals are to blame for specific illnesses, or how those chemicals interact and manifest in a person's specific genetic makeup. At this moment in time, our only choice is to avoid as many toxins as possible.

The question isn't if we are toxic, it's a question of just how toxic we are. The following list of symptoms is indicative of several "diseases," as well as symptoms of toxicity.

- ADD and ADHD
- ALD (Adrenoleukodystrophy - the progressive destruction of the insulation around the brain's nerves)
- Arthritis and related conditions
- Bi-polar disorder
- Birth defects

- Brittle nails
- Cancer (prostate, pancreatic, kidney, liver)
- Cardio Dysfunction (angina, palpitations, hypertension, arrhythmia, valve prolapse)
- Chronic fatigue and related chronic symptoms
- Cognitive disturbances (brain fog, memory problems)
- Cold intolerance
- Decreased cognitive function ("brain fog"), memory recall, initiative
- Dementia, including Alzheimer's Disease
- Diabetes
- Dizziness
- Dry skin
- Eczema
- Enlarged liver (hepatomegaly), pancreas, etc.
- Fibromyalgia
- Gastrointestinal disorders
- Hair loss
- Headaches
- Hearing disturbances (sound sensitivity, buzzing, ringing, ear pain)
- Hypospadias
- Hypothyroidism
- Immune deficiency
- Increased cholesterol

- Loss of stamina
- Low sperm count
- Lupus
- Malaise (a general feeling of unwellness)
- Multiple Sclerosis
- Muscle pain and weakness
- Neuralgia (nerve pain)
- Neuritis (nerve inflammation)
- Numbness
- Parkinson's
- Psoriasis
- Rheumatic conditions
- Spontaneous abortion
- Tingling or burning sensations
- Tiredness and lethargy
- Tumors (lung, kidney, breast, brain)
- Vision problems including cataracts, glaucoma, blurry vision
- Weight gain

After collecting all of this information, Lichen Sclerosis was no longer an auto-immune disease of "unknown cause" to me. It belonged right up there with all of the other symptoms of toxicity. For me, the magnitude of how I was being insidiously poisoned, and the sheer magnitude of chemicals I was unwittingly applying to my skin and consuming every single day was astonishing and depressing. I felt abused by Big Industry, but ashamed of my own prior ignorance and culpability in developing LS. The scope of collusion, corruption, and ineffectiveness of our government to protect us made me feel disappointed, disillusioned, and extremely angry.

I'd come to the conclusion that I'd have to think about, examine, and analyze every single aspect of my life and no longer could I grab a box, bag, can, jar, or bottle of *anything* off a store shelf, even if it is marked "organic," without scrutinizing the ingredients first. I could no longer place *anything* in my shopping cart without analyzing it and no longer could I sit at someone's table and eat their non-organic food without thinking about the chemical toxins I'd be consuming or how they'd bio-accumulate inside my body, and how simply eating that food could lead me down the path to disease once more. Because I had learned so much, I could no longer look at a plate of food, or anything else for that matter, the same way ever again.

Since I have educated myself, I'll now eat before leaving home or bring food with me if organic food is not available when I'm dining out. This has not made me popular at some friends' homes, but my health is of the utmost importance to me. If people can't understand that, it is not my problem but theirs. On rare occasions when I do eat at a restaurant, I'll choose seafood such as mussels, king crab, or calamari because they cannot be faked, king crab and calamari are always wild caught, and although mussels are farmed, they are the most environmentally friendly aquaculture.

I now live on toxin-alert at all times. Although it may sound that way, I'm not paranoid about it. After all, with every breath, I've inhaled more than clean air and this is a fact of life. But I can limit the number of toxins in my home, and try to eliminate as many as possible when I'm away from home.

Now, not only do I bring my own filtered water wherever I go, I make more of my food from scratch. I've also begun growing my own organic food and organically raising my own free-range chickens.

Despite all of these changes in my life, and even though other maladies began to disappear when I switched to organic products, I still had Lichen Sclerosis.

Although there wasn't a dramatic or immediate positive result from switching to filtered water or eating organic food aside from the great taste, these changes alone didn't alleviate my LS.

By the end of December 2009, I'd just embarked on what would become Part 2 of my overall healing protocol and it would take nearly a year before I was able to see the internal, external, and obvious evidence of improved health.

Sources:

USDA/National Organic Program (NOP). Pdf. [65 FR 80657, Dec. 21, 2000, as amended at 68 FR 61993, Oct. 31, 2003, and 68 FR 62217, November, 2003]

American Museum of Natural History, "National Survey Reveals Biodiversity Crisis – Scientific Experts Believe We are in Midst of Fastest Mass Extinction in Earth's History", www.amnh.org/museum/press/feature/biofact.html. Accessed 11/06/2010

Burrow, Marian, "Options to Organic Produce," May 22, 2002, www.mercola.com

GreenBiz Staff, "EPA Plans to List 'Chemicals of Concern,'" GreenBiz, January 4, 2010. www.greenbiz.com

Gupta, Sanjay M.D., "Toxic America," CNN, June 2, 2010

Gupta, Sanjay, M.D., "Toxic Childhood," CNN, June 3, 2010

Rangan, Urvashi, Ph.D., "Consumers Union Derides Dark-of-Night Weakening of Organic Law," Consumers Union, October 27, 2005. www.consumersunion.org

Sharpe, Richard, "Men Under Threat: The Decline In Male Reproductive Health and the Potential Role of Exposure to Chemicals During In-Utero Development," Briefing by ChemTrust. www.chemtrust.org.uk/Press and Media.php

Artificial Sweeteners Sources:

Brackett, Cori, Sweet Misery: A Poisoned World, 2005. DVD. http://www.amazon.com/Sweet-Misery-Poisoned-Cori-Brackett/dp/B000BQ5IWS/ref=sr_1_2?ie=UTF8&qid=1302536477&sr=8-2

Consumer Federation of America, Letter to US Food and Drug Administration Re Docket No. FDA-2010-P-0491. http://www.foodinstitute.com/CFAcommentHFCS.pdf

Wikipedia, "Fructose." http://en.wikipedia.org/wiki/Fructose

What's In That Fruit Juice? Sources:

USFDA Commodity Food Fact Sheet for Schools & Child Nutrition Institutions, "A343 - Apples, Fresh," Updated 05-30-07. http://www.fns.usda.gov/fdd/schfacts/FV/A343_ApplesFresh.pdf

Buhler, Dr. Donald R. and Dr. Cristobal Miranda, "*Antioxidant Activities of Flavonoids,*" The Linus Pauling Institute, Oregon State University, Department of Environmental and Molecular Toxicology, November 2000. http://lpi.oregonstate.edu/f-w00/flavonoid.html

Hamilton, Alissa, Ph.D., "*Squeezed: What You Don't Know About Orange Juice,*" Yale University Press, May 2009

Hamilton, Alissa, Ph.D., "*Freshly Squeezed: The Truth About Orange Juice in Boxes,*" Civil Eats, May 6, 2009. http://civileats.com/2009/05/06/freshly-squeezed-the-truth-about-orange-juice-in-boxes/7

Mott's: http://www.motts.com/products/familyhealthyfavorites/mottsoriginal100 applejuice.aspx

Self Nutrition Data, "*Apples, Raw, With Skin,*" Nutrition Facts. http://nutritiondata.self.com/facts/fruits-and-fruit-juices/1809/2

The George Mateljan Foundation, "How Does Fruit Juice Compare to Whole Fruit?" http://www.whfoods.com/genpage.php?tname=george&dbid=24

Welch's: http://www.welchs.com/products/100-percent-grape-juice

Wysong, Dr. Randy, "*Fructooligosaccharides.*" www.wysong.com

Chocolate Sources:

Center for Science in the Public Interest, "Chemical Cuisine: Learn About Food Additives." http://www.cspinet.org/reports/chemcuisine.htm#blue2

Honey Sources:

Mercola, Dr. Joseph, "The Honey You Should Never Buy: It May Be Tainted with Lead and Antibiotics," January 28, 2012. http://articles.mercola.com/sites/articles/archive/2012/01/28/bees-death-destroy-food-supply.aspx

MSG Sources:

Blaylock, Russell L., MD, "Excitotoxins: The Taste That Kills", Health Press, 1997. www.healthpress.com

Schwartz, George R., MD, "In Bad Taste: The MSG Symptom Complex", Health Press, 1999. www.healthpress.com

Pesticides Sources:

U.S. EPA Report, "About Pesticides," 2000-2001. http://www.epa.gov/pesticides/pestsales/01pestsales/usage2001.htm

U.S. FDA, "Pesticide Residue Monitoring Program for Years 2004-2006." http://www.fda.gov/Food/FoodSafety/FoodContaminantsAdulteration/Pesticides/ResidueMonitoringReports/ucm125183.htm

Bennett, K.P. et al. "Rice Pesticides Monitoring in the Sacramento Valley, 1995," Environmental Hazards Assessment Program, State of California Environmental Protection Agency, Department of Pesticide Regulation, Environmental Monitoring and Pest Management Branch. February 1998. www.cdpr.ca.gov/docs/emon/pubs/ehapreps/eh983execs.pdf

Beyond Pesticides, "Despite Industry Claims, Herbicide Use Fails to Decline with GE Crops," June 3, 2011. www.byondpesticides.org/dailynewsblog/?p=5414

Beyond Pesticides, "What's in a Pesticide?" Safety Source for Pest Management, Beyond Pesticides.org. http://www.beyondpesticides.org/infoservices/pcos/ingredients.htm

Costello, Dr. Sadie, et al., "Parkinson's Disease and Residential Exposure to Maneb and Paraquat From Agricultural Applications in the Central Valley of California," American Journal of Epidemiology, January 6, 2009. aje.oxfordjournals.org/cgi/content/abstract/169/8/919

Curl, C.L., et al. "Organophosphorus Pesticide Exposure of Urban and Suburban Preschool Children With Organic and Conventional Diets," Environmental Health Perspectives. 2003 March; 111(3):377-82.

Environmental Working Group, "Overexposed: Organophosphate Insecticides in Children's Food," 1998, pp. 1-3. www.ewg.org/reports/ops

Environmental Working Group, "Body Burden." 2003. www.ewg.org/reports/bodyburden2/execsumm.php

Environmental Working Group, "2012 Shopper's Guide to Pesticides in Produce™." June 29, 2012. http://www.ewg.org/foodnews/summary/

"Hazards of Pesticides Used on Potatoes: Table 2", Journal of Pesticide Reform/Winter 1997 – Vol. 17, No. 4 – Northwest Center for Alternatives to Pesticides/NCAP. www.pesticide.org, potatoes.pdf

Lu, Ce, et al. "Organic diets significantly lower children's dietary exposure to organophosphorus pesticides", Environmental Health Perspectives, Vol. 114, No. 2:260-263. 2006. abstract: ehp.niehs.nih.gov/docs/2005/8414/abstract.html

McCullum-Gomez, Christine, C., and Riddle, J., "Promoting Sustainable Food Systems through Organic Agriculture: Past, Present and Future," Hunger and Environmental Nutrition Practice Group of the American Dietetic Association, Spring 2009. www.hendpg.org

Mercola, Joseph, M.D., "Organic Pesticides Not Always Best Choice," July 17, 2010. http://articles.mercola.com/sites/articles/archive/2010/07/17/organic-pesticides-not-always-best-choice.aspx

Schafer, Kristin, "Nowhere to Hide: Persistent Toxic Chemicals in the U.S. Food Supply", Pesticide Action Network North America, 2000. http://www.panna.org/sites/default/files/NowhereToHide2001.pdf

Smith, Jeffrey M., "The Scary Truth about Genetically Engineered Insect Control", August 9, 2007. http://articles.mercola.com/sites/articles/archive/2007/08/09/enjoy-pesticides-in-every-bite-of-gmo-food.aspx

GMO Sources:

U.S. Department of Veterans Affairs, Agent Orange and Vietnam Veterans – Health Issues. http://www.vba.va.gov/bln/21/benefits/herbicide/

U.S. Environmental Protection Agency, "Polychlorinated Biphenyls." http://www.epa.gov/epawaste/hazard/tsd/pcbs/index.htm

U.S. Environmental Protection Agency, "Polychlorinated Biphenyls: "Health Effects of PCBs." http://www.epa.gov/epawaste/hazard/tsd/pcbs/pubs/effects.htm

U.S. Environmental Protection Agency, "Dioxin." http://cfpub.epa.gov/ncea/CFM/nceaQFind.cfm?keyword=Dioxin

U.S. FDA, Agency Response Letter GRAS Notice No. GRN 000283 to Raymonnd C. Dobert, Ph.D., Monsanto Company, Re Stearidonic Acid Soybean Oil (SDA), September 4, 2009. http://www.fda.gov/Food/FoodIngredientsPackaging/GenerallyRecognizedasSafeGRAS/GRASListings/ucm185688.htm

Veterans of the Vietnam War, Inc., Information Packet. http://www.vvnw.org/educational_material/agent_orange.htm

Brändli, Dirk and Sandra Reinacher, "Herbicides Found in Human Urine," *Ithaka,* English Translation translated by Thomas Rippel, January 7, 2012. http://www.ithaka-journal.net/herbizide-im-urin?lang=en

Burns, John M., "13-Week Dietary Subchronic Comparison Study with MON 863 Corn in Rats Preceded by a 1-Week Baseline Food Consumption Determination with PMI Certified Rodent Diet #5002," December 17, 2002. http://www.monsanto.com/monsanto/content/sci_tech/prod_safety/fullratstudy.pdf,

The Cornucopia Institute, "GMO Apples?" December 6, 2013. http://www.cornucopia.org/2013/12/crushed-nutsrotten-apples-pasteurized-nuts-gmo-apples-tell-fda-usda/

Dow AgroSciences News Release, "New Unique Colex-D™ Technology Announced From Dow AgroSciences, *Innovative Technology Designed for Growers, Key Component of the New Enlist™ Weed Control System*," March 4, 2011. www.enlist.com.

Dow AgroSciences News Release, "Dow AgroSciences Announces Name of Enlist™ Weed Control System Herbicide Component, *Enlist Duo™ Herbicide Will Provide Growers Exceptional Weed Control*," August 31, 2011. PDF. www.elist.com.

Foucart, Stéphane, "Controversy Surrounds a GMO," Le Monde, 14 December 2004. http://www.blackherbals.com/controversy_surrounds_a_gmo_.htm

Hopkinson, Jenny and Evich, Helena Bottemiller, "Food Industry to Fire Preemptive GMO Strike," The Cornucopia Institute. January 8, 2014. http://www.cornucopia.org/2014/01/food-industry-fire-preemptive-gmo-strike/

Huber, Don M., COL (Ret), Letter to USFDA Secretary Vilsack, January 17, 2011. http://thebayougardener.com/smf/index/php?topic=5849.0

Monsanto Inc., "Food Safety." www.monsanto.com/newsviews/Pages/food-safety.aspx

Smith, Jeffrey M., *"Monsanto's Roundup Triggers Over 40 Plant Diseases and Endangers Human and Animal Health,"* Institute for Responsible Technology, January 14, 2011. http://www.responsibletechnology.org/posts/monsanto%E2%80%99s-roundup-triggers-over-40-plant-diseases/

Smith, Jeffrey M., "Dow Launches Multi-Herbicide Tolerant GM Soy," Institute for Responsible Technology, September 6, 2011. http://www.responsibletechnology.org/newsletters/09012011spillingthebeans.html

Smith, Jeffrey M., "10 Reasons to Avoid GMOs," Institute for Responsible Technology. http://www.responsibletechnology.org/10-Reasons-to-Avoid-GMOs

Smith, Jeffrey M., "Genetically Modified Corn Study Reveals Health Damage and Cover-up," Institute for Responsible Technology, June 2005. http://www.seedsofdeception.com/Public/Newsletter/June05GMCornHealthDangerExposed/index.cfm

Smith, Jeffrey M., "Introduction," *Seeds of Deception*, page 3. seedsofdeception.com/pdf/118.pdf

Smith, Jeffrey M., *"Scrambling and Gambling with the Genome,"* Institute for Responsible Technology, July 2005. http://www.responsibletechnology.org/gmo-dangers/Scrambling-and-Gambling-with-the-Genome-July-2005

Smith, Jeffrey M., "Monsanto's Roundup Triggers Over 40 Plant Diseases and Endangers Human and Animal Health," Institute for Responsible Technology, October 2011. http://action.responsibletechnology.org/o/6236/t/0/blastContent.jsp?email_blast_KEY=1150514

Weatherby, Craig, "Monsanto's Fishy 'Omega-3' Soy," Vital Choices Newsletter, April 11, 2011. http://www.vitalchoice.com/shop/pc/articlesView_old.asp?id=1376

Weatherby, Craig, "Gene-Modified Food Fears Fueled by Secrets," Vital Choices Newsletter, March 10, 2011. http://www.vitalchoice.com/shop/pc/articlesView_old.asp?id=1323

Labeling Sources:

USDA/National Organic Program (NOP), Title 7-Agriculture, Part 205–National Organic Program, Subpart D–Labels, Labeling, and Market Information. Updated January 7, 2002. www.ams.usda.gov/AMSv1.0

Wiles, Richard et al. "Overexposed: Organophospate Insecticides in Children's Food," The Environmental Working Group, Executive Summary, January 1998. http://www.ewg.org/report/overexposed-organophosphate-insecticides-childrens-food

Irradiated and Microwaved Food Sources:

Agency for Toxic Substances & Disease Registry, "Toxic Substances Portal – Toluene." February 2001. http://www.atsdr.cdc.gov/toxfaqs/tf.asp?id=160&tid=29

Agency for Toxic Substances & Disease Registry, "Toxic Substances Portal – Benzene." CAS ID #: 71-43-2. http://www.atsdr.cdc.gov/substances/toxsubstance.asp?toxid=14

National Institute of Environmental Health Sciences, "Dioxins." http://www.niehs.nih.gov/health/topics/agents/dioxins/index.cfm

US Department of Labor, Occupational Safety and Health (NIOSH), "Occupational Safety and Healthy Guideline for Xylene." http://www.osha.gov/SLTC/healthguidelines/xylene/recognition.html

Douglas Laboratories, "Amino Acid Functions." L-Lysine product label

Dulberg, Andrew Scott, *"The Popcorn Lung Case Study: A Recipe for Regulation?"* N.Y.U. Review of Law & Social Change, February 17, 2011. Vol. 33:87, pages 87-126. http://socialchangenyu.com/2012/09/26/the-popcorn-lung-case-study-a-recipe-for-regulation/

Mercola, Dr. Joseph, *"Isn't That Non-Stick Coating in Your Microwave Popcorn?"* December 8, 2006.
http://articles.mercola.com/sites/articles/archive/2006/12/08/isnt-that-nonstick-coating-in-your-microwave-popcorn-part-two.aspx

Mercola, Dr. Joseph, "Why Did the Russians Ban an Appliance Found in 90% of American Homes?" May 18, 2010.
http://articles.mercola.com/sites/articles/archive/2010/05/18/microwave-hazards.aspx

Raul, F., et al. Food-borne Radiolytic Compounds (2-alkylcyclobutanones) May Promote Experimental Colon Carcinogenesis, Laboratoire d-Oncologie Nutritionnelle, F-6000 Strasbourge, France, Nutrition Center 2002; 44(2): 189-91. Abstract.
http://www.ncbi.nlm.nih.gov/pubmed/12734067

Thomas, Carolyn, "Microwave Popcorn: (Still) Bad for You," January 9, 2010. http://ethicalnag.org/2010/01/09/micro-popcorn/

Valentine, Tom, Interview with Dr. Hans Hertel, Nexus Magazine, Volume 2, #25 (April-May 1995)

Wysong, Dr. Randy, "Food's Dangerous Middle," 100 Pet Truths Newsletter, April 29, 2011. www.wysong.net

Factory Farming Sources:

U.S. FDA Summary Report, "Antimicrobials Sold or Distributed for Use in Food-Producing Animals," 2009.
www.fda.gov/downloads/ForIndustry/UserFees/AnimalDrugUserFeeActADUFA/UCM231851.pdf

USDA Food Safety and Inspection, *"Minnesota Firm Recalls Turkey Burger Products Due to Possible Salmonella Contamination,"* FSIS-RC-028-2011.
http://www.fsis.usda.gov/News_&_Events/Recall_028_2011_Release/index.asp

USDA Food Safety and Inspection, "Arkansas Firm Recalls Ground Turkey Products Due to Possible Salmonella Contamination," FSIS-RC-060-2011.
http://www.fsis.usda.gov/News_&_Events/Recall_060_2011_Release/index.asp

USDA Food Safety and Inspection, "Arkansas Firm Recalls Ground Turkey Products Due to Possible Salmonella Contamination," FSIS-RC-071-2011.
http://www.fsis.usda.gov/News_&_Events/Recall_071_2011_Release/index.asp

USDA Food Safety and Inspection Service, "Current Recalls and Alerts," November 13, 2011.
www.fsis.usda.gov/Fsis_Recalls/Open_Federal_Cases/index.asp

Poultry Sources:

U.S. FDA News Release, URGENT Nationwide Egg Recall, "Eggs in Their Shells May Put Consumers at Risk for Salmonella," August 19, 2010. www.fda.gov/newsevents/newsroom/pressrelease.

IRS "Poultry Industry Market Segment Specialization Program," Training 3123-013 (03/2002). www.smallbusinessnotes.com/pdf/poultry.pdf

Davis, Sandy, Davis Farm, Colebrook, New Hampshire

DeNoon, Daniel J., "New Egg Recall Due to Salmonella," WebMD Health News, November 2010. http://www.webmd.com/food-recipes/food-poisoning/news/20101109/new-egg-recall

Food, Inc., DVD

Gittins, Jennifer, "The Life Cycle of a Chicken." www.ehow.com/about_5316141_life-cycle-chicken.html

Meat Sources:

USDA Food Safety and Inspection Service, Recall Notification Report FSIS-RC-056-2011. www.fsis.usda.gov/Fsis_Recalls/RNR_056_2011/index.asp

USDA Food Safety and Inspection Service, "California Firm Recalls Ground Beef Due to Possible *E.Coli* 0157:H7 Contamination." www.fsis.usda.gov/News_& Events/Recall_080_2011_Release/index.asp

USFDA, "2009 Summary Report on Antimicrobials Sold or Distributed for Use in Food-Producing Animals." www.fda.gov/downloads/ForIndustry/UserFees/AnimalDrugUserFeeActA DUFA/UCM231851.pdf

USDA, Food Safety and Inspection Service, "Food Ingredients and Sources of Radiation Listed and Approved for Use in the Production of Meat and Poultry Products," Docket No. FSIS-2011-0018, Federal Register Volume 78, Number 45, Pages 14636-14640, March 7, 2013. http://www.gpo.gov/fdsys/pkg/FR2013-03-07/html/2013-05341.htm

Center for Science in the Public Interest, "Chemical Cuisine, Learn about Food Additives." http://www.cspinet.org/reports/chemcuisine.htm#caramelcolor

Center for Science in the Public Interest, "Chemical Cuisine, Learn about Food Additives." http://www.cspinet.org/reports/chemcuisine.htm#artificialcolorings

Food Inc., DVD

How Stuff Works, *"How Do Artificial Flavors Work?"* Accessed July 25, 2011. http://science.howstuffworks.com/question391.htm

Huff, Ethan A., "USDA Caves to Food Industry Pressures, Approves Three New Toxic Meat Preservatives," Natural News, April 5, 2013.
http://www.naturalnews.com:80/039792_USDA_meat_preservatives_chemicals.html

Janquart, Philip A., "FDA Approves Three Meat Preservatives," Courthouse News Service, March 12, 2013.
http://www.courthousenews.com/2013/03/12/55664.htm

Lohse, Rodney, "Dangerous Meat Deceptions", TodayTonight, Australia. Video.
http://au.todaytonight.yahoo.com/article/9190450/consumer/glued-meat-widespread

Mercola, Joseph, MD, "The Meat You Should Never, Ever Eat, May 4, 2011.
http://articles.mercola.com/sites/articles/archive/2011/05/04/has-your-meat-been-glued-together-why-you-need-to-know-and-avoid-this-dangerous-process.aspx

Mercola, Joseph, MD, "If You Eat Processed Meats, Are You Risking Your Life?" January 22, 2011.
http://articles.mercola.com/sites/articles/archive/2011/01/22/if-you-eat-processed-meats-youre-risking-your-life.aspx

Wikipedia, "Transglutaminase."
http://en.wikipedia.org/wiki/Transglutaminase

World Cancer Research Fund/American Institute for Cancer Research, "2007 Expert Report, Food, Nutrition, Physical Activity and the Prevention of Cancer: a Global Perspective," Press Release, May 23, 2011.
http://www.wcrf-uk.org/audience/media/press_release.php?recid=153

World Cancer Research Fund, "WCRF Criticises Meat Industry Over Misleading Public Statement." Press Release, February 12, 2010.
http://www.wcrf-uk.org/audience/media/press_release.php?recid=97Accessed 01-25-2011

Fish Sources:

Farmed and Dangerous, Coastal Alliance for Aquaculture Reform.
http://www.farmedanddangerous.org/salmon-farming-problems/

Food & Water Watch, "What's on Your Fish? Sodium Tripolyphosphate: Another Chemical to Avoid," Fact Sheet, June 2010.
http://www.foodandwaterwatch.org/factsheet/whats-on-your-fish/

Hartnell, Randy, "Fishy Con Game Continues," Vital Choices Newsletter, March 10, 2011.
http://newsletter.vitalchoice.com:80/e_article002254829.cfm?x=bkc2779,bmfq12DK

Weatherby, Craig, "Fish Fraud Marches On," Vital Choices Newsletter, December 13, 2012.
http://www.vitalchoice.com/shop/pc/articlesView.asp?id=1966

Weatherby, Craig, "Fishy Bait & Switch Continues," Vital Choices Newsletter, February 21, 2013. http://www.vitalchoice.com/shop/pc/articlesView.asp?id=1991

Milk Sources:

Baum, Rob, "The Importance of Colostrum," Baum Farm, Canaan, VT, September, 2011

Baum, Rob, "A1 vs. A2 Milk," Baum Farm, Canaan, VT, September 4, 2011

Craig, Patricia, "Proper Handling of Goat Milk," Apple Haven Farm, West Stewartstown, NH, July 6, 2011

Crewe, J. R., MD, "The Milk Cure: Real Milk Cures Many Diseases", *Certified Milk Magazine*, January 1929. Weston A. Price Foundation. www.realmilk.com/milkcure.html,

Jonsson, Randolph, *"Homogenization: A Closer Look,"* Raw-Milk-Facts.com. http://www.raw-milk-facts.com/homogenization_T3.html)

Kung, Limin, Jr., Ph.D., "The Importance of Colostrum for Calves," Ruminant Nutriton & Microbiology Laboratory. http://ag.udel.edu/anfs/faculty/kung/articles/importance_of_colostrum_for_calv.htm

Granite State Dairy Promotion, "NH Dairy Timeline." www.nhdairypromo.org/indexTimeline.htm

Mercola, Dr. Joseph, "The Cancer Time Bomb Sitting in Your Refrigerator – Will You Stop Consuming It?" October 23, 2011. http://articles.mercola.com/sites/articles/archive/2011/10/23/rbgh-in-milk-increases-risk-of-breast-cancer-aspx?e_cid=20111023_SNL_Art_1

Mercola, Dr. Joseph, "The Witch-Hunt That's Taking It to One of America's Healthiest Food Choices," December 31, 2010. http://articles.mercola.com/sites/articles/archive/2010/12/31/us-government-sneakily-subsidizes-milk-industry.aspx

Smith, Jeffrey M., "10 Reasons to Avoid GMO's," Institute for Responsible Technology, August 25, 2011. www.responsibletechnology.org/blog/1619

State of California and A.G.Kawamura, Secretary of California Department of Food and Agriculture vs. Organic Pastures Dairy Company, LLC and Claravale Farm, Inc., Reporter's Transcript of the Proceedings, April 25, 2008. http://www.realmilk.com/documents/expert-testimony-0508.pdf

Woodford, Keith, "The Devil in the Milk: A1 or A2? How Beta Caseins Are Changing the Dairy Industry," 60:65, Acres USA, December 2009, Vol. 39, No. 12. http://www.acresusa.com/toolbox/reprints/Dec09_Woodford.pdf

Wysong, Dr. Randy L, "Immunoglobulins," Wysong 100 Pet Truths Newsletter. www.Wysong.net

Wysong, Dr. Randy L., *"The Cholesterol Myth: Believe It to Your Peril,"* Inquiry Press, 2010

Milk Substitutes Sources:

Cohen, Robert, "Stomach Aches Caused by Carrageenan." www.notmilk.com

Infant Formula Sources:

Vallaeys, Charlotte, "Replacing Mother – Imitating Human Breast Milk in the Laboratory", January 5, 2008, updated April 15, 2011. www.cornucopia.org/2008/01/replacing-mother-infant-formula-report/

What Else May Be Hiding in Milk Products? Sources:

Federal Register, "Flavored Milk; Petition to Amend the Standard of Identity for Milk and 17 Additional Dairy Products," February 20, 2013. https://www.federalregister.gov/articles/2013/02/20/2013-03835/flavored-milk-petition-to-amend-the-standard-of-identity-for-milk-and-17-additional-dairy-products

Regulations.gov, Docket FDA-2009-P-0147, Amend the Standard of Identity for Milk, 21 C.F.R. 131.110, to Include Optional Characterizing Flavoring Ingredients With any Safe and Suitable Sweetener." http://www.regulations.gov/#!searchResults;rpp=25;po=0;s=Docket%252BNo.%252BFDA-2009-P-0147;fp=true;ns=true

Chlorination Sources:

Aquasana, "What is MTBE?" http://view.s4.exacttarget.com/?j=fe961771776c007f70&m=fea11570746 5067a77&ls=fdfd17717063077b75137077&l=fec015787d630779&s=fe571 1767763037a7314&jb=ffcf14&ju=fe5310767c640d7b7613&r=0

Conacher, Duff and Associates, *"Troubled Waters on Tap: Organic Chemicals in the Public Drinking Water Systems and the Failure of Regulation*, Center for Study of Responsive Law. January 1988, v, 114 p.; 28cm

Fluoride Sources:

Centers for Disease Control and Prevention, Emergency Preparedness and Response, "Facts About Hydrogen Fluoride (Hydrofluoric Acid)." http://www.bt.cdc.gov/agent/hydrofluoricacid/basics/facts.asp)

Centers for Disease Control and Prevention, "My Water's Fluoride." http://apps.nccd.cdc.gov/MWF/Index.asp.

Centers for Disease Control and Prevention, "Background: Infant Formula and the Risk for Enamel Fluorosis," May 28, 2010. http://www.cdc.gov/fluoridation/safety/infant_formula.htm#top#top

Centers for Disease Control and Prevention, "Overview: Infant Formula and Fluorosis, January 7, 2011. http://www.cdc.gov/fluoridation/safety/infant_formula.htm#top#top

Centers for Disease Control and Prevention, Morbidity and Mortality Weekly Report, "Engineering and Administrative Recommendations for Water Fluoridation", September 29, 1995. Vol. 44, No. RR-13. http://apps.nccd.cdc.gov/MWF/Index.asp

U.S. Department of Health & Human Services, "HHS and EPA Announce New Scientific Assessments and Actions on Fluoride", News Release, January 7, 2011. http://www.hhs.gov/news/press/2011pres/01/20110107a.html

U.S. Department of Labor, "Occupational Safety and Health Guidelines for Hydrogen Fluoride." http://www.osha.gov/SLTC/healthguidelines/hydrogenfluoride/recognition.html

U.S. Department of Labor, OSHA Regional News Release, "US Labor Department's OSHA Proposes $119,000 in Fines to Honeywell International in Metropolis, Ill., for Safety Violations Following Hydrogen Fluoride Vapor Release," June 22, 2011. http://www.osha.gov/llsl/loshaweb/owadisp.show_document?p_table=NEWS_RELEASES&p_id=20130

U.S. Department of Labor, "Silicon Tetrafluoride." http://www.osha.gov/dts/chemicalsampling/data/CH_267175

U.S. Environmental Protection Agency, "Hydrogen Fluoride," Technology Transfer Network Air Toxics Web Site, November 6, 2007. http://www.epa.gov/ttn/atw/hlthef/hydrogen.html

U.S. Environmental Protection Agency, Office of Water, "Questions and Answers on Fluoride", EPA 815-F-11-001, January 2011. http://water.epa.gov/lawsregs/rulesregs/regulatingcontaminants/sixyearreview/upload/2011_Fluoride_QuestionsAnswers.pdf

The National Academies, National Research Council, "Fluoride in Drinking Water: A Scientific Review of EPA's Standards", March 22, 2006. Http://www.nap.edu/webcast/webcast_detail.php?webcast_id=325

Cooper C., et al. "Water fluoride concentration and fracture of the proximal femur." Journal of Epidemiology and Community Health. 1990; 44:17-19.

Jacobsen, S. J. et al. "Regional Variation In The Incidence Of Hip Fracture: US White Women Aged 65 Years And Older. JAMA . 1990; 264:500-502.

Mercola, Dr. Joseph, "One of the Biggest Health Frauds EVER Perpetrated on the American People," May 11, 2010. http://articles.mercola.com/sites/articles/archive/2010/05/11/toxic-fluoride-contaminates-iceland-volcanic-ash-and-is-killing-animals.aspx

Pesticide Action Network North America (PANNA), "Sodium fluoride – Identification, Toxicity, Use, Water Pollution Potential, Ecological Toxicity and Regulatory Information." http://www.pesticideinfo.org/Detail_Chemical.jsp?Rec_ID=PC34385

Riggs, B.L., et al. "Effect of Fluoride on the Fracture Rate in Postmenopausal Women with Osteoporosis," New England Journal of Medicine. 1990; 322:802-809

The Fluoride Action Network, "Why You Need to Avoid These 'Healthy' Fruits and Nuts," August 11, 2011. http://www.fluoridealert.org/

Air Fresheners Sources:

Centers for Disease Control and Prevention, "Benzothiazole in Asphalt Fume", National Institute for Occupational Safety and Health (NIOSH), Manual of Analytical Methods (NMAM), Issue 1: 15 January 2998. www.cdc.gov/niosh/docs/2003-154/pdfs/2550.pdf

National Toxicology Program, Department of Health and Human Services, CAS Registry Number: 140-11-4 Toxicity Effects. http://ntp.niehs.nih.gov/index.cfm?objectid=E87DA8C3-BDB5-82F8-F685ED7A7F920F9C

Pontillo, Patrick, Chemical Sensitivity in Mainstream Medical Documentation, "The 80+ Chemical Ingredients in Febreze", July 26, 2011. http://www.chemicalsensitization.com/2011/07/80-chemical-ingredients-in-febreze.html

Mercury Source:

US EPA, "Mercury in Dental Amalgam." http://www.epa.gov/mercury/dentalamalgam.html

Aluminum Sources:

General Chemical USA, "Aluminum Sulfate (Alum)." www.generalchemical.com

Pepi, Dr. Anita, "Aluminum Poisoning." www.drpepi.com/aluminum-poisoning.php

Chapter 4
Diet & Exercise

"Let thy food be thy medicine and thy medicine be thy food." Hippocrates

DIET

While I had eliminated toxic products and foods, I still had LS and wondered if altering my diet, as my doctor had suggested, would eliminate my LS.

But some LS sufferers had eliminated gluten and dairy from their lives, and while they reported that these changes seemed to help control their symptoms, it didn't cure their LS.

I decided to look into some of the popular diets, such as the Paleo Diet, and obscure diets based upon personality or blood type. I purchased a book, *Eat Right For Your Type*, by Dr. Peter J. D'Adamo, which lists foods to eat and the ones to avoid based upon blood type.

For my blood type, I was disappointed that many of my favorite foods, such as melons, cabbage, nuts, plus all meats and poultry were things I should avoid. In essence, for my blood type, I should become vegetarian. This was not a pleasant prospect for me as I enjoy all food groups.

The one thing I found in common with all of these "diets" is that they are based upon elimination. It just didn't seem logical to me, especially since I love and have been consuming nuts and melons for my entire life and hadn't suffered ill effects. Thus I put aside the idea that a diet of denial might help me, and instead concentrated on how my diet, even if it was organic, might still contain elements contributing to my LS.

What I learned about some of the foods I was still eating made me alter my diet again, but not in the way you might think.

By diet I'm not talking about losing weight, diet food, or diet plans, although I will discuss them briefly. There are definite allergens within many food groups and some people are allergic to an entire food group, while others to a food type within a food group. And still others may have no known allergic reactions to any food groups or food types. This discourse assumes that the reader has minimal or no food allergies.

Many people today have food allergies, thanks to environmental toxins, genetically modified food, leaky guts from prescribed and over-the-counter pharmaceuticals, all combined with genetic makeup.

I have a lifelong deadly allergy to scallops, although I have no problem eating shellfish and any other type of seafood. Doctors find this specific allergic reaction unusual as it does not include the entire shellfish food group. But even though I must avoid scallops, it doesn't mean I've eliminated *all* seafood, and this is the premise of this section, which focuses on diet.

People assume when we use the word *diet*, it means they must eliminate things such as gluten, dairy products, meat, carbohydrates, and so on. But when humans appeared on the scene, "no" was not part of our vocabulary. We ate whatever nature presented for us to thrive and evolve. We probably didn't have food allergies then, either. We are omnivores and our digestive systems evolved to allow us to eat an enormous variety of foods.

Know that when I use the word *diet*, I'm strictly talking about food *types*: the *types* we need to consume, and the *types* that we need to avoid. The bottom line for me is that the *type* of food we need in order to be healthy *must be* organic, whole, and raw as much as possible. The *types* of food we *need to eliminate* are processed foods, genetically modified foods, and foods that are not organic.

People find it difficult to stay on typical diets of denial and elimination because they are depriving themselves of the food groups their human body needs. The diet I refer to is not one of denial or elimination and nothing is left out—it includes everything. The only stipulation is that it *must* be 100% organic, right down to the salt and pepper, and it must be as raw, as whole, and as close to the way nature made it as possible.

Food is medicine. Ancient civilizations have always used food that way. Healthy food, that is. Look at nature. Give plants soil rich in nutrients and they are healthy and thrive, able to fend off disease and enemies. But give them poor soil and they'll do poorly until they eventually fail. Healthy food should not make people sick. That's not the way nature works.

Rather, it's the *types* of foods that are making us sick that we need to cut out, and by types I am *not* referring to grains, meats, dairy, or vegetables. Instead, I mean processed foods, foods with artificial ingredients, and foods that are genetically modified and drenched in chemical pesticides and herbicides. In fact, they can't even be called food. Real food, the type that nature has perfected over many millions of years, is what nourishes us. Fake food makes us sick.

When people ask me what I eat, I tell them I am on a "see food diet." I see food, I eat it. I have not eliminated any food groups whatsoever. What I have eliminated are foods that are not organic and those that are highly processed, organic or not.

That doesn't mean I won't eat a slice of my own homemade organic bread or a small portion of my homemade organic ice cream. But I don't eat large portions and I don't eat them every day. To paraphrase Paracelsus, the poison is in the dose.

One food staple in our home has been a homemade mixture of organic brown rice and organic wild rice. Wild rice is not rice at all, but instead is a grass seed. I do not eliminate this food item from my diet because carbohydrates are important for proper brain and nervous system function. However, we favor baked potato (sweet or regular) or other legumes, and have the rice mixture occasionally.

Instead of junk/processed food (and that includes organic junk/processed food), I eat as much raw and whole foods as possible. My snack foods include a glass of whole raw milk, a handful of raw nuts, or raw seeds, such as pepita or sunflower, which are very filling. I'll turn to organic jumbo flame raisins from Braga Farms to squelch a craving for something sweet, or a teaspoon of organic raw honey. If I'm really desperate for a decadent treat, a couple of organic bittersweet wafers or an organic peanut butter cup from Mama Ganache Artisan Chocolates will do the trick. I do not deny myself anything, not even a bit of processed sugar now and then, the key phrase being now and then. But it must be organic.

Processed potato chips, candy bars, ice cream, cookies, crackers, or other commercial snack products do not enter my home, even if they are "organic." Fresh organic popcorn popped on the stovetop in a stainless steel popper with a little Himalayan pink salt and organic virgin coconut oil is a favorite whole food snack for us.

In an effort to rid themselves of Lichen Sclerosis, and other auto-immune symptoms, some people have gone the elimination route of avoiding gluten or dairy products, have switched to a vegetarian regimen, or eat according to blood type. But to me, this is worrisome. In Chapter 8, Preliminary Testing, I discuss cholesterol levels and inflammation. It is the small triglycerides from processed foods that are a major cause of inflammation in our body. So reducing or eliminating processed foods will reduce inflammation because most processed foods start out as flour (enriched or whole grain), which results in small triglycerides (fats) that are the main culprits in causing inflammation.

It may not be that gluten in and of itself is the culprit, but the fact that modern grains, as opposed to ancient grains, have been hybridized and that may be the main contributor to wheat allergies. This means that avoiding gluten or any other food group simply because they've received a bad rap is missing the point. Unless someone has real allergies to gluten, dairy, or meat, eliminating these foods may cause even more harm than good in the long run.

Meats (and by that I mean beef, lamb, pork, poultry, and fish), dairy, eggs have all received bad press, just as fats have. By badmouthing entire groups of foods, people forget about differentiating between the *types*.

Processed dairy foods are deadly for no other reason than the fact that they are processed, which includes just about every dairy product in the grocery aisles. They are not whole foods because processing foods destroy nutrients, turning them into toxins that work against us. Unless it is *raw*, then it is processed, and therefore has had all of the nutritional value removed. Typically, these processed dairy products are also made from A1 protein type milk, which is an allergen in and of itself. That is another reason that these types of processed dairy products are bad for us. On the other hand, raw dairy products made using A2 protein type milk, such as raw cheese or raw milk and yogurt, have all of the nutrition the human body requires still intact; these nutrients include probiotics, antibodies, and whole vitamins. This means that eliminating *all* dairy products does the body a great disservice.

By eliminating all fats, people have also eliminated essential fatty acids, which are crucial for reducing inflammation, and preventing disorders such as arthritis, cataracts, and macular degeneration. Our body is like any machine where all the parts have to be oiled or they will eventually dry out and seize.

Turning to a vegetarian diet in order to shed disease also can have disastrous results due to the lack of essential nutrients that only meat, poultry, and fish provide. As a result, inflammation in the form of arthritic and other auto-immune conditions can arise. I worry about this trend of elimination because other ailments may turn up at the same time but people fail to see the correlation.

Each food group presents its own unique set of vitamins, minerals, enzymes, fatty acids, and the like. By eliminating just one food group, people can become deficient in zinc, vitamin B12, and other essential nutrients that are not only key, but also act as co-factors for cellular metabolism, the structure of proteins and cell membranes, cell signaling, apoptosis (gene-directed cell death), the absorption of nutrients such as copper, iron, calcium, folic acid, and vitamin A. Zinc deficiency manifests as weakened immune system function, impaired wound healing, and visual disorders. Yes, you can take supplements, but unless they are whole food, they often are synthetic knockoffs and cannot compare to what nature provides in a whole, readily bio-available form.

We are omnivores who evolved by eating what nature provided in its purest form. We require specific nutrients that can only be derived from eating whole grains, dairy, meat, poultry, and fish. But the nutrients provided depend on the type of food that is eaten. Indigenous peoples catch, kill, and eat meat or fish, while developed societies factory farm it and may pollute it with growth hormones, antibiotics, and other chemicals.

For this reason, I believe a safe, healthy diet consists of organic food, especially meat from free range, pasture- (grass) and/or alfalfa-fed animals, with very little in the way of grain, and absolutely no corn silage. Animals raised and fed as they were evolved to eat will have very little fat and their meat will have a high nutritional value.

I don't use a lot of beef, lamb, or pork when I cook and we mostly eat poultry and fish. But a couple times a month we eat whole, unprocessed meats such as bison, lamb, and heirloom pork (meaning they're not in the form of burgers or hotdogs), perhaps a small steak (4 oz or less) or lamb, with chicken, turkey, or wild caught fish most of the time. The point is I haven't needed to eliminate any food *groups* from my diet to get well.

I recognize that some readers may be vegetarians. But if anyone has stopped eating certain food groups to get well because that particular food group has been vilified, this is unnecessary and quite possibly harmful as it may mean starving the body of extremely important nutrients and quite possibly could allow disease to continue to manifest. For this reason, I do not recommend that a food group be eliminated based upon current popularity. While traveling on the road to health a varied diet will be beneficial.

Some people who have issues with being overweight may have developed the problem from eating empty, nutrition-depleted calories, chemical additives, and pesticides found in processed and non-organic foods. These unhealthy foods affect the way the body creates and stores fat. To lose weight, some people try food combining diets that deprive them of certain foods on specific days or require combinations of specific foods. This makes no sense to me because our body isn't going to negate a specific food's nutrients because we didn't eat it on the right day or with the right combination of other foods.

I found most prepackaged diet food plans unacceptable because the food is processed, prepackaged, not organic, and most likely include GMO ingredients. Homemade diet food recipes call for "high quality ingredients" using boxed cake mixes. It's not possible for boxed cake mixes to be "high quality" for the same reasons discussed above, and even worse is the spray oil often used in these cases.

It is very important to examine what's in our food if we want to eat a healthy, nutritious diet and it means eliminating packaged foods. In the past, I used packaged products, including boxed cake mixes, but when I was trying to restore my health, I began looking at the ingredients list on one of my former favorite mixes. It contains not only sugars in many forms (probably from GMO sources), but also enriched and bleached flours, an anti-caking agent, hydrogenated oils that include lots of trans fats, emulsifiers, texturizers, synthetic vitamins, artificial flavors, and a pinch of heavy metals in the form of aluminum. How can these ingredients be considered high quality? I've also never used a food release pan spray that is often recommended in baking because of the ingredients. Here's what one of the most popular non-stick pan sprays contains:

- **Canola Oil** –Actually, canola oil is made from rapeseed, and unless it is organic rapeseed, most of this oil is derived from genetically modified, Roundup-Ready® rapeseed engineered to contain lower erucic acid (omega-9 fatty acid). Genetically modified rapeseed was developed in Canada and the name "canola" is derived from **CAN**adian **O**il, **L**ow **A**cid. High levels of erucic acid are considered a contributor to heart disease, but only if it was consumed by the gallons. The sole purpose of creating canola oil was to produce a cheap cooking/frying oil that could be used in nearly every food product on supermarket shelves and in fast food chains. But it had to be modified so people wouldn't consume too much Omega-9 fatty acid in proportion to their consumption of Omega-3 and Omega-6 fatty acids. Naturally occurring erucic acid is found in kale, broccoli, and Brussels sprouts and combined with Omega-3 oil's oleic acid, is crucial in protecting the myelin (insulation) around our brain's nerves.

- **Grain Alcohol** – This is another name for ethanol, a corn derivative that's most likely genetically engineered and pesticide/herbicide ready, and which is widely known as an additive to gasoline.

- **Lecithin** – Used as an emulsifier; if it's not organic, it's made with genetically modified soybean oil, which animal studies show to cause birth defects and fetal death.

- **Isobutane** – Used as a propellant, it is also known as methylpropane, which is most widely used as a refrigerant in freezers and air conditioning. It is a petrochemical derivative and an isomer of butane.

- **Propane** – Used as a propellant, it is a liquefied petroleum gas and a byproduct of gasoline processing and petroleum refining.

Cooking spray cans include warning labels that the contents are extremely flammable and that inhaling the fumes can be extremely harmful, if not fatal. There's no way I'd want to spray a pan with it and then cook in it. But my husband uses it to grease the augers of our snowblower.

Rather than using dangerous canned cooking sprays, I now use only organic, non-GMO oils that are free of pesticides and other processing contaminants such as hexane, as was discussed in Chapter 3.

In addition to never using cooking sprays, I also have never liked or used coated, non-stick pans. For starters, they are made of aluminum, which is highly reactive, especially for cooking acidic foods. In 1985, after my mother died of Alzheimer's disease, my husband insisted that we get rid of all of our aluminum pots, pans, and other aluminum cookware and utensils in favor of stainless steel because he'd heard of studies showing high concentrations of aluminum in the brains of Alzheimer victims. If you look at your recommended daily vitamin and mineral requirements, aluminum is not one of them, but manufacturers include aluminum in many products, including baking powder and deodorant.

In addition to aluminum, non-stick pots, pans, and utensils are coated with polytetrafluoroethylene (PTFE), the technical name for the synthetic otherwise known as DuPont's trademarked brand, Teflon™. Teflon™ is a member of the perfluorinated chemical (PFC) group. According to the U.S. Environmental Protection Agency PFC's pose "persistence, bioaccumulation, and toxicity properties to an extraordinary degree." PFC's are also found in stain and grease repellants in food wraps, carpeting, furniture, and clothing (stain guard).

In 2003, the Environmental Working Group commissioned tests that showed that in just 2-5 minutes on a conventional stove-top, the non-stick coating began to break apart and emit toxic particles and gases. In addition, flu-like symptoms of headache and fever, also referred to as "Teflon™ flu," results from breathing in the fumes of those emissions. Long-term effects of routine exposure to Teflon™ have not been adequately tested.

Getting back to the topic of the chapter, which is diet, I believe that commercial liquid diets are the worst choice of all to lose weight because they contain no natural fiber, no whole foods, and no whole micronutrients that the body requires to be healthy and to function optimally. Instead, commercial liquid diets are made up of chemicals and synthetic vitamins, with "fiber" that quite often consists of cellulose, which we cannot digest or use. You might as well consume a scouring pad for all the nutritional value your body will derive from a commercial liquid diet to lose weight. (This does not mean that people who have had gastric surgery of any kind should avoid a liquid diet; it means I do not recommend conventional liquid diets merely to lose weight).

For anyone who wants a shake or other form of liquid meal, it would be much better to put organic raw milk, raw egg yolk, banana, fresh blueberries, sweet black cherries, and vanilla extract into a blender and drink the shake. This would be real fiber, protein, natural whole sugar, and a multitude of micro-nutrients, and doesn't take much time to make.

But like with any dietary option, you must decide what works for you.

RAW FOOD

We are the only species that cooks our food. Raw food is full of complete vitamins, minerals, amino acids, enzymes, and essential fatty acids that will be destroyed by cooking, or else significantly reduced. Also, subjecting foods to high temperatures can turn their vital nutritional elements into toxins, especially when grilling or broiling.

While I'll probably never eat truly raw meat, I try to make it as rare as possible. Baking at low temperature or steaming meats and fish have become my standard cooking methods. But I eat most of my vegetables and all of my fruits raw. Sulfur-rich vegetables, especially raw, boost the body's immune master molecule, glutathione, which enables the antioxidant properties of micronutrients to become bio-available. Without high levels of glutathione, vitamins and minerals would go unused. When we have low levels of glutathione, we become disease-prone and people with chronic illnesses, including auto-immune disorders, tend to be deficient in glutathione.

Cruciferous vegetables such as broccoli have high sulfur content and are rich in glutathione. Examples of glutathione-boosting vegetables include:

- Garlic
- Onions
- Broccoli
- Kale
- Collard greens
- Cabbage
- Cauliflower
- Watercress
- Brussels Sprouts
- Kohlrabi
- Mustard
- Rutabaga
- Turnip
- Bok Choy
- Chinese Cabbage
- Horse Radish
- Radish
- Wasabi

But as good for us as these vegetables are, we shouldn't overdo them because too many cruciferous vegetables can result in hypothyroidism if there is insufficient iodine in one's diet. Unfortunately, today's modern diet of non-organic, processed and genetically modified foods is insufficient in natural iodine and selenium, which is vital for T4 and T3 conversion. This is just one more reason why eating a balanced diet of whole organic raw foods is advisable.

Juicing is a popular way to consume raw vegetables and fruits, and this makes a sweet potato easier to eat raw than biting into an uncooked one. Although I have not turned to juicing, I like to blend some raw foods into a delicious smoothie or shake, and my favorite morning "fruit shake" concoction consists of entirely raw protein and raw fruit. I recommend this **only** if you know exactly where the ingredients come from, and all **must be organic.** The ingredients include:

1	Ripe	Banana peeled
1	Cup	Blueberries (fresh or frozen)
15	Cherries	Bing/Sweet (fresh or frozen)
½	Cup	Raw whole goat or raw cow milk
1	Egg	Raw yolk only
½	teaspoon	Vanilla Extract

Combine in blender and blend until everything is reduced to a thick mixture. Pour into a glass and drink.

By now it should be clear why I specify using only organic ingredients. The other point is that it is imperative for the raw milk (from goats or Jersey cows) and raw eggs to come from independent local farms. The eggs **must** come from chickens that are healthy, truly free-range and are able to forage for the majority of their food. These chickens must be organically raised and free of vaccines and routine antibiotics. Healthy chickens will *not* produce salmonella-contaminated eggs. If the only eggs available to you are sold in supermarkets, even though they may be labeled as organic or free-range I would not recommend eating them raw. The raw milk **must** come from cows that are organically raised, pastured and grass fed, non-GMO hay (alfalfa) fed, not fed corn silage or GMO corn that will produce E.coli in their intestines, and which are not given rBGH or rBST that will cause mastitis and add pus into their milk.

If obtaining raw milk is unavailable (selling raw milk is against the law in many states), you certainly may use organic pasteurized milk, but understand that all pasteurized milk is dead milk that has had the life cooked out of it. It also is devoid of the nutritional value of raw milk.

Our diet now includes as many raw foods as possible. I eat raw nuts, raw seeds, raw fruits and raw vegetables. My husband loves peanut butter, and we buy organic peanut butter that contains nothing but ground organic peanuts, without any sugar, preservatives, or additional oil. My organic daily salad has several staples: chopped celery, sliced red and green cabbages, grated carrot, diced red and green leaf lettuce, romaine, broccoli, spinach, sun-dried tomatoes, and organic flame raisins. When available, especially during summer months when they can be locally grown and fresh picked, I add bell peppers (red, yellow, orange), tomatoes, and sugar snap peas. When in season I add avocado. Recently I began sprouting organic seeds for our salads.

For dressing, I use a 50/50 mix of organic cold pressed extra virgin olive oil, organic pepper, Himalayan pink salt, maxi-flake nutritional yeast, a 50/50 mixture of organic spirulina/chlorella powder, and organic balsamic or organic unfiltered apple cider vinegar, mixed well.

- **Nutritional Yeast** is yellow, somewhat crunchy, has a mild cheese-like flavor, is very high in B12 and B-complex vitamins and is sold in health food stores and food co-ops, as well as on-line. I buy maxi-flake nutritional yeast in 5-pound batches.

- **Spirulina** is a whole superfood that is rich in nearly every vitamin and mineral the human body needs. Aside from my daily whole-food vitamins and minerals, I believe that spirulina in my nightly salad increases my daily intake of essential nutrients.

- **Broken Cell Wall Chlorella** is an algae that binds with heavy metals, especially mercury and aluminum, and aids the body in their removal. In addition to drinking detox tea to cleanse my liver and kidneys, taking molybdenum to detoxify my liver, and using healing soaks to remove toxins from my body, I take *broken cell wall* chlorella daily to naturally help my body to further eliminate toxins.

Spirulina and chlorella can be found on-line in pill form, but I prefer to use the individual powders and combine them myself, which allows me to add as much, or as little of each as I desire. Buying the powdered form is also less expensive. Note that the powder is lightweight and can become airborne when mixing. For this reason, I mix them outside.

I usually purchase organic nutritional yeast, spirulina, and chlorella in bulk and store in air-tight, food-safe containers. Health food stores and food co-ops purchase bulk foods in these containers, and discard them when they are empty. If there is a health food store or co-op near you, if you ask, most likely they will give them to you at no cost. Some may not. (See the appendices for where to purchase food safe containers.)

COOKING OILS

Although too much oil can be a problem, especially for those trying to lose or maintain their weight, we need fats in our diet, especially essential fatty acids, the Omega- 3, 6, and 9 fats contained in natural oils such as olive, flaxseed, and fish oils. These fats act as a natural anti-inflammatory and also aid in brain and immune function. In order for the body to convert and maximize beta-carotene into Vitamin A, essential fatty acids are required, and a deficiency in essential fatty acids can lead to cancer, cataracts, and macular degeneration.

However, these essential fatty acids are very fragile, and when exposed to even low heat, their nutritive value is destroyed and they become rancid, which changes them so they'll actually work against us. Olive oil has a shelf life of only 6 months maximum and it must be kept in a cool, dark, air-tight environment. Cold pressed flax seed oil must be kept refrigerated.

Cooking with Virgin Coconut Oil

So what's a cook supposed to do? What oil can we use that has a decent shelf life, won't become toxic when exposed to high heat, and one that isn't GMO? The answer is organic virgin coconut oil. When I first purchased organic virgin coconut oil, I was shocked that it was solid, not liquid. I was also delighted, as I'd pondered over what to use to replace the solid hydrolyzed and most likely GMO vegetable oil I'd formerly used. Ever since, I've used Nutiva organic virgin coconut oil for just about everything. It's a healthy way to create your own non-stick cookware. Whenever I bake, whether using a stainless steel or glass pan, I coat the surface with organic virgin coconut oil. I also use the oil to brown meats, and to pop popcorn. I enjoy spreading coconut oil, instead of butter, on breads. An added benefit is that any residual coconut oil left on utensils is applied to my skin.

WHOLE BUTTER vs MARGARINE

Whole butter is just that...whole. It's made from raw milk/cream, a bit of salt, and churned until it solidifies and has just those two ingredients, unless it's salt-free, and then it has only one.

On the other hand, margarine is a concoction of hydrolyzed oils, artificial color and flavor. Don't let the term *natural* or even *organic* fool you. Some margarine manufacturers tout that their oils are expeller pressed. Don't be fooled by this, either. An expeller may be used to derive the oils, but oils are liquid and for them to become a thick spread, they have to be hydrogenated. Margarine is a highly processed laboratory concoction containing as many as eleven ingredients, which shows it's not a whole food, unlike butter. Margarine is imitation food and nothing more. Maybe you can't tell it's not real butter, but your body can.

I'll be honest and tell you that for a while, I gave up butter in favor of an organic margarine. The ingredients were organic expeller-pressed palm, soybean, canola and olive oils, filtered water, salt, natural flavor (derived from corn), soybeans, soy lecithin, lactic acid, and colored with annatto extract. I'm embarrassed to admit it, but that was before I learned about the dangers of chemicals in food. Now I look at that ingredients list and wonder what I was thinking!

Let's take a closer look at that "buttery spread," and see what it contains:

- **Trans Fats** – Even though the fake butters are purported to have zero trans fats in them, that fact is based only on the serving size. If there's less than 0.5% per serving, the manufacturer can legally claim 0% trans fats on the label. But during hydrogenation, which turns liquid vegetable oils into spreadable solids, trans fats are made. This means that no margarine, or any other hydrogenated product, is really trans-fat free; it's just a technicality because of the amount included. Man-made trans fats contribute to heart disease, cancer, osteoporosis, hormonal imbalance, skin disease, infertility, reproductive disorders, low birth weight, and growth and learning disabilities in children.

- **Free Radicals** – All biochemicals are bound in some way, either by electrons, proteins, or some other conducting element. Free radicals are electron-starved elements that search the body, looking for electrons to steal. Once they've robbed these electrons, the result is free radicals that damage whatever they come into contact with; they are health-robbing free agents that are considered carcinogenic and contribute to heart disease. In our diet, free radicals are found when most oils are heated during cooking as well as from high heat industrial processing.

- **Synthetic Vitamins** – They are incomplete, artificial, and man-made.

- **Emulsifiers** – Soy lecithin (which can be GMO if it's not organic) is synthetic, not natural; it gives hydrogenated oils their "creamy" texture.

- **Preservatives** – Most imitation-butter vegetable spreads contain preservatives such as BHT (butylated hydroxytoluene) and others.

- **Solvents** – Non-organic spreads can be contaminated with hexane or other solvents used during the oil extraction process.

- **Bleach** – Oils that have been hydrogenated or partially-hydrogenated are naturally grey and are bleached white.

- **Annatto Color** – Color is added to make imitation butter spreads appetizing after hydrogenation and bleaching. The coloring is extracted using solvents and derived from the Achiote tree. Annatto is linked to food allergies.

- **Artificial Flavor** – Hydrogenated oils have a distinctly fake flavor compared to the real thing. Whether the label states that the flavor is artificial or claims to be "natural", it is still a fake butter taste.

- **Mono- and Di-glycerides** – These fats, from the oils used to make margarine, are high in trans-fats as a result of processing.

- **Soy Protein Isolate** – This is a highly processed powder that acts as a texturizer to give "body" or substance to the product. It has been linked to thyroid dysfunction, digestive disorders, among other health issues.

- **Sterols** – These are estrogen compounds added to spreads to give them cholesterol-lowering qualities. These compounds can impair normal endocrine function.

Butter has been a staple of civilization since man milked his first mammal and churned it into butter. There is no valid reason to create a substitute for it. What does butter have that margarine doesn't?

- **Fat Soluble-Vitamins** – Butter, especially when it is raw, includes iodine, lecithin, selenium, vitamins A, D, K2, E, and many other co-factoring nutrients that protect against heart disease, maintain good vision and endocrine system function.

- **The "Wulzen" Factor** – Researcher Rosalind Wulzen discovered a compound in raw animal fat, along with Vitamin K2, that protects against calcification in joints (arthritis) and the pineal gland, as well as against cataracts and hardening of the arteries. It is also referred to as the "anti-stiffness" factor.

- **Conjugated Linoleic Acid (CLA)** – A compound that contains strong anti-tumor properties and encourages muscle building rather than fat storage.

- **Fatty Acids** – These compounds support immune function, boost metabolism, and have anti-microbial properties that help control pathogenic micro-organisms in the intestinal tract.

- **Omega-3 and Omega-6 Essential Fatty Acids** Butter contains the perfect balance between Arachidonic Acid (ARA) and Docosahexaenoic Acid (DHA), both instrumental in maintaining brain function, skin health, and prostaglandin balance. Prostaglandins are instrumental for muscle contractions and relaxation, blood vessel dilation and constriction, blood pressure control, and controlling inflammation.

- **Saturated Fats** – Saturated fats are healthy fats that are saturated with hydrocarbons, making them a stable form of fat. They are found in plants and animals, are critical to lung function, and actually help protect against asthma.

- **Glycosphingolipids** – These are lipids found in butterfat that aid digestion by protecting against gastrointestinal infections, especially in the very young and very old. Children who drink pasteurized skim milk from A1 type cows will have diarrhea 3-5 times more often than children who drink whole milk from A2 type cows or goats.

- **Lecithin** – This whole form of lecithin is totally different from synthesized lecithin used as an emulsifier in foods. Raw, whole, complete lecithin found in raw butter aids in the assimilation and metabolizing of cholesterol and other fat molecules. It is a critical nutrient in every cell membrane, and is a key to maintaining neurological health.

- **Cholesterol** – Cholesterol derived from pastured, grass-fed animals is not the same as the artery-clogging cholesterol that comes from processed foods. Cholesterol from organic and raw sources is highly digestible. The natural *sterols* found in cholesterol are integral to the production of the natural steroids our bodies make, which help protect us against cancer, heart disease, and mental illness.

- **Trace minerals** – The body needs only minute amounts of trace minerals, but they are required for many biochemical processes that are critical for optimal health. They are found in butterfat globules and include manganese, zinc, chromium, copper, iodine, and selenium.

Unfortunately, in the U.S. raw butter is not allowed to be sold commercially. While there is no law against it, the fact that the USFDA has no guidelines regarding raw butter has been interpreted by food safety regulators that it can't be sold. Some producers of organic raw milk make raw butter for themselves and may be willing to share some with you if you ask.

I purchase raw organic cream from my local dairy farm and make my own butter. It is time consuming but knowing that it is a whole food is worth the effort.

If ready-made pasteurized butter is all that is available to you, I recommend avoiding the name brand industrial farm produced butters that line your grocer's shelves. Instead, at the very least look for organic brands wherever possible, but beware that some organic butters often include colorants. If your supermarket doesn't carry organic butter, try a health food store or food co-op. Organic butter produced from pastured cows or sheep is superior because the animals are not given antibiotics, synthetic growth hormones, or pesticides, and should include only sweet cream, salt, and microbial cultures. Organic butter is rich in conjugated linoleic acid (CLAs) and Omega-3 fatty acids. Once you try it, you will never want to use any other butter or margarine.

SPROUTED FLOUR

Cakes, cookies, and other sweets are rare to non-existent in our household now, but I still make my own hand-made breads (no bread machine) using only organic sprouted flours.

Why sprouted flour?

- Digestibility - Grains contain starches and sprouting makes those starches more digestible by breaking down a portion of the starches and converting them to simple sugars similar to those of vegetables.

- Enzyme Production - The process of sprouting produces digestive enzymes.

- Vitamins – Sprouted flour has increased Vitamins C, B-complex, especially B_2, B_5, and B_6, as well as a dramatic increase in carotene.

- Reduced Anti-nutrients – Whole grains contain enzyme inhibitors (anti-nutrients) and phytic acid, which is a substance that inhibits the absorption of calcium, magnesium, iron, copper, and zinc. Sprouting neutralizes phytic acid and enzyme inhibitors.

- Neutralized Aflatatoxins – These are carcinogens that are found in grains and sprouting neutralizes them.

While flours made from sprouted grains are healthier than regular grain flour, they still contain gluten. For those with gluten sensitivity, organic sprouted gluten-free flours are also available and include amaranth, black bean, buckwheat, oat, quinoa, lentil, and more. My favorite place for organic sprouted stone ground flours is To Your Health Sprouted Flour Company.

EXERCISE

Hippocrates said that *"Walking is man's best medicine."* And I agree. Aside from removing toxic foods and products from my life, and eating smaller but more frequent portions, the other healthy change in my life was losing weight. While I have always been physically active (I was running every other day when I was diagnosed with Lichen Sclerosis), I began hiking every day, except in the rain (I hate getting wet).

When I was diagnosed with Lichen Sclerosis in 2009, I weighed 169 pounds. I was overweight, but not obese. A year later, now free of the disease, I weighed 130. Two months after that I was down to 120 lbs. While I was happy that I could now fit into my skinniest jeans from when I was 25 years old, I looked gaunt and almost sickly. At 5' 4", my best weight is between 125-130 pounds, but I don't always maintain my best weight.

It took me a year to lose the weight and I did it without diet pills, diet food, or a formal diet plan. I didn't eliminate food groups and ate everything I usually ate; I just stopped eating non-organic food, processed food (even though it was organic), and cut down on the amount I ate using portion control. I started to keep track of everything I put into my mouth and was astonished to find out how many calories I'd been consuming. Once I started paying attention, instead of going back for seconds, I cut back to one reasonably sized serving that I measured and weighed. For each portion, I counted the calories, cholesterol, and fat content, and set 900 calories or less per day as my goal unless I was involved in very physical activity. I allowed myself no more than 200 grams of cholesterol and no more than 50 grams of fat per day.

To calculate my intake of calories, cholesterol, and fat, I used two readily available calorie/nutrient booklets. Because I make most of my food from scratch, I knew how much of each ingredient I was using and calculated the totals divided into portions. This meant I knew the counts for every meal I made. But my focus was more on making better, healthier choices in the foods I ate. The calories don't add up to much in a bowl of raw vegetables.

My doctor had suggested I eat more small meals in a day rather than a few large ones. She explained that by only eating 2-3 meals per day, my body was hanging onto fat because it didn't know when it would be fed again. She said that by eating smaller meals more often my metabolism would speed up, and it made sense to me.

I began eating all day long, approximately every two hours. Some of the meals would consist of ½ of a baked organic sweet potato (59 calories) or a handful of raw organic nuts. I'd limit myself to one poached organic egg, or make an organic fruit shake, or have some organic yogurt made from raw whole milk. I also ate slower and actually felt full. In addition, I started drinking more water, which is also important in losing weight as it helps flush out and eliminate fat we are losing and helps us to feel full.

While I no longer count calories, I still eat small portions, rarely eat sugary foods such as cake, pie, cookies, etc., I do not eat processed foods, and I am still very physically active and do a lot of walking/hiking. As a result, I am usually able to maintain my ideal weight, or close to it.

As discussed in earlier chapters, the skin is the body's largest organ of elimination. When we sweat, we are eliminating a much greater percentage of toxins than all of our other organs and systems combined. If we don't sweat enough, the burden of waste and elimination falls on our other organs of elimination (liver, kidneys, lymphatic system) and taxes them more than if we also sweat.

This is the reason that aside from diet, exercise is so important in losing weight and in our overall health. Next to healthy food and eliminating toxins from food, personal care products, etc., exercise is the major key to good health. Exercise increases the oxygen levels in our blood and sends it to our brain, and it strengthens the immune system by increasing the production of glutathione.

THE PEDOMETER

In addition to changing what and how I ate, and eliminating toxic products, I also began to exercise. To do this I didn't have to spend a ton of money by joining a gym or health club, and I didn't have to drive anywhere to do it. I just clipped on my pedometer, put on my walking shoes, and headed out the door.

In fact, the only thing I actually bought was a pedometer based on reviews and features I wanted that tracks distance, the length of time it took, the number of aerobic steps (I aim for 10,000 aerobic steps minimum but then I've been hiking for a couple of years), and the number of calories and grams of fat burned.

I live in a mountainous area with almost no flat roads, and I chose a route with the most hills to climb, and also the least traveled by motorized vehicles to avoid inhaling exhaust. When I started, at first I could barely make it halfway up one hilly part of the route. My legs would feel like wet noodles, my heart would be pounding, and I'd be gasping for breath. But as I continued to walk every day, I gradually got further and further up the hill, until one day I made it to the top without having to stop to catch my breath even once. Now it takes me just 1 hour and 20 minutes to walk the hilly 5 miles without having to stop to rest or catch my breath. I do this every day, regardless of the weather or temperature, unless it's raining. Like I said, I hate walking in the rain. But when I'm done, I am soaked anyway...with sweat.

I've noticed that when I start walking my sweat has a strong odor, which indicates that waste is being removed from my body. By the end of my hike, there's no odor because my body has purged itself. Someone told me that if you aren't overloaded with toxins, then you won't have stinky sweat. I'm not sure if this is true, but it seems to be in my case.

Walking doesn't cost anything, aside from a new pair of walking/hiking shoes every year. And because I don't have to do anything other than walk out my front door, I'm more inclined to keep at it. If I had to travel somewhere in order to exercise, I'd be less inclined to go.

If you want to exercise, whether to lose weight or just become healthier, start slowly and pick an easy goal, even if you only go around the block the first day. Build up your stamina gradually. Then, once you're used to walking, you may want to try a route that's more challenging and includes some hills. If you live near a beach, walking in sand is a great workout. Once you're comfortable exercising, go at a pace that will increase your heart rate. When you're healthy and strong, try to reach the point where you're breathing heavy and soaked with sweat by the time you are done. Also pick an area as far away from traffic as possible to avoid the toxic and heavy metal emissions from automobiles.

I used to take long hikes, sometimes as far as 13 miles. But then I found out that we derive as much benefit from more frequent exercise of a shorter duration, and now my daily routine is 5 miles. But keep in mind that it took nearly a year to work up to 5 hilly miles a day.

The key to sticking with an exercise program is to figure out when doing it works best for you. I'm a morning person and wake up full of energy. I get up early, feed the animals, drink 13 ounces of water, put on my hiking gear, and out the door I go for 1 ½ hours of time to myself and my thoughts. When I come home, I shower and am ready for the day. By late afternoon or dinnertime, I'm winding down and by then I'm not in the mood for any form of exercise. If I left exercising for later in the day I'd never stick to an exercise program.

My husband, on the other hand, is a night person who goes to bed very late and gets up late. It takes him a long time to get going, but by mid-afternoon, he's full of vim and vigor, just when my body starts to wind down. Sometimes I'll grudgingly take a hike with him (my second for the day), but most often he'll go by himself, and for him, exercising in the afternoon is the time that works best.

For other people, an evening workout is best. It's up to you to determine when to schedule your exercise program to fit with your optimal time of day, if that's possible. If you work and afternoons are best for you to exercise, see if you can take a late lunch hour and go then. If your work schedule doesn't make exercise possible at your optimal time of day, pick the next-best time for you.

Exercise will get you into great shape and take or keep the pounds off. Any exercise that increases your heart rate and causes you to sweat helps you detoxify. Getting oxygen into your bloodstream also will create a hostile environment for pathogens, making you healthier. So go for it—you have nothing to lose and you'll feel great.

ELECTROLYTES

Electrolytes are electrically charged minerals that help maintain a proper fluid balance needed for healthy biochemical interactions. When we sweat, we lose not only toxins, but also electrolytes. They are referred to as *electro*lytes because they are minerals that conduct an electrical charge. Electrolytes are micronutrient minerals that are essential for nerve impulses, muscle contractions, and physiological functions. There are many micronutrients lost during sweating, but the major ones are sodium, chloride, calcium, magnesium, and potassium. Water cannot replace these lost elements, and the average athlete can lose in excess of 4500 mg of salt per liter of sweat. Depending upon external conditions such as heat or temperature and athletic conditioning, an athlete may lose 2.2 liters of fluid per hour.

Low electrolyte symptoms include:

- Weakness
- Nausea
- Vomiting
- Muscle Cramping
- Dizziness/Fainting
- Confusion

When they have low electrolyte symptoms, people often turn to sports drinks, which typically have a lot of sugar, usually in the form of high fructose corn syrup, along with artificial flavors, colors, and synthetic mineral replacements. Some people believe that during strenuous exercise, the body will immediately burn up and eliminate the toxins from these drinks. I don't agree because I believe that just like any other food item, the artificial ingredients are not readily bio-available, meaning the body will not be able to utilize them easily or at all. First they must be metabolized, bound, and then eliminated, which takes time. Since exercise makes the body convert fat to energy quickly, it'll be too busy doing so to dispose of newly ingested toxins, which will not pass out of our body so readily.

My favorite all-natural electrolyte replacement, both during or after physical exercise, is organic watermelon with a pinch of Himalayan pink salt added. Himalayan pink salt is preferable because it contains over 80 trace minerals including calcium, copper, natural iodine, potassium, magnesium and more. White salt, including white sea salt, is processed sodium chloride and does not contain micronutrients, which is why it needs to be iodized to avoid developing goiter. After a workout, I sit down with a huge bowl (about 4 cups) of sliced watermelon. After eating it, not only am I cooled down, but I also feel completely refreshed. For very long and strenuous workouts, I'll slice up as much as 8 cups of watermelon (preferably seedless), toss it into the blender to liquefy it, add a pinch of salt, and take it along in a glass or BPA-free stainless steel container.

Another very good, hydrating source of electrolytes, if you can find it, is coconut water (not to be confused with coconut milk). You will most likely find it in a refrigerated section of a health food store. It comes from an immature green coconut. Other food items to bring along during a long, strenuous workout include organic grapes, organic granola bars made with raw honey, raisins, toasted oats, raw peanut butter, and raw nuts and/or seeds such as sunflower, sesame, flax or pumpkin (pepita). I make in advance batches of my own raw organic granola bars using the ingredients listed above, wrap them with untreated parchment or waxed paper and then freeze them in a food- and freezer-safe container. They can be eaten frozen, or allowed to thaw slightly before eating them.

With toxic products and foods out of my life, I believed I was on the road to recovery. But I wondered if there was some other connection to LS. What was I *missing*?

Sources:

Blaylock, Dr. Russell L., "The Case for a Link to Autism Spectrum Disorders," March 14, 2008.
http://articles.mercola.com/sites/articles/archive/2008/03/14/the-danger-of-excessive-vaccination-during-brain-development.aspx

Drake, Victoria J., Ph.D., "Zinc," Linus Pauling Institute, Micronutrient Information Center, Oregon State University, February 2008.
http://lpi.oregonstate.edu/infocenter/minerals/zinc/

Fallon, Sally and Enig, Mary G., Ph.D., "Why Butter is Better," The Weston A. Price Foundation, January 1, 2000.
www.westonaprice.org/food-features/why-butter-is-better)

Houlihan, Jane et al., "Canaries in the Kitchen: Teflon Toxicosis," Environmental Working Group Research, May 2003. http//www.ewg.org/reports/toxicteflon

Wikipedia, Polymer Fume Fever, accessed May 18, 2010. http//en.wikipedia.org/wiki/Polymer_fume_fever

Chapter 5
The Missing Link?

I felt like a walking toxic time bomb. It was obvious to me that the products I'd used daily, the food I'd ingested, had increasingly destroyed my body until it could no longer keep up the fight, and it showed in the gradual destruction of my skin. It horrified me to think that I had unwittingly contributed to the irreparable damage done to my body, and starting from each day forward, the best I could hope for was to make better educated choices. After all of my research of how toxins destroy the human body, it only made me feel more scared than ever, and hopeless.

It was the very end of November 2009 that I summoned the courage to speak to a friend about the exact nature of my diagnosis and describe my research, along with the steps I'd taken to eliminate all the things I thought had contributed to my disease.

She had been undiagnosed, misdiagnosed, and suffered from Lyme disease for years until she became disabled from the disease. In her search for a cure she stumbled upon a naturopath, Dr. David Jernigan, who had cured himself of Lyme disease, and had also resolved his daughter of West Nile Virus. His Lyme detoxification protocol was still new at the time, but through the use of only a handful of Dr. Jernigan's botanicals, my friend's Lyme disease was eliminated and she regained her health. One day she asked me: *"Do you think your disease could be Lyme related?"* She knew that my husband had taken antibiotics for Lyme in 1992 and that I had been tested for Lyme at the time as well, but that the test results were "inconclusive" for both Lyme disease and Lyme antibodies. There was nothing in my lab report to warrant treatment and I never exhibited symptoms of Lyme.

The Lyme infection occurs when a microscopic spirochete is transmitted to humans via insect bite, typically from a tick, but spiders and other biting insects also carry infectious spirochetes. The spirochete enters the body and infects every part of it by producing toxic bacteria. Couples exchange bodily fluids, so it made sense that I might have become infected with Lyme bacteria antibodies.

But the idea that Lyme disease had anything to do with my Lichen Sclerosis still seemed far-fetched to me, and I told my friend that I didn't think one had anything to do with the other. That's when she sent to me two dermatology reports.

The first described a chronic form of the Lyme infection called borreliosis that is in fact sometimes shared by Lichen Sclerosis patients, and the report further proposed that the spirochete that causes human Lyme may also be a factor in Lichen Sclerosis. The report stated that tissue samples from 61 cases of Lichen Sclerosis were tested for Lyme antibodies and 62% of them tested positive for Lyme antibodies. The report further stated that the Lyme Borrelia infection was far more significant in the early stages of Lichen Sclerosis than in the late phase. Of the 61 Lichen Sclerosis tissue samples, only 38% did *not* involve Lyme disease antibodies.

The second report, by Dr. Giusto Trevisan, professor and chairman of the Institute of Dermatology, University of Trieste, Italy, points out the proven skin manifestations of Lyme borreliosis, and describes Lichen Sclerosis and other skin disorders such as Scleroderma as further manifestations of Lyme borreliosis infection.

Still, there are Lichen Sclerosis sufferers all over the world, and not all have a connection to Lyme disease or even access to Lyme infectious ticks or other such insects, and not every Lichen Sclerosis tissue sample in the study showed a positive relation to Lyme. And what about very young children seemingly born with Lichen Sclerosis? Most haven't yet been exposed to tick-infested areas or bitten by other Lyme-infected insects, so what correlation to Lyme disease could they possibly have?

But what if there *is* a link between Lyme infection and Lichen Sclerosis? What if it *is* the missing link that causes these mysterious cases of LS? I felt that if there was even a remote chance that this could be the cause for my disease, it was worth investigating.

I purchased a copy of Dr. Jernigan's book, *Beating Lyme Disease*. I found the book full of valuable information, much of which confirmed that eliminating toxic products and foods from my life were steps in the right direction. Jernigan's book describes how the body interacts with its internal and external environment in both positive and negative ways, and I found his description of "The Perfect 7 Treatment and Detox Protocol™ to be very interesting, although it's an intense one that includes 14-day fasting, organ flushing, enemas, a regimen of botanicals, and numerous other therapies like infrared sauna. Although the Jernigan protocol sounded like it could work, I also knew one LS sufferer who had tried several rounds of intense detoxification but still had Lichen Sclerosis, and it made me hesitate.

Primum non nocer, Latin for First Do No Harm. Being a cautious person, I usually start slowly with most new things I try and watch for results before fully committing myself. In the case of the Jernigan protocol, I decided to err on the side of caution and try just the botanicals. If they didn't work, I could always try the more intense aspects of the protocol to see if they would relieve my LS. For instance, a more invasive aspect of the "Perfect 7 Treatment and Detox Protocol™" calls for a 14-day fast during which only one "superfood" drink is taken. When I investigated this "superfood" elixir, I was disturbed to find that it contained sodium benzoate as a preservative. The fact it contained a preservative at all was a disappointment, but that it was sodium benzoate, a known carcinogen linked to cancer, was even more distressing and a definite turn off. That's when I decided this protocol was not for me.

But the botanicals appealed to me. They are partially based upon Traditional Chinese Medicine and are not only Lyme specific, but also broad enough to target bacteria, viruses, plus chemical and heavy-metal toxicity. In other words, whether my Lichen Sclerosis was related to Lyme or simply a result of toxic overload, these botanicals would cover all the bases. Specific botanicals would help restore my body's ability to reduce and regulate microbial and environmental toxins on its own. The remaining botanicals help the body eliminate all types of heavy-metal and chemical toxins by binding with them and flushing them out.

While I was considering the botanicals, I began studying how supplements can help with overall detoxification and alleviate the toxicity caused by chemicals such as sodium lauryl sulfate and sodium laureth sulfate molecules.

By this point, I had come to realize that the symptoms of Lyme disease and the symptoms of toxic overload are identical, and that to our bodies, a toxin is a toxin in terms of how it deals with them. It doesn't matter if the toxins are originated by a spirochete, virus, bacteria, chemicals, or all of them combined. How our body reacts to them, and how they affect us physically is dictated by our genetic makeup and will lead those of us with a similar genetic makeup down the path to Lichen Sclerosis. For people with a different set of genetic markers, the toxic burden will manifest as any number of other auto-immune disorders, including Fibromyalgia, Lupus, Arthritis, and so forth.

To me, this meant that by eliminating toxic products and foods, along with taking supplements and botanicals, the healing process could begin.

Sources:

    Jernigan, David A., B.S., *"Beating Lyme Disease,"* Somerlyton Press, 2nd Edition, 2008

    Selim, Angelica, M.D, "Lichen Sclerosus and Borrelia burgdorferi: Are We Missing the Link?" Journal Watch Dermatology, July 11, 2008. http://sci.tech-archive.net:80/Archive/sci.med.diseases.lyme/2008-07/msg00052.html

    Trevisan, Giusto, M.D., "Atypical dermatological manifestations of Lyme borreliosis," Dermatovenerologica Alpina, Pannonica et Adreiatica (acta), Vol. 10, No. 4, 2001. http://ibmi.mf.uni-lj.si/acta-apa/acta-apa-01-4/trevisan.html

Chapter 6
Allopathic versus Alternative Medicine

"You can't medicate yourself out of a disease that you've behaved yourself into." Dr. Roby Mitchell

The population of the United States makes up only 5% of the total world population, but we use 70% of the world's total prescription drugs. Why are we the sickest nation on the planet? Is it because conventional, mainstream, or Western medicine is allopathic medicine?

The term *allopathic* was coined in the early 19th century by the founder of homeopathy, Dr. Samuel Hahnemann and is derived from the Greek: "állos" meaning other, or different. Allopathic medicine treats "other than the disease" because this form of medicine treats symptoms, rather than treating the body as a whole. Under allopathic medical treatment, we are given drugs to treat our symptoms; the symptoms sometimes go away and we have an illusion of health. But often, if we stop taking the medicine, the symptoms return because the root cause of the disease has not been addressed. Conventional medicine assumes that the human body is stupid and doesn't know what it is doing. It fails to understand and appreciate why the human body does what it does.

In treating symptoms, allopathic medicine disrupts the entire balance of the human body, resulting in side effects, both expected and unexpected. These side effects often require even more prescriptions to counter them. It is not uncommon for people to be on multiple prescriptions, in some cases 31 or more! Additionally, allopathic medicine tends to be made of synthesized chemicals, as opposed to alternative medicine, which is derived from nature. In fact, many medicines, even allopathic medicine, were originally plant based. For instance, aspirin was originally made from the bark of the white willow tree. Today it is instead synthesized by the pharmaceutical industry.

We in the United States (New Zealand is the only other country that allows direct consumer advertising by the pharmaceutical industry) are bombarded with drug commercials, always depicting people living fabulous lives in spite of their diseases. The ads show actors in pastoral settings. Meanwhile, a soothing voice-over runs down the litany of side effects, many of them far worse than the disease itself.

Pharmaceutical drugs are readily prescribed for even the most easily treatable problems. For example, several years ago, I injured my right index finger, which became swollen and when I bent it, I heard and felt a "snap." My doctor diagnosed tendonitis and handed me a sample bottle of Celebrex.

Suspicious of allopathic "medicine" even then, I went home and studied the ingredients, along with the side effects listed on the pamphlet. The "mild" side effects listed for Celebrex include constipation, diarrhea, dizziness, gas, headache, heartburn, nausea, sore throat, upset stomach, and stuffy nose.

But the "severe" side effects include rash, hives, itching, trouble breathing, tightness in chest, swelling of the mouth, face, lips, and/or tongue, bloody or black, tarry stools, change in urine production, chest pain, confusion, dark urine, depression, fainting, fast or irregular heartbeat, fever, chills, persistent sore throat, hearing loss, mental or mood changes, numbness of arm or leg, one-sided weakness, red, swollen, blistered, or peeling skin, ringing in the ears, seizures, severe headache or dizziness, severe or persistent stomach pain or nausea, severe vomiting, shortness of breath, sudden or unexplained weight gain, swelling of hands, legs, or feet, unusual bruising or bleeding, unusual joint or muscle pain, unusual tiredness or weakness, vision or speech changes, vomit that looks like coffee grounds, and yellowing of the skin or eyes. The statistical gastrointestinal side effects of Celebrex include nausea (up to 9%), upper abdominal pain (7.32% to 10.4%), dyspepsia (2.8% to 8.8%), abdominal pain (1.3% to 8.5%), vomiting (± 7.3%), diarrhea (4.9% to 10.5%), acid reflux (4.7%), and flatulence (2.2%).

In less than 2% of patients taking Celebrex, the following side effects occurred: constipation, diverticulitis, dry mouth, dysphagia, eructation, esophagitis gastritis, gastroenteritis hemorrhoids, hiatal hernia, melena, stomatitis, tenesmus, tooth disorder, intestinal obstruction, intestinal perforation, gastrointestinal bleeding, colitis with bleeding, esophageal perforation, pancreatitis, cholelithiasis, and ileus. Rare but also reported side effects include serious gastrointestinal disorders including toxicity, hemorrhage and intestinal anastomotic ulceration.

And then there's the ultimate side effect: Death. Five of 10 reported deaths for people taking Celebrex were attributed to pre-conditions, such as stomach, gastrointestinal or bleeding ulcers, interaction with other drugs, kidney disease, and heart attack. But one has to ask, "Would those people still have died then had they not taken Celebrex?"

After considering these possible side-effects and negative outcomes, I decided that no matter how weird my finger seemed, I didn't want or need any of those side effects. It was overkill for my swollen, snappy finger. Besides, hot, steamy shower water soothed my finger and temporarily stopped the snapping when I bent it. So, rather than take my chances with Celebrex, I treated my finger three times a day by wrapping my finger with a cloth soaked in hot water and then allowed to cool enough so I could stand the heat. Soon my finger returned to normal, and the only side effects I suffered was the extra time and effort my "treatment" took.

As consumers and patients, we are suckered by carefully crafted TV commercials to tune out the side effects. We assume that they can't possibly happen to us, and that we won't have that "rare" adverse reaction. Besides, the U.S. Food and Drug Administration wouldn't have approved a drug if it were that lethal, would they? Our doctor wouldn't prescribe them for us if they were that harmful, would he/she? The commercials reassure us that a magic cure comes in a bottle, and that when you go to your doctor, you expect him/her to dispense that magic in the form of a prescription. How many times have you heard the phrase, "Ask your doctor about...."? Yes, *ask* your doctor about poison in a bottle.

OVER-THE-COUNTER AND PRESCRIPTION DRUGS

"Pharmaceutical drugs are largely allopathic in nature, meaning that they are aimed at addressing and counteracting the symptoms of the illness and disease, but not the underlying cause(s). They attempt to force the body into submission but by so doing create their own stresses, imbalances, and diseases. Pharmaceuticals are a last resort if health is the goal."

Dr. Randy Wysong

Prescription and over-the-counter drugs seem so harmless, but do we know what is in them? Do we understand what all of the ingredients actually do? Do we have any idea what body function they are preventing? Do we ever read the pamphlets that come with medications? Do we heed the warnings?

If you, the reader, are like just about everyone else, you've answered "no" to all or most of the questions above. We should not rely on those "soothing" commercials, or the belief that the FDA wouldn't approve a dangerous drug, or our doctor wouldn't offer us anything that could potentially harm us.

If we take these seemingly harmless prescription and over-the-counter medications frequently, what are they masking, and how are they harming us? And how do they interact with other prescribed or OTC meds? When we take prescription medications, often we are blocking and masking symptoms, along with the warnings our bodies are trying to send us.

What many of these drugs have in common is that they are neuro-transmitter blocking agents. This means that they block the signals from our brain that tell us something is wrong.

Many of the drugs we take to stop symptoms of pain, stomach upset, or other day-to-day problems contain anti-cholinergic properties, meaning they "inhibit activity of the neurotransmitter acetylcholine," which plays a critical role in memory and cognitive function. Continued use of these medications can create mild cognitive impairment, and may even create or aggravate Alzheimer-like symptoms, especially in older people. Additionally, they can cause nervousness, confusion, disorientation, hallucinations, restlessness, irritability, dizziness, drowsiness, blurred vision, and light sensitivity.

Swallowed or injected, these anti-cholinergic drugs can have systemic effects. Dr. Leo Galland's partial list of over-the-counter and prescription drugs containing anti-cholinergic properties includes antihistamines, acid blockers, and antidepressants. The list of common drugs containing anti-cholinergic properties is very long, and includes, but is not limited to:

Antispasmotics: These are taken for stomach cramps or bladder problems and can be found in prescription medications as well as over-the-counter cold and cough remedies. A partial list of products includes:

- Atropine – A prescription drug for stomach cramps, vomiting

- Detrol (Tolterodine)

- VesiCARE (Solifenacin) – Prescribed for overactive bladder

- Atrovent® (Ipratropium Bromide) – Used in asthma inhalers

- Spiriva® (Tiotropium Bromide) – Used in asthma inhalers

- Oxivent® (Oxitropium Bromide) – Used in asthma inhalers

- Colidrops Pediatric (Hyoscyamine) – Treats bowel and bladder muscle cramps, symptoms of Irritable Bowel Syndrome (IBD), colitis, pain caused by kidney or gall bladder stones, stomach ulcers, and Parkinson's disease muscle problems.

- Oxytrol (Oxybutynin Transdermal) – Used in the treatment of overactive bladder

- Toviaz (Fesoterodine fumarate) – Used to treat overactive bladder

- Urispas (Flavoxate) – Used to treat frequent and painful urination associated with infections of the prostate, bladder, or kidneys

Antihistamines: Used alone or in combination with other drugs in numerous over-the-counter and prescription medications relieving symptoms of allergy, cold, dizziness, or sleep aids. The following is a list of some, but certainly not all, of the brands that include antihistamines:

- Benadryl (Diphenhydramine)
- Claritin (Loratadine)
- Contac (Clemasine)
- Dramamine (Dimenhydrinate)
- Tavist (Clemasine)
- Unisom (Doxylamine)

Antacids: Used to relieve heartburn and stomach pain. Some examples are:

- Pepcid (Famotidine)
- Tagamet (Cimetidine)
- Zantac (Ranitidine)

Antidepressants: These drugs are used to combat mild to severe depression. Some examples include:

- Cymbalta (Duloxetine)
- Elavil (amitriptyline)
- Lithium
- Paxil (Paroxetine)
- Prozac (Fluoxetine)

Muscle relaxants:

- Flexeryl (Cyclobenzaprine
- Norlex (Orphenadrine)
- Soma (Carisoprodal)

Antiarrythmics: Used to treat cardiac arrhythmias, or erratic heartbeat. Some examples include:

- Digoxin
- Norpace (Disopyramide)
- Procainamide
- Quinaglute (Quinidine)

Antiemetics: Used to suppress nausea and vomiting. The following are some of the most common:

- Compazine (Prochlorperazine)
- Phenergan (Promethazine)
- Seroquel (Quetiapine)

Eye Medications in Drop Form: Opthamalic drops are used or prescribed by a physician for a variety of reasons; to dilate the pupils of the eye before an eye exam, before or after eye surgery, to treat eye inflammation (uveitis), and as lubrication to combat dry eye. The following are a few examples:

- Cyclopentolate – Ophthalmic eye drops used to dilate the eye before exam or surgery

- ISOPTO® (Homatropine Hydrobomide) – Used to dilate the eye before or after surgical procedure or to treat eye inflammation such as uveitis

- Tropicamide – Used to dilate the pupils of the eye before eye examination and before or after surgery. Brand names include Mydral, Mydriacyl, Ocu-Tropic, and Tropicacyl

Miscellaneous Medications: The following list includes examples of drugs that are used as painkillers, diuretics, to control stomach acid, as antidepressants, and as antidiarrheal medication:

- Celebrex (Celecoxib) – anti-inflammatory pain relief

- Keflex (Cephalexin) – an antibiotic

- Lasix (Furosemide) – a diuretic to reduce fluid retention

- Lomotil (Diphenoxylate) – controls diarrhea

- Prevacid (Lansoprazole) – used to reduce stomach acid
- Restoril (Temazepam) – a sleep aid
- Topamax (Topiramate) – a drug for preventing migraine headaches and to control epileptic seizure
- Valium (Diazepam) – a tranquilizer
- Vicodin (Hydrocodone) – a narcotic pain reliever

There are many more neuro-transmitter blocking drugs, and far too many to list here. But even if a medication or over-the-counter drug is not listed here, it does not mean it is free of anti-cholinergic ingredients. For a comprehensive list, and for more information on drug interactions, go to Dr. Leo Galland's Pilladvised website http://pilladvised.com.

An example of exactly how deadly this form of drug can be is the drug Topamax (intended to treat epilepsy and migraine). According to the FDA, as well as the Topamax press release, oral cleft, otherwise known as cleft palate, occurs 11 times higher than the general population in babies born to mothers who took this drug during the first trimester of pregnancy. The list of possible and quite severe side effects is extremely long. Many adverse reactions can become permanent.

- Vision problems including:
  - Acute myopia (nearsightedness)
  - Secondary angle closure glaucoma
  - Permanent blindness
- Increased risks of suicide
- Neurological problems
- Breathing difficulties

According to the U.S. Food and Drug Administration, the list of drugs that have reported adverse reactions is quite long, alphabetically listed from A to Z. Here are only a handful:

- Accutane
- Avandia
- Darvocet, Darvon and Propoxyphene
- DES
- Fosamax
- Levaquin
- Meridia
- Nuvaring
- Prempro
- Reglan
- Yaz/Yasmin

Researching drugs in print ads, commercials, information pamphlets from the pharmaceutical companies, U.S. government websites such as the FDA, and court testimony, there is a very long list of hazardous side effects for every pharmaceutical drug. According to Gwen Olsen, a former pharmaceutical industry sales representative, *"All drugs are toxins. There is no safe drug."* There isn't one that doesn't come with side effects ranging from mild to life threatening. One television drug commercial lists "lymphoma" as a side effect! Why take a chance on contracting a deadly disease?

The drug, Avandia, caused over 100,000 heart attacks before it was taken off the market. Even as the mounting evidence stacked up, the drug was still touted as safe and it took the FDA four years to remove it from the list of approved drugs. Why do so many people have to suffer or die before a drug is taken off the market? Perhaps this happens because the very same people who approve the drugs are the same ones to remove them. Sadly, the same can be said for every single pharmaceutical drug on the market, or about to come to market. The buying public becomes the guinea pigs.

How do these drugs get approved in the first place, and why are doctors so quick to prescribe them? In the past, the FDA used to conduct testing before deciding whether or not to approve a product for market. This is no longer the case, and typically, the USFDA merely relies on whatever testing the manufacturer presents.

It is a fact that Big Pharma "funds" the FDA with application fees that are paid for every single pharmaceutical drug application. According to the Federal Register, the 2012 fee schedule was an astonishing $1.8 million for new drug applications requiring clinical data. It was a bit less for applications not requiring clinical data, but they were still a whopping $920,750. As a result, according to testimony by two former FDA scientists, the pharmaceutical industry *expects* their drugs to be quickly approved (fast-tracked) with little FDA scrutiny.

BIG PHARMA'S INFLUENCE ON DOCTORS

Pharmaceutical companies influence physicians long before they ever receive their license to practice medicine. The pharmaceutical industry spends millions donating to medical schools. In 2008, Harvard University received more than $11.5 million for "research and continuing education classes." In addition, pharmaceutical insiders often lecture at medicals schools, touting the benefits of their specific miracles in a bottle. Out of Harvard's 8,900 professors, 1,600 admitted that they or family members had ties to the industry.

By the time medical students graduate, they have not only been educated about the human body and its workings; they also are fully versed in the benefits of pharmaceutical drugs. Unfortunately, they have no training in nutrition or alternative healing.

An ongoing investigation revealed that in the years 2009-2011, twelve pharmaceutical companies paid over $761 million to physicians for consulting, speaking, research, and expenses.

Doctors who have long since graduated medical school rely on studies and reports about specific drugs written by highly respected physicians. But what actually happens is that pharmaceutical industry ghostwriters create glowing reports that include industry-sponsored positive studies. The drug manufacturer then pays well-respected doctors to read the reports and put their stamps of approval on them. Pharmaceutical company sales representatives give these bogus reports to physicians, who see the well-respected physician's name, and assume that the drug must be beneficial.

Doctors and researchers who produce unfavorable studies lose research funding, are subject to having their research teams disbanded, and their results buried. In such cases, their credibility is undermined and their careers ruined.

Another way in which Big Pharma influences doctors is by controlling the medical journals they rely on. As examples:

- In 2003 the pharmaceutical industry spent $448 million in medical journal advertising, making up 97-99% of the journals' advertising revenue

- Often pharmaceutical companies will place ads in journals only if, in return, their products are favorably editorialized in the journals

- In 2008, a careful review of six leading medical journals revealed that nearly one quarter of all the research articles published were likely written by pharmaceutical industry ghost writers

- Pharmaceutical companies will pay medical publishers to create mock "medical journals" that contain collections of ghost-written articles that are favorable to their company's products. There is no disclosure that the professional looking mock "medical journals" are totally fabricated and paid for by Big Pharma. An example is the *Australasian Journal of Bone and Joint Medicine,* which is a collection of reprinted articles (most likely ghost-written) praising Merck's repertoire of pharmaceuticals. The "journal" was published by Elsevier and paid for my Merck.

ALLOPATHIC MEDICATIONS SIDE-EFFECTS

Allopathic medicine quite often has a cascading or domino effect of treating symptoms and causing disease. Allopathic medicine can rob the body of nutrients it needs in order to function properly. Take statins, for instance, which block cholesterol production. Unfortunately, this is also the same route the body uses to produce Coenzyme Q10, the enzyme critical for brain function as well as building muscle, and as a result, Coenzyme Q10 is depleted.

With so many people taking so many different drugs, prescription and/or over-the-counter, the chances of an overdose or adverse reactions have escalated. Just recently, a major OTC pain relief drug manufacturer pulled their product from the shelves; they are relabeling their product to advise users to take a smaller dosage than the previously recommended dose. The main ingredient is acetaminophen, which is an ingredient in many other over-the-counter drugs and using too much of it can cause serious liver damage or liver failure. People who cannot avoid taking pain medications are advised to alternate between over-the-counter drugs that include acetaminophen (Tylenol) and ibuprofen (Advil, Motrin IB).

It is estimated that in the United States alone, 450,000 medication-related hospitalizations and deaths occur annually due to adverse reactions to single or combined drugs.

PROBLEMS CAUSED BY ALLOPATHIC MEDICINE AND DRUGS

A group of researchers painstakingly reviewed and fully referenced statistical evidence of the huge number of problems caused by allopathic medicine and drugs. Their findings revealed that each year there are approximately:

- 2.2 million adverse reactions to prescribed drugs in-hospital

- 20 million annual unnecessary antibiotic prescriptions given to people with viral infections for which the drugs are useless

- 8.9 million unnecessary hospitalizations due to complications from medical treatment

- 7.5 million unnecessary medical and surgical procedures performed

- 783,936 iatrogenic deaths, meaning they are inadvertently caused by a physician, surgeon, medical treatment, or diagnostic procedure

According to former pharmaceutical industry sales rep Gwen Olsen, when a pharmaceutical is approved for market, they don't even know half of the adverse reactions the drug will cause. There isn't a single drug or vaccine on the market that doesn't cause some sort of reaction ranging from mild to fatal.

HOW ALLOPATHIC MEDICINE HAS CHANGED

Doctors practicing allopathic medicine went from being general practitioners who dealt with illnesses of the entire human body and its functions and interactions to a field of specialists who focus on only one area of the anatomy or bodily systems. Allopathic medicine treats the human body as a bunch of parts that have no relationship to each other.

When will doctors, and their patients, realize there is no allopathic magic bullet, no magic in a bottle? Health or a cure does not come from a drug that merely masks symptoms and has worse side effects than what it is supposed to be treating.

In research for this book, I was amazed to find an enormous amount of documentation for current pharmaceutical drugs that are known to have side effects, some of which are fatal. I also found pages of adverse reaction lawsuits, trial testimony, research studies, and documentation from the pharmaceutical makers themselves. It is shocking to see how many of these harmful drugs are still on the market, still being prescribed, and still being taken by consumers who believe them to be safe.

It raises the question: How many more allopathic drugs that harm consumers daily will it take before people demand *real* medicine that's not cooked up in laboratories? After all, there are safer alternatives, including some in existence for thousands of years, including Traditional Chinese Medicine (TCM), which has been used for more than 5,000 years.

One must look to nature for the answer to *real* health and *real* healing. Health comes from food grown the way nature intended, without chemicals; and products consisting of nature-made ingredients only. The medicines we take should be equally as pure.

Allopathic medicine at first looked to nature, using medicinal herbs from the Deadly Nightshade family, Foxglove (Digitalis), and white willow bark for pain relief. But somewhere along the way, allopathic medicines became synthesized from a mishmash of chemicals, and some containing viruses, bacteria, or fungi. Each of us responds differently to these drug cocktails.

Unlike allopathic pharmaceutical drugs, alternative medicines are derived from nature. The botanicals are grown in fields, the tinctures either from cold pressed or steam distilled oils. They are a whole medicine that works synergistically with the whole body. They do not treat or cure any disease; they merely aid the human body in restoring itself.

Today, there is a pharmaceutical pill for just about every malady. But to me, the real and safest remedy comes from removing toxic ingredients from our lives, and natural healing. Nature has provided everything we need to be healthy.

VACCINES

"I think that vaccines have to be considered the bargain basement technology for the 20th century."

Dr. Maurice Hilleman, former head of Merck's Vaccine Division

Vaccines have become a controversial tool that some researchers believe cause a great deal of harm to some of those who receive them. For example, Dr. Andrew Wakefield, a gastroenterologist who published a study linking the onset of autism and inflamed bowels in very young children after receiving the MMR vaccine, says *"Medicine, presented with the possibility of an iatrogenic catastrophe, has boarded a dissonant bandwagon and has gone after those who have concerns – genuine concerns – that childhood vaccines may be responsible, at least in part, for the autism epidemic. The relevant science has been grossly misrepresented, crushed beneath the wheels of a Public Relations 16-wheeler that is out of control. In the meantime a relentless tsunami of damaged children claims this land."*

Today, our genes are being mutated by the onslaught of toxins. Diseases that didn't exist 50 years ago are common-place now, and diseases that rarely existed, such as autism, are now prominent. Worse, we seem to accept infection, disease, and auto-immune disorders such as arthritis and other kinds of ill health as normal or expected aspects of aging.

In the early 1980's, the growing number of lawsuits against the pharmaceutical industry and health care providers became so great that many vaccine producers got out of the business. This created such a fear that there wouldn't be enough vaccines manufactured to serve the public that in 1986, Congress stepped in and created the National Childhood Vaccine Injury Act (P.L.99-660), establishing the National Vaccine Injury Compensation Program (NVICP). To discourage further defection from vaccine manufacture, the program grants the pharmaceutical industry and healthcare providers immunity from lawsuits stemming from harm caused by vaccines. The program is administered jointly by:

- The U.S. Department of Health and Human Services (HHS);
- The U.S. Department of Justice (DOJ);
- The U.S. Court of Federal Claims (the Court)

The NVIPC is a type of "no-fault" alternative that includes a trust fund totally paid for with taxpayer dollars. Every time a single dose vaccine is given to "prevent" one disease, a small excise tax of seventy-five cents goes to support the fund. When a multiple-dose vaccine is given to "prevent" multiple diseases such as the MMR vaccine for measles-mumps-rubella, the excise tax rises to $2.25. To date, U.S. taxpayers have paid millions of dollars into the trust fund and vaccine manufacturers are not liable financially.

Not surprisingly, my research of government information on vaccines produced claims that there is no valid link, no valid studies, and no scientific research to prove that vaccines aren't safe. And yet, as early as February 1999, in a report to the chairman of the U.S. Senate Committee on Health, Education, Labor and Pensions the United States General Accounting Office stated the number of injury claims against vaccines since the reporting system's inception was 5,355. The report further stated that the trust fund had grown to $1.3 billion from excise taxes paid, versus awards handed out. By 2012, according to the CDC "approximately 30,000" vaccine adverse reaction reports (VAERS) are filed annually."

Research shows that half of the awards made since the NVIPC program's inception were for neurological injuries. Because of the way the program is structured, the burden of proof of injury falls on the petitioner, making it difficult to qualify for compensation. Timing of vaccine injury is critical. For example, if a child becomes ill and dies several days after vaccination, the program does not recognize the vaccination as the cause, even when all other causes of death have been ruled out, whereas if the child had died within minutes or a couple of hours after vaccination, the program administrators *might* consider vaccine injury as a *possible* cause.

The report further stated that the trust fund had grown to $1.3 billion due to excise taxes paid versus awards handed out and that according to the U.S. Accounting Office Report, the government "borrows" from this surplus. Since the government uses the trust fund as its private piggy bank, it is no wonder then that more and more vaccines are being mandated.

Meanwhile, vaccines are money makers for the pharmaceutical industry. In 2010, Unicef bought $747 million worth of vaccines for 58% of the world's children. As of 2009, drug companies sold in excess of $1.5 billion worth of swine flu shots, in addition to the $1 billion in annual flu shots, which are part of an ever increasing $20 billion global vaccine market. Is it any wonder Big Pharma keeps rolling out new vaccines for every conceivable illness, and the federal government is more than happy to mandate the current schedule of 69 doses of 16 vaccines for children from the moment of birth to the age of 18? Is it surprising then, that every American from the age of 6 months until death should receive an annual flu vaccine? Apparently vaccine developers are working on vaccines to prevent obesity, to be administered in the fetal stage. That means children would be vaccinated even before birth! Is the health of our children really at stake, or is it the health of the pharmaceutical industry's bottom line?

Who else financially benefits from vaccines? Anyone who administers them benefits financially, including doctors, hospitals, drugstores, schools, to name a few. Here's how it works:

- A set fee of 10% to 25% above the purchase cost for each vaccine is set by contract with a managed care organization (HMO, Medicare, etc.). As an example, if 1,000 doses of a vaccine are purchased at $10 each, the fee collected from the managed care organization will be $1,000 to $2,500 per 1,000 doses administered.

- Vaccine administration fees ranging from $14 to $30 may be collected by physicians, hospitals, or other facilities that charge patients for vaccination. If 1,000 patients are given single dose vaccinations, the administration fee profit would be between $14,000 and $30,000.
- Add to that, if 1000 patients call for a flu shot, a physician may also schedule a "well visit."

Let's use the 2012-2013 flu season as an example of just how profitable a single vaccine jab can be for the medical community. One doctor estimated that physicians' vaccine profits could be $25,000 to $42,500 or more depending upon the number of patient visits. A major drugstore chain reported that it administered 5.5 million flu vaccine doses (up 200,000 doses from the previous year) for a minimum $55 million profit. Add to that the additional purchases a customer might make during the flu shot visit and you can begin to understand why many drugstore chains are so eager to "give away" flu shots.

Is it any wonder then that allopathic medicine is so anxious to inject us with vaccines?

If you *really* want to do some research on vaccines, there is a mountain of studies available on non-recoverable adverse vaccine reactions and death written by eminent doctors and medical specialists, as well as testimony by pharmaceutical insiders who became whistleblowers. There are also websites such as SaneVax.org, or NVIC.org. The National Vaccine Information Center (NVIC) is spearheaded by parents of children who have been injured by vaccinations and is devoted to vaccine education. Other such websites not only call for greater scrutiny of vaccines, but also a halt to the massive childhood vaccination campaigns. As with NVIC, these websites provide testimony written by parents of perfectly healthy children who have been irreparably damaged, or died, following vaccination.

Eminently qualified individuals including Dr. Andrew Wakefield, and Dr. Russell Blaylock, a retired neurological surgeon, among many others, have spoken out about the dangers of vaccines.

The big question is: Do we really need so many vaccines, especially the mega-doses children are given today? Most infants born in the 1950s received three separate injections of the DTP (diphtheria, tetanus, pertussis) vaccines. They were given boosters just before starting kindergarten. Then, children in the early 1960's were given one dose of the Salk polio vaccine, followed by additional doses of the Sabin oral polio vaccine. Children were also vaccinated for small pox at that time

Today's children are being vaccinated for childhood illnesses that are not typically life threatening, including chicken pox, measles and other relatively harmless illnesses. Somehow it's become unacceptable for a child to develop and recover from a childhood illness.

The Centers for Disease Control and Prevention estimates that from 1990 to 2007 out of 3-4 million cases of chicken pox annually, there were about 50 chicken pox associated children's deaths per year (0.00142%).

According to the Federal Vaccine Adverse Events Reporting System (VAERS), between March 1995 (when the chicken pox vaccine was introduced) and July 1998, in just three years there were 6,574 reports of vaccine injury, which translates to 67.5 adverse reactions per 100,000 doses. Approximately 1 out of every 33,000 vaccinations (about 4%) resulted in vaccine injury including shock, encephalitis (brain inflammation), thrombocytopenia (a blood disorder), cellulitis (bacterial skin infection), transverse myelitis (inflammation of the spinal cord), Guillain-Barré syndrome (nervous system disorder), and 14 deaths (0.042%).

Every vaccine comes with a long list of possible side effects ranging from mild to fatal, but what happens when children are administered multiple vaccines at once? A recent study tracking adverse events reported in VAERS from 1990 to 2010 shows a correlation between increased hospitalizations and mortality rates of infants in relation to the number of vaccine doses given at one time. For example, only 11.0% of children receiving 2 vaccine doses per medical visit were hospitalized, whereas 23.5% of children receiving as many as 8 vaccine doses in one medical visit required hospitalization. Likewise, the death rate among children receiving 1-4 vaccine doses per medical visit was 3.6%, while mortality increased 5.5% among children receiving 5-8 doses all at once. Meanwhile, the majority of reported vaccine injury cases involve the Hepatitis B vaccine which is administered at birth. Between 1992 and 2005 there were 36,788 reported cases of adverse reactions to the Hepatitis B vaccine. Of those cases, 14,800, more than 40%, required hospitalization and there were 781 deaths. The Hepatitis B vaccine has been linked to Sudden Infant Death Syndrome (SIDS).

Our bodies do a good job of protecting us from viruses we encounter, even in childhood. Each virus strain contains a specific shape. Each time we come into contact with a new virus strain, we create antibodies that mold themselves to that particular pathogen's specific shape. In scientific literature, this is referred to as the "lock and key" system, where the virus shape is the lock, and the antibody is the key. For every virus strain we come into contact with, our immune system produces a matching antibody. This is the body's way of recognizing the virus if it ever comes into contact with it again, and it already has the means to eliminate that virus by the antibody's secretion that penetrates the membrane and either destroys the virus outright, or the secretion "tags" the virus so that our body's killer cells will attack it. Antibodies, like all cells in the body, age and die or expire via gene-directed cell death, and so whenever the body comes into contact with a virus it has previously "met," new antibodies are created. This is the body's natural booster shot, without the vaccine, and why the body's natural immunity can last a lifetime.

With vaccination, allopathic medicine bypasses the body's own defense mechanisms by injecting us with a virus to stimulate an immune response. Since this is precisely what our immune system does whenever it comes into contact with a new pathogen, but without the added "adjuvants" of mercury, aluminum, and foreign DNA that vaccines may contain, the question has to be: "Why do we need a vaccine?"

It's bad enough to be vaccinated once, but children now are routinely vaccinated multiple times with multiple doses of various vaccines, in some instances soon after birth, before they have even begun to develop their immune systems. In fact, the average child is given 69 vaccines in multiple doses for nearly 20 diseases by the time they reach 18 years of age, with the majority of vaccines administered before a child is 2 years old.

What does all this vaccine do to them? How does this harm them? Why do children need to be vaccinated so frequently, especially against diseases that aren't typically life threatening?

Do healthy people really need a flu shot every year? If they do, then the vaccines aren't doing their job properly because they are not activating our body's own immune defenses.

Flu Vaccines

In fall of 2011, the Centers for Disease Control and Prevention announced that flu vaccines were effective only 60% of the time *when all age groups were combined*. When all age groups aren't combined, the effectiveness for one single group drops dramatically. There is one statement on the CDC's web page that defines the effectiveness of the flu vaccine: *"In general, the flu vaccine works best among young, healthy children and older children. Lesser effects of flu vaccine were often found in studies of young children (e.g., those younger than 2 years of age) and older adults."*

This isn't surprising in that children younger than age two do not yet have fully developed immune systems. Older adults are the most likely to have health challenges, and compromised immune systems so the vaccine is less likely to be effective. This is why the CDC states that flu vaccines are less effective for these two groups. *"Success,"* according to the CDC, is *"among healthy adults and older children."* In other words, if you're not healthy to begin with, the vaccine may not offer protection against the flu.

It is important to understand that annual flu vaccines are based on previous years' strains, and depending upon which vaccine strain most closely matches the current year's strain of influenza, that is the vaccine that is manufactured for the current flu season. Keep in mind that viruses are living organisms that constantly mutate, which makes it impossible to predict and manufacture an effective vaccine a year in advance.

It is estimated that the 2012-2013 flu vaccine worked a mere 1% of the time with the elderly (the group the CDC states is the least benefited by the flu vaccine but regardless are urged to get a flu shot), and many of those who had already been vaccinated contracted the flu anyway.

The conclusion is that vaccines work best if you're already healthy. But in that case, chances are your immune system will naturally be able to fend off disease without the flu vaccine.

We've already learned about genetically modified food and the possible dangers they pose. Now genetically modified vaccines are being injected into us.

The FDA has approved a new flu vaccine called Flublock targeted for people between the ages of 18-49. According to the package insert, this vaccine will contain genes from three different virus strains (H1N1, H3N2, B/Wisconsin/1/2010), as well as a baculovirus (*Autographa californica* nuclear polyhedrosis). It will also contain residual DNA from the vaccine's host, the fall armyworm (*Spodoptera frugiperda*).

The insect-incubated vaccine is then extracted using Dow Chemical Company's Triton™ X-100. According to Dow's product sheet, Triton™ X-100 is a "surfactant with excellent detergency" and is used in household and industrial cleaners, paints and coatings, pulp and paper, textiles, metalworking fluids, agrochemicals, and oilfields.

The vaccine dose is suspended in sodium chloride, monobasic sodium phosphate, dibasic sodium phosphate, and polysorbate 20, which is an emulsifying agent used in many topical cosmetics and skin care products, as well as a fragrance ingredient.

With insect DNA, genes from three different viruses, and several chemicals thrown in, *what could possibly go wrong?*

According to clinical studies that were conducted by the manufacturer, the vaccine is less than 50% effective and side effects include:

- Injection site pain
- Headache
- Fatigue
- Joint aches and pains
- Lip and tongue swelling

Severe side effects may include

- Anaphylaxis
- Eye infection, facial swelling, breathing difficulties (Oculorespiratory syndrome)
- Guillain-Barré syndrome
- Inflammation of the lungs and heart (Pleuropericarditis)

As previously explained, the body develops *lifelong* antibodies when subjected to childhood illnesses and it is rare for someone who has had these illnesses to get them again. If this is how our immune system works, then why must the flu vaccines have to be repeated annually? Obviously, then, flu vaccines must not stimulate the body to create even year-long antibodies. Doesn't this make it clear that flu vaccines are an abject failure? And in that case, why does the CDC push for "seasonal" flu vaccination?

For me, the answer is easy: follow the money. Vaccines in general, and the flu vaccine in particular, reap profits for the pharmaceutical and the allopathic medicine industries. And thanks to the tax paid on every vaccine that goes directly to the National Vaccine Injury Compensation Program, which rarely pays out to the multitudes who are permanently injured by vaccines, government agencies profit as well.

Grace Stuart, MD, a retired physician, explained to me that bad reactions to vaccines are the result of high titer. Titer measures how much of an antibody has formed in blood for a specific antigen such as a specific virus or a form of bacteria. A simple blood test can show whether antibodies are present and whether the body already has enough immunity to a specific virus or bacteria or other pathogen. In the case of sufficient immunity, "booster" shots are not only useless, but potentially harmful.

Dr. Russell Blaylock, a retired neuro-surgeon, has described the dangers of the large number of childhood vaccines now administered, as well as problems stemming from vaccines in general. Thermographic images show the inflamed brains of children following multiple vaccinations and there is well-documented and heartbreaking trial testimony of parents whose children have never recovered from vaccine-induced brain inflammation and who have suffered irreparable damage or death. According to the National Vaccine Information Center (NVIC), as well as the U.S. Department of Health and Human Services, typical adverse reactions include:

- Pronounced swelling, redness, heat or hardness at the injection site
- Body rash or hives
- Shock/collapse
- Screaming or hours of persistent crying
- Extreme sleepiness or long periods of unresponsiveness
- Twitching or jerking of body, arm, leg or head
- Crossed eyes
- Weakness or paralysis
- Loss of eye contact, social withdrawal
- Inability to roll over, sit or stand up
- Loss of vision or hearing

- Restlessness, hyperactivity, or inability to concentrate
- Sleep disturbances or changes in wake/sleep patterns
- Head banging or onset of repetitive movements
- Joint pain
- Muscle weakness
- Disabling fatigue
- Memory loss
- Chronic ear or respiratory infections
- Violent or persistent diarrhea or chronic constipation
- Violent or persistent vomiting
- Breathing problems
- Excessive bleeding or anemia
- Epileptic seizures
- Signs of autism
- Death

What's In Vaccines?

Vaccines are cultivated in living "hosts" and contain all the foreign DNA and RNA of their hosts. These components may prompt allergies and auto-immune diseases from bacteria, fungi, viruses, yeast, bovine fetal serum, human aborted fetal serum, egg protein, and monkey kidney tissue. The CDC's *Ingredients of Vaccines Fact Sheet* lists the following vaccine ingredients:

- **Aluminum** to "stimulate a better response"
- **Antibiotics** to "prevent bacterial growth during vaccine production and storage"

- **Formaldehyde** to "inactivate bacterial toxins" as well as "kill unwanted viruses and bacteria" and that "*most* formaldehyde is removed" before the vaccine is packaged
- **MSG** "to stabilize and prevent changes when a vaccine is exposed to heat, light, acidity or humidity"
- **2-phenoxy-ethanol** "to stabilize and prevent changes when a vaccine is exposed to heat, light, acidity or humidity" (it's also a chemical used in insecticides)
- **Mercury** as a "preservative added to vials containing more than one vaccine"

Both aluminum and mercury are toxic heavy metals, formaldehyde is a carcinogen, and MSG is an excitotoxin. Doesn't it make sense that the body's immune response is from having these heavy metals and chemicals injected into it rather than the virus the vaccine contains?

But there are even worse and more serious implications. According to an interview with Dr. Maurice Hilleman, the former head of Merck's Vaccine Division, he states, "*The yellow fever vaccine had the leukemia virus in it. There are 40 different viruses in these vaccines.*" He went on to say that people who were given polio vaccine in the 1950's received a vaccine that was tainted with a monkey kidney virus, SV-40, that is linked to cancer. The reason being that monkey kidneys were used to cultivate the vaccine. That virus has been linked to lung, brain, and bone cancers in humans, with the rare SV-40 virus inexplicably showing up in cancer tumors.

And it isn't just those who received the polio vaccine in the 1950's who are developing cancers with this SV-40 link; cancers in younger people have also revealed the SV-40 virus. One theory is that the virus may have been passed on from one generation to the next, while another is that humans are continuing to be exposed to this rare virus because all subsequent polio vaccines are "seeded" from the original batch.

These heavy metals, viruses, bacteria, and foreign matter are injected into us every time we are vaccinated. Toxicity in mercury and aluminum, especially in children, can be the result of multiple vaccinations.

The body produces the peptide, Glutathione, which is the master binding agent that bonds with and removes heavy metals and provides a natural detoxification process. Unfortunately, poor diets of processed and unhealthful non-organic foods, medications, and toxins in personal and home care products deplete this critical detoxifier. Some individuals are genetically predisposed to a glutathione deficiency.

However, when *inorganic* heavy metals such as aluminum or mercury are injected into the body via vaccines, these inorganic compounds deactivate the binding proteins of glutathione, disabling the body's ability to detoxify heavy metals, especially mercury. The body's inability to eliminate these compounds results in heavy metal toxicity as these substances lodge in organ tissues, particularly in the heart, liver, and brain.

Disorders attributed to heavy metal poisoning include, but are not limited to:

- Chronic fatigue syndrome
- Heart disease
- Cancer
- Chronic infections
- Auto-immune disorders
- Diabetes

- Autism
- Alzheimer's Disease
- Parkinson's Disease
- Multiple Sclerosis
- Asthma
- Arthritis
- Liver disease
- Kidney disease

Gardasil Human Papilloma Virus (HPV) Vaccine

While many of these vaccine toxicity problems started over 60 years ago, not much has changed. Vaccines are just as contaminated and just as deadly. The only difference now is that there is a vaccine for almost everything. And now the latest example is the vaccine Gardasil (marketed as Cervarix in Europe), which has been heavily promoted for both boys and girls to be used in protecting against the spread of cervical cancer, which is caused by certain strains of the Human Papilloma virus.

There are over 150 different strains of the Human Papilloma virus. A handful cause genital warts, and around a dozen strains can lead to cervical cancer. Fortunately, the immune system usually overcomes the HP virus within 1-2 years. A small percentage of strains may linger that *might* trigger cancer, but it may take more than 20 years for cellular changes to develop into pre-cancerous lesions. These are usually detected with annual PAP smears and are easily treated.

Unfortunately, Gardasil doesn't protect against all the possible pathogens that cause cervical cancer, and PAP smears are still required later on for girls who get the vaccine.

Although initially seeming to be a worthwhile vaccine, in the U.S. alone there have been over 28,000 documented adverse reactions or side effects from Gardasil that have required emergency room visits and the number is still climbing. Some children receiving the vaccine have become permanently incapacitated or have died. Studies reveal that the HPV vaccine causes adverse reactions 5 to 20 times more often than any other vaccine.

It is difficult to pinpoint statistics because many side effects don't appear immediately after vaccination, and as a result, many healthcare practitioners rule out the vaccine as the cause. As a result, it is estimated that only 1-10% of vaccine injuries are submitted to VAERS, including those from Gardasil. Following are VAERS statistics for Gardasil adverse events in the U.S.:

GARDASIL ADVERSE REACTIONS	TOTAL AS OF OCTOBER 2011	TOTAL AS OF JANUARY 2013
TYPE	TOTAL	TOTAL
Disabled	763	924
Deaths	103	130
Permanently disabled	4,777	5,736
Abnormal PAP smear	430	515
Cervical Dysplasia	157	203
Cervical Cancer	41	61
Life Threatening Event	444	543
Emergency Room	9,115	10,225
Hospitalization	2,307	2,911
Extended Hospitalization	201	229
Serious Adverse Reaction	3,111	3,901
Total Adverse Events	23,388	28,661

Gardasil is a genetically modified vaccine that has been linked to permanent neurological disorders and death following vaccination. That's because our immune system evolved to bind with and remove toxins that we ingest, and the "blood brain barrier," which is made up of highly specialized cells that line brain capillaries, protects the central nervous system by preventing harmful chemicals such as aluminum and mercury, viruses, bacteria, and foreign DNA from entering the brain. But our immune system has not evolved to have these potentially harmful toxins injected into us, and as a result, ingredients toxic to the central nervous system have crossed the blood-brain barrier, causing permanent neurological damage.

The Gardasil vaccine contains "virus-like particles" (VLPs) HPV-6-L1, HPV-11-L1, HPV-18-L1 and HPV-16-L1, which are referred to as the vaccine's "fingerprints."

In a recent breakthrough study, HPV-16-L1 particles were discovered in the brains of two teenage girls, each from a different country. Both had died from cerebral hemorrhage following injection of the HPV vaccine. The study suggests that the virus particles entered the brain via absorption by attaching to the aluminum adjuvant used in the vaccine, and the virus particles had bound to the walls of cerebral blood vessels, triggering an auto-immune response where the immune system, sensing foreign invaders in the brain, attacked the cerebral blood vessels, resulting in fatal brain hemorrhaging.

This may explain other neurological symptoms following Gardasil injection reported in VAERS as follows:

- Persistent migraines
- Fainting
- Seizures
- Tremors and tingling sensations
- Myalgia
- Motion abnormalities
- Psychotic symptoms
- Cognitive impairment

- Death

In a separate recent study, HPV-16-L1 particles were found in the blood and spleen of a teenage girl who died in her sleep six months after her third Gardasil injection. HPV-16-L1 particles do not show up in typical testing methods or autopsy.

Now, a doctor who was instrumental in the development and marketing of Merck's vaccine has begun speaking out about the benefits and health risks surrounding the vaccine. In an interview on a major television network, the doctor suggested that because of the way statistics are calculated, there may be *higher* incidences of serious side effects from the vaccine than there are annual deaths from cervical cancer. She bemoaned the vaccine's short-term effective immunity of only 5 years, and felt it should last for at least 15 years instead. She also questioned whether the health risks of the vaccine outweighed taking a vaccine for a disease that can be easily detected through annual PAP smears and very effectively cured. What was most revealing was her concern that the use of Gardasil would end up being "the most costly public health experiment in cancer control."

Public health *experiment*? Do parents realize they are volunteering their innocent, healthy children as part of a giant clinical study for this untested vaccine with potentially tragic side effects? Unfortunately not enough of them do.

Are Vaccines Responsible for the Decline in Infectious Diseases?

It is a common belief that vaccines are the primary reason that rates of infectious diseases have dropped. According to the World Health Organization and UNICEF, seven serious illnesses (smallpox, diphtheria, tetanus, yellow fever, whooping cough, polio, and measles) have been brought "under control" through the use of vaccines.

However, the National Health Federation compiled data on the mortality rates in the United States from measles, scarlet fever, typhoid, whooping cough (pertussis), and diphtheria from 1900 through 1965. The data tracks the death rates of each disease per 100,000 people. For each of these infectious diseases the graphs show a steady decline in mortality rates long before a vaccine for some of these diseases was introduced. And in each case where a vaccine was introduced, mortality rates spiked. For example, the graphs show that the mortality rate from diphtheria in 1900 was 40 per 100,000 people, but the mortality rate had continuously and naturally declined over two decades and by 1920, only 15 per 100,000 had died from the disease. After the diphtheria vaccine was introduced in 1923, the mortality rate spiked to nearly 20 deaths per 100,000 people, followed by a continued decline in deaths. The charts show this natural decline in all five of these infectious diseases, with all of them reaching their lowest levels (2 or less deaths per 100,000 people) around 1940, after which the death rates for all of these diseases flat line.

Another example is measles, which had declined from less than 15 deaths in 1900 to less than 2 per 100,000 people by 1940. The measles vaccine wasn't introduced until 1963.

This natural decline can also be seen in both typhoid (over 30 deaths per 100,000 in 1900 to less than 2 by 1940) and scarlet fever (over 10 deaths per 100,000 in the 1900's versus less than 2 by 1942) There was never a vaccine developed for Scarlet Fever, and the first Typhoid vaccine licensed in the U.S. was in 1989.

So then how do we explain the decline in mortality rates from these infectious diseases long before a vaccine was developed, or not introduced at all? One answer is the introduction of antibiotics, but that didn't occur until 1945. That still doesn't explain the continued drop in mortality rates prior to the introduction of antibiotics.

According to some researchers, scientists and doctors, the answer lies in greater access to clean water, enhanced food distribution, and improved sanitation and sewage disposal. Many other diseases that stem from unsanitary conditions and poor nutrition could be eased through the use of proper hygiene, sanitation and an improved diet rather than vaccines.

There are many pro's and con's surrounding the vaccine debate, and there may be even more vaccine side effects that are not attributed to vaccines at all. Results of a German study released in September 2011, *KiGGS – The German Health Interview and Examination Survey for Children and Adolescents,* compared health issues of over 17,000 vaccinated and unvaccinated German children. Using that study as a comparison, a similar study was begun in December 2010 and within a year, over 11,000 survey questionnaires were submitted (mostly from the U.S.). While this ongoing study is not a controlled study and depends upon answers to a questionnaire, the results so far are quite interesting:

Health Issue	% of US Vaccinated	% of KiGGS Unvaccinated
ADHD	7.9	2.0
Allergies (at least 1)	22.9	10.6
Asthma/Chronic Bronchitis	18.0	2.4
Autism	1 in 55	4 out of 17,000
Diabetes Mellitus	0.1	0.1
Ear Infections	11.0	2.0
Epilepsy/Seizures	3.6	0.3

Health Issue	% of US Vaccinated	% of KiGGS Unvaccinated
Hay fever	10.7	2.6
Herpes	12.8	0.2
Migraine	2.5	1.1
Neurodermatitis	13.2	7.0
Scoliosis	5.3	0.5
Thyroid Disease	1.7	0.1

The use of vaccines is controversial, with proponents arguing that vaccines are responsible for the decline of many infectious diseases and are completely harmless, while others claim the opposite.

I don't believe any drug or vaccine studies are 100% unbiased and impartial. Many are funded by the very industry that is looking for a positive outcome for their product. Like any data, the information can be skewed, with the more positive figures made prominent, while the negative results are downplayed or buried. Even with "independent" studies, where does the research money come from? Does the scientist performing the study have his or her own bias, and if so, can he or she put aside that opinion to come to an unbiased conclusion?

Even with supposed clinical, independent, unbiased, unmassaged studies, chances are that there's a flaw somewhere. Take, for instance, the Denmark Study, which the CDC has used as their benchmark to defend the safety of vaccines. The study states that the rates of autism rose despite the removal of Thimerosol (mercury preservative) from vaccines, and in one group, no vaccine was given at all. Unfortunately, the scientist who spearheaded the study has been charged with tax evasion, fraud and money laundering in connection with the study. While the CDC claims this has no bearing on the study, these charges cast a shadow on his integrity. Can we assume he didn't cheat with the study results?

Dr. Andrew Wakefield, an eminent gastroenterologist, was vilified and eventually lost his license to practice medicine in England for bringing to light the possible link between the mumps, measles, and rubella vaccine (MMR) and autism.

Rupert Murdoch's media empire was connected to this effort to discredit Dr. Wakefield. One pharmaceutical company that makes the MMR vaccine, GlaxoSmithKline, has James Murdoch on its board. Murdoch, who is Rupert's son, also manages the British newspaper, *The Sunday Times,* which published many slanderous articles about Dr. Wakefield.

If that's not enough of a connection, the reporter who was instrumental in bringing the case against Dr. Wakefield on his fitness to practice medicine received his information from an agency funded by the Association of the British Pharmaceutical Industry, which may have had a vested interest in protecting a drug company's vaccine products. And, to top it off, a very close blood relative of the High Court Judge who denied the parents of children treated by Dr. Wakefield to have their claims against vaccine manufacturers brought to trial, is also on the board of GlaxoSmithKline, and he serves as an executive board member of the publisher of the *Lancet*, which first published, and then removed, Dr. Wakefield's 1988 findings about the dangers of vaccines for children. The head of Reuters News service, which also promoted the crucifying of Dr. Wakefield, serves on the board of Merck, Inc. And finally, a prominent writer for the UK's *Daily Mirror*, another publication that wrote numerous denigrating articles about Dr. Wakefield, just happens to be married to the former chairman of GlaxoSmithKline.

These kinds of conflicts of interest are not unusual in our food, pharmaceutical, healthcare, chemical/bio-tech industries and government. An examination of the list of people serving on advisory boards, executive boards, appointees at the USFDA, the EPA, members of special government committees, and even advisors to the President of the United States shows conflicts of interest. While I haven't cross-referenced who is on every board of directors, I wouldn't be surprised if these same individuals also serve on the boards of television, radio, and newspaper conglomerates, which may explain why media rarely discloses anything negative about these industries.

It would seem that the continued development of vaccines for treatable illnesses fall under the "Problem-Reaction-Solution" strategy. Under this theory:

1. A problem is manufactured or created – For example under this scenario the public is alerted to impending dire consequences from treatable illnesses such as chicken pox or the flu

2. The public reacts – The public becomes fearful and demands protection

3. The problem is resolved in a way that completes your own agenda – In this resolution the healthcare industry benefits from the creation and perpetual administration of chicken pox and flu vaccines for illnesses that the vast majority of the population would naturally recover from and develop lifelong antibodies

This strategy can be applied not only to every vaccine currently on the market, but also to the nearly 400 new vaccines being developed for health issues such as obesity, acne, smoking, and alcoholism to name a few.

Unfortunately none of the billions of dollars spent on the research and development of never-ending drugs and vaccines is ever applied to disease prevention through elimination of environmental toxins that are making us sick in the first place.

Allopathic medicine, which merely treats or suppresses symptoms, disrupts the functioning of the human immune system and in some instances bodily functions, creating a cascade of other symptoms that require even more prescriptions. With the almost unlimited variety of drugs and vaccines, you would think we'd be the healthiest society on the planet. Instead, we actually are one of the sickest.

With more vaccines being fast tracked and mandated, it is becoming increasingly difficult to avoid being subjected to vaccines, especially for children. Children are being denied an education if they don't submit to federal, state or school mandated vaccinations, and parents' objections are being overruled.

Every state has a policy regarding healthcare exemptions based on religious or philosophical beliefs. To find your state's exemption regulations, go to http://www.nvic.org/Vaccine-Laws/state-vaccine-requirements.aspx

So who and what do you trust? Again I have to turn to logic and nature. Fifty-plus years ago, children didn't receive nearly 70 vaccinations and they turned out pretty darn well. Yes, they got sick, but most survived with strengthened immune systems and antibodies that would last a lifetime. If a vaccine really worked as well as the human body's lifelong antibodies, why do we need repeated vaccinations? Why do we need flu shots every year? Do we really believe the "flu" is only circulating around the globe during "flu season?" Knowing what is included in vaccines, do we really want "foreign" matter, heavy metals, and preservatives injected into us? Do we want to take risks like the ones that came with the polio vaccine, for example?

If there are voices of opposition, I'd rather err on the side of caution. I believe that *less is more*. I've never had a flu shot and I haven't had a cold in so long I can't remember when I had one last. I take whole-food vitamins, exercise, and eat whole organic raw foods whenever possible. If my immune system is weak and I get sick and die, it is natural selection and survival of the fittest. They'd have to strap me down, kicking and screaming before I'll voluntarily be injected with any vaccine.

Only you can decide for yourself who to trust.

ANTIBIOTICS AND THE IMMUNE SYSTEM

Antibiotics, which have been overused for decades, actually weaken the immune system. The concept of "use it or lose it" applies here. Antibiotics take over, actually replacing the immune system's function. Building the immune system is like building muscle tissue. The more you exercise or build it up, the stronger it becomes. Just as exercise keeps the body in top condition, the immune system also needs to be strengthened through exposure to pathogens such as bacteria and viruses. This exposure makes a healthy immune system develop antibodies.

In a conversation with Dr. Paul G. King from the Coalition for Mercury-free Drugs, he explained to me that with each repeated or new exposure to a particular strain of virus or bacteria, the immune system continues to create antibodies and receives a natural "booster" shot. This is how we develop life-long immunity. If we are not continuously exposed to these pathogens, old antibodies eventually die and no new ones are created. This leaves us wide open to the very bacterial and viral diseases we are trying to avoid.

People also are told to avoid crowds during cold and flu season when they actually should be exposing themselves to these strains to exercise their immune systems and naturally boost them against these specific pathogens.

Once again, conventional allopathic medicine will not allow nature to take its course and antibiotics are routinely given, even for illnesses caused by a virus, such as a cold. Unless an illness is bacterial, it can't be treated with antibiotics, so it makes no sense to prescribe them otherwise, especially for viral infections like the flu. Beyond being prescribed for viruses for which they have no effect, antibiotics are also given repeatedly for the same bacteria, resulting in "superbugs," or bacteria that are resistant to commonly used antibiotics. This happens because even though antibiotics do kill most of the target bacteria, some survive and mutate, becoming stronger and antibiotic resistant. This also results when patients do not complete a full course of antibiotics.

In the factory farming of animals, antibiotics are routinely given to animals in their feed as a preventative measure. According to the FDA, in 2009 alone, 29 million pounds of antibiotics were given to factory farm animals. Those antibiotics stored in their tissues end up on your dinner plate unless you eat organic meats. The animals also excrete antibiotics and the manure is used to fertilize crop fields. This results in additional consumption of antibiotics when those crops also land on your dinner plate. This practice of routinely giving animals antibiotic-laced feed has also resulted in mutated bacteria that affect both humans and animals. In addition, municipal water filtration systems do not filter out antibiotics that we have excreted, and as a result, we consume them via our drinking water. It's a wonder we need any antibiotics at all.

There are several antibiotic-resistant bacteria:

- MRSA USA300 - Ethicillin-Resistant Staphylococcus Aureus
- MRSA ST398 – The "pig strain" that affects swine and factory farm workers.
- Acinetobacter – A soil- and water-borne bacteria affecting extremely ill hospitalized patients.
- Gonorrhea
- Klebsiella pneumonia
- Neisseria meningitides
- Streptococcus pneumoniae
- Tuberculosis
- Typhoid fever
- VRE (Vancomycin-Resistant Enterococci)
- VISA/VRSA (Vancomycin-Intermediate/Resistant Staphylococcus Aureus)

A healthy immune system will eventually overcome and destroy the "bad" bacteria, preventing it from proliferating. But chemical environmental toxins in food, personal care products, air, water, etc. impair the immune system, which leads to inflammation from fighting off these invaders. The result is that immunity becomes weakened. When the immune system is so overwhelmed by environmental toxins, other pathogens can get a foothold.

Bacteria, like viruses, are living organisms and communicate with and learn from each other. They also are able to change shape, which they do to camouflage themselves to hide from the immune system.

Another problem with excessive use of antibiotics is that they kill off both bad and good bacteria. Our bodies are full of beneficial bacteria, from our skin to our digestive system, which carries about 5 pounds of bacteria. It is our immune system's first line of defense. Good digestive bacteria destroy bad bacteria in our gut from the foods we eat and are also responsible for the digestive process, breaking down the food in the gut so that the body can absorb and use it.

By killing off good bacteria with antibiotics, the body's natural balance is thrown off, allowing bad bacteria to proliferate. It is why people on repeated doses of antibiotics often suffer yeast infections and users are advised to eat yogurt or take a probiotic supplement to replace the beneficial bacteria. People prone to bacterial infection do not have enough good or beneficial bacteria present in the digestive system. It is also a sign that the underlying cause has not been addressed. Unfortunately, conventional medicine will keep administering round after round of antibiotics, treating symptoms without finding and treating the root cause. When young children are routinely given multiple doses of antibiotics per year, this weakens their immune systems before they've had a chance to fully develop.

The human body is designed to heal itself and doctors aren't omnipotent. In reality, doctors can't heal a simple cut or bruise. It's the body that heals itself. Doctors can cut us open and remove body parts, but it is the body that recovers and heals us. The human body is self-contained and equipped to battle microbes and viruses, or mend a simple wound. It does everything it can to heal and protect itself to its last dying breath. The body performs all these functions perfectly until we abuse it, intentionally or unintentionally. When we stop abusing it and nourish it properly, most of the time it will spring back to life.

We are brainwashed into believing Lichen Sclerosis and so many other diseases came out of nowhere. People don't try to figure out what precipitated it or how to mitigate it. Instead, all they want is a magic cream or pill, and the pharmaceutical companies are more than willing to supply them, often at the expense of our health.

Conventional allopathic medicine describes an auto-immune disorder as "the body turning against itself." But the human body wasn't designed to do that. Rather, it was designed to protect itself at all costs. Compare it to an animal with its leg caught in a trap and will gnaw off its leg to save itself. One way to view it is that the animal turned against itself by destroying its limb, but in reality it is trying to save its own life.

The human body does the same thing. It increases cholesterol output to protect its cells against inflammation from toxic overload. It destroys cells mutated by chemical infiltration. It's not turning against itself, it's trying to preserve itself.

We've all heard or seen how missing rivets, or weakened metal at key supports have caused buildings to collapse. And so it is with the human body. When pathogens invade and take up residence anywhere, the body becomes weakened. When toxins are stored in our tissues, our organs become weakened. Eventually the body collapses under the weight of toxic overload, just like a building with a weakened structure.

The human body can also be compared with a massive network of highways. Every minute of the day, bodily roads are congested with "vehicles" delivering proteins, enzymes, vitamins, minerals, and molecules to every cell. Some make a return trip, carrying used molecules, cellular debris, and other waste to our organs for cleaning, and elimination. But along the way, toxins, such as sodium lauryl and sodium laureth sulfates build chemical bridges in our cells, creating a roadblock. The body then must take an alternate route to deliver the needed nutrients. When another toxin appears, blocking the body's path to delivering key nutrients, yet another detour must be made. As each detour is taken, the delivery time is slowed down and sometimes stops. When this happens, the body does what it can with too little of something it needs, depending upon what can get through the toxic traffic jam. And this is how we end up with disease.

This is also why diseases recur: because once we have cured ourselves, we repeat the same behavior of toxic exposure that caused the original problem. This will result in a recurrence when the body has been forced to make the same detours.

Alternative medicine seeks to treat the human body as a whole. The idea is not to mask symptoms, create new symptoms, or blast the disease out of the body. Instead, the goal is to remove the roadblocks that have caused the body to dysfunction in the first place. Alternative medicine gives our body the biological information and rebuilding blocks it needs to heal itself. This type of medicine does not have the side effects of conventional or allopathic medicine, some of which can be fatal, because alternative medicine works by optimizing our body's own natural healing capacity. Alternative medicine works synergistically with the body and it uses what is already found in nature, substances that the body recognizes and can use.

I found a good explanation of how alternative medicine works by Dr. Randy Wysong. He described chondroitin as *"A protein-carbohydrate complex derived from cartilage, which promotes the health of bones, joints, tendons and cartilage. Regular supplementation with chondroitin promotes the health of bones, joints, tendons, and cartilage."*

When making soup stock, I simmer bones until joint cartilage liquefies. This liquefied substance is natural, not synthesized, chondroitin the body recognizes and can use. This made clear to me how alternative medicine works, and in particular, how nutraceuticals would help me to overcome Lichen Sclerosis.

Despite my criticisms, allopathic medicine has its place. For example, cancer survivors rightfully acknowledge the fact that they are alive because of the allopathic medical intervention they received and I have no argument with that. I've benefited from foot surgery myself, which could not have been corrected any other way. Today, some 30+ years later, my foot is still perfect, with no pain whatsoever. Could alternative medicine have accomplished this outcome? No.

Even though it may seem that I have trashed conventional allopathic medicine and ruled it out, that is not the case. In saving lives from gunshot wounds, or putting people back together after horrific accidents, modern allopathic medicine *is* amazing. But in the end, it is the human body that heals itself after these miraculous interventions. This is why people with the same diseases receiving the same treatments can have opposite outcomes. It all depends on the individual's body.

In many instances, conventional and alternative medicine can work together. But unfortunately, most doctors look upon alternative medicine with skepticism and in conventional medical schools they are not trained to use it. Only doctors who take an interest in alternative medicine become open to working with it. This kind of combined effort of the two approaches to medicine can greatly benefit a patient.

An example of how well this combination can work is seen in how the elderly uncle of a friend in China was treated for a serious illness. The uncle contracted Severe Acute Respiratory Syndrome (SARS), which is an acute form of pneumonia that afflicted thousands in 2003 and resulted in at least 750 deaths in China. The uncle was hospitalized and treated with western medicine to "knock the virus down," followed by Traditional Chinese Medicine (TCM) treatment to nurture him back to health.

Conventional medicine has made great strides in saving lives treating cancer, and many cancers now have a high survival rate. But "curing" people almost always involves pumping patients full of chemicals that not only kill the disease, but destroy just about everything else in their bodies. Conventional medicine also is miraculous when it can cut out a tumor or remove a diseased limb or organ, or replace it with a transplant or mechanical device.

In other words, if you can be blasted with chemicals or radiation, or be sliced and diced to obtain a cure, conventional medicine works. And I'll be the first to admit that if I lost a limb or organ and received a prosthesis or transplant that allowed me to continue a "normal" life, I'd be very grateful to conventional medicine. There *is* cutting edge technology being developed at this moment, including regrowth of organs and body parts, and this is truly miraculous.

But in terms of preventing disease in the first place, or curing chronic diseases and illnesses, conventional medicine's track record isn't very good. In those cases the most conventional medicine can offer is maintenance.

Conventional medicine offers no cure for a host of chronic or fatal illnesses, including Lichen Sclerosis, ALS (Amyotrophic Lateral Sclerosis aka Lou Gehrig's Disease) Alzheimer's, Arthritis, Autism, Emphysema, Fibromyalgia, Multiple Sclerosis, Parkinson's, or any of the other, ever-increasing number of auto-immune disorders too numerous to list. In those cases, allopathic medicine can offer only drugs that suppress symptoms and/or suppress the immune system to slow the disease's progression, along with pain maintenance. Unfortunately, none of that is miraculous.

Some believe that alternative medicine and a healthier lifestyle is not only the cure for disease, but also its prevention. And yet there is no guarantee either way. People choose allopathic medicine and die anyway, and it happens with the alternative medicine route, too. And maybe some of it comes down to luck in finding the right path that will work for a given individual.

For me, conventional medicine did not hold out any hope for curing my LS; it could only offer the suppression of my symptoms by suppressing my immune system, and that's why I searched for an alternative solution. I wanted to find an approach that treated my body as a whole, interconnected organism, making my body stronger so it could overcome the disease on its own, rather than merely trying to treat my symptoms. I was also forced to adopt a new outlook and way of living.

I'd felt hurt and angry when my husband blamed me for my Lichen Sclerosis, but in a way he was right. For my entire life, I'd used products that contained an ever-growing list of ingredients that not only could I not pronounce, but had no idea what they were. I'd had some misgivings about them, but never bothered to research them. The same thing applied to food. As

Dr. Mitchell said, I had behaved myself into having a disease.

To truly heal requires an about-face in mindset and lifestyle, and a change in philosophy and behavior. What I present in this book is a radically different approach to LS compared to conventional medicine. And by drastically altering my lifestyle, no longer being too lazy to examine and investigate everything before allowing it to enter my life, I was able to behave myself out of that disease.

My approach is nothing like what Lichen Sclerosis sufferers have been led to believe by conventional medicine. We are told LS is incurable because allopathic medicine tells us so. That means we don't search for, or even demand, answers. Because it's an auto-immune disorder, it sounds scary, mysterious, and unconquerable. We have been told to smear toxic substances on our bodies for the rest of our lives that won't cure us or get to the root of the disease, and just might make it worse. Every allopathic medication used in treating LS is immuno-suppressive. So, when our bodies are telling us something is wrong, conventional medicine treats our body like a protestor and tries to medically silence it.

For me, applying a toxic cream for the remainder of my life to treat my LS was unacceptable. I didn't agree with that approach, so I developed one of my own.

Sources:

U.S. Department of Health and Human Services, Health Resources and Services Administration (HRSA), National Vaccine Injury Compensation Program. http://www.hrsa.gov/vaccinecompensation/

U.S. Department of Health and Human Services, Health Resources and Services Administration (HRSA), National Vaccine Injury Compensation Program Fact Sheet.
http://www.hrsa.gov/osp/vicp/fact_sheet.htm

U.S. Department of Health and Human Services, Vaccine Injury Compensation Trust Fund.
http://www.hrsa.gov/vaccinecompensation/VIC_Trust_Fund.htm

USFDA, Protein Sciences Corp. Flublok Package Insert, "Contraindications, Warnings and Precautions." http://www.fda.gov/BiologicsBloodVaccines/Vaccines/ApprovedProducts/ucm335836. htm, STN_125285.0_Package_Insert.pdf

USFDA, "Vaccines, Blood & Biologics: Flublock®, Updated February 12, 2013. http://www.fda.gov/BiologicsBloodVaccines/Vaccines/ApprovedProducts/ucm335836htm

USFDA, Protein Sciences Corp. Summary Basis for Regulatory Action, January 16, 2013. http://www.fda.gov/BiologicsBloodVaccines/Vaccines/ApprovedProducts/ucm335836. r_Flublok_Corrected_SBRA_125285_0_508_2.pdf

USFDA 2009 Summary Report: Antimicrobials Sold or Distributed for Use in Food-Producing Animals, December 9, 2010. http://www.fda.gov/AnimalVeterinary/NewsEvents/CVMUpdates/ucm236143.htm. PDF

U.S. General Accounting Office, Report to the Chairman, Committee on Health, Education, Labor and Pensions, U.S. Senate, "Vaccine Injury Compensation: Program Challenged to Settle Claims Quickly and Easily, December 1999. www.gao.gov/new.items/he00008.pdf

Centers for Disease Control and Prevention, "Seasonal Influenza (Flu) Questions & Answers, Vaccine Effectiveness – How Well Does the Flu Vaccine Work?" www.cdc.gov/flu/about/qa/vaccineeffect.htm)

Centers for Disease Control and Prevention, 'Ingredients of Vaccines – Fact Sheet." www.cdc.gov/vaccines/vac-gen/additives.htm

Centers for Disease Control and Prevention, Vaccine Adverse Event Reporting System (VAERS), Updated 2012. http://www.cdc.gov/vaccinesafety/Activities/vaers.html

Centers for Disease Control and Prevention, "Fact Sheet: Basic Information About Severe Acute Respiratory Syndrome SARS." http://www.cdc.gov/ncidod/sars/factsheet.htm

Federal Register, Table 11 - Fee Schedule for FY 2012, Vol. 76, No. 147, August 1, 2011, Notices, Page 45837. http://www.gpo.gov/fdsys/pkg/FR-2011-08-01/pdf/2011-19332.pdf

Attkisson, Sharyl, "Gardasil Researcher Speaks Out", CBS News, August 29, 2009. www.cbsnews.com/stories/2009/08/19/cbsnews_investigates/main5253431.shtml?tag=re1.channel

Baker, S. L., "FDA Approved Big Pharma Drugs Without Effectiveness Data," Natural News, May 4, 2011. http://www.naturalnews.com:80/032279_Big_Pharma_fraud.html

Belkin, Michael, "Belkin's Testimony to Congress Concerning Hepatitis B Vaccine," May 18, 1999. Abstract. http://www.medicalveritas.com/images/00007.pdf

Belkin, Michael, Testimony Before the Advisory Committee On Immunization Practices -- Centers for Disease Control and Prevention, February 17, 1999. http://www.nvic.org/vaccines-and-diseases/Hepatitis-B/michaelbelkin.aspx

Dow Chemical Company, Triton™-100 Product Sheet. http://www.dow.com/products/market/oil-and-gas/product-line/triton/product/triton-x-100/

Eli Lilly Faculty Registry, Payments to Individuals and Grants to Organizations. http://www.lillyfacultyregistry.com/pages/lilly-registry-report.aspx

Erickson, Norma, "Gardasil Fingerprints Found in Post-Mortem Samples," S.A.N.E. Vax, Inc., October 23, 2012. http://sanevax.org/breaking-news-gardasil-fingerprints-found-in-post-mortem-samples/

Estate of Tambra Harris vs Secretary of the Department of Health and Human Services, United States Court of Federal Claims, Stipulated Damages Decision, No 01-499V, March 23,2011. http://www.uscfc.uscourts.gov/sites/default/files/CAMPBELL-SMITH.HARRIS032311.pdf

Galland, Dr. Leo, Pill Advised. http://pilladvised.com/

Galland, Dr. Leo, "Memory Loss Can Be Caused By Over-The-Counter Drugs," The Huffington Post, March 19, 2011. www.huffingtonpost.com/leo-galland-md/memory-loss-drugs-_b_822245.html

GlaxoSmithKline, Fees Paid to US Based Healthcare Professionals for Consulting and Speaking Services, 4th Quarter 2009. http://gsk-us.com/docs-pdf/responsibility/hcp-fee-disclosure-2q-4q2009.pdf

Goldman, G.S. and N.Z. Miller, *"Relative Trends in Hospitalizations and Mortality Among Infants by the Number of Vaccine Doses and Age, Based On the Vaccine Adverse Event Reporting System (VAERS), 1990-2010."* Sage Journals, Human & Experimental Toxicology, 2013. http://het.sagepub.com/content/31/10/1012.full

Health Sentinel, "United States Disease Death Rates." http://www.healthsentinel.com/joomla/index.php?option=com_content&view=article&id=2654:united-states-disease-death-rates&catid=55:united-states-deaths-from-diseases&Itemid=55

Heyes, J. D., "The True Story of SV40, the Cancer-Causing Virus Hidden in Polio Vaccines," Natural News, June 29, 2011. http://www.naturalnews.com:80/032854_SV40_polio_vaccines.html

Hilleman, Dr. Maurice, Edward Shorter interview with Dr. Maurice Hilleman in conjunction with WGBH Public Television and Blackwell Science. http://www.youtube.com/watch?v=edikv0zbAIU. Uploaded by Dr. Leonard Horowitz

Hoffer, Dr. Abraham et al. *"Hospitals and Health: Your Orthomolecular Guide to a Shorter, Safer Hospital Stay."* Basic Health Publications. February 28, 2010

Hyman, Mark, M.D., "Glutathione: The Mother of All Antioxidants," The Huffington Post, April 10, 2010. http://www.huffingtonpost.com/dr_mark_hyman/glutathione-the-mother-of_b_530494.html

Jernigan, David A. Jernigan, B.S., *Beating Lyme Disease*, Somerleyton Press, 2008

King, Paul G., Ph.D.,"A Critical Review of Medscape Medical News Article: 'Evidence Suggests Vaccines Do Not Cause Autism," Coalition for Mercury-Free Drugs (CoMeD), October 21, 2005. http://mercury-freedrugs.org/docs/051101_Thimerosal(49_55_%20Hg)CausesHgPoisoning_III_DrOrensteina.PDF

Leape, Lucian L., M.D., "Error in Medicine," JAMA, December 21, 1944. Vol 272. No. 23.
gawande.com/documents/ErrorinmedicineWhathavewelearned.pdf

Lee, Sin Hang, "Detection of Human Papillomaviurs L1 Gen DNA Fragments in Postmortem Blood and Spleen After Guardasil Vaccination – A Case Report," Advances in Bioscience and Biotechnology. 2012, 3, 1214-1224. https://www.dropbox.com/s/46m4o78mybhsz9f/ML%20-%20Lee%202012%20Advances%20in%20Bioscience%20and%20Biotechnology%20-%20Detection%20of%20human%20papillomavirus%20L1%20gene%20DNA%20fragments%20in%20postmortem%20blood%20and%20spleen%20after%20G.pdf

Loudon, Manette, "The FDA Exposed: An Interview with Dr. David Graham, the Vioxx Whistleblower," Natural News, August 30, 2005. http://www.naturalnews.com/011401_Dr_David_Graham_the_FDA.html

Madsen, K. M. et al, "Thimerosal and the Occurrence of Autism: Negative Ecological Evidence From Danish Population-Based Data," U.S. National Library of Medicine, National Institutes of Health, Pediatrics. 2003, Sep: 112(3Pt 1):604-6. http://www.ncbi.nlm.nih.gov/pubmed/12949291

Meeting of the Immunization Practices Advisory Committee (ACIP) of the Centers for Disease Control, Atlanta, Georgia, May 12, 1986. www.nvic.org/cmstemplates/nvic/pdf/acip-may-12-1986-transcript.pdf,

Merck, Fees Paid to US Based Healthcare Professionals for Consulting and Speaking Services, 4th Quarter 2009. http://us.gsk.com/docs-pdf/responsibility/hcp-fee-disclosure-2q-4q2009.pdf

Mercola, Dr. Joseph, "Flacking for Big Pharma," February 14, 2013. http://articles.mercola.com/sites/articles/archive/2013/02/14/big-pharma-tricks.aspx?e_cid=20130214_PRNLv1_art_2&utm_source=prmrnl&utm_medium=email&utm_campaign=20130214

Mercola, Dr. Joseph, "How to Tell if Your Doctor is on the Drug Industries' Payroll," January 14, 2012. http://articles.mercola.com/sites/articles/archive/2012/01/14/medical-experts-paid-off-by-drug-companies.aspx

Mercola, Dr. Joseph, "Always Question This Advice – Facts Which Will Make Your Blood Boil," May 12, 2011.
http://articles.mercola.com/sites/articles/archive/2011/05/12/modern-medicines-fatal-flaw-death-by-propaganda-part-i-the-paradoxical-paradigm.aspx

Mercola, Dr. Joseph, "Average Drug Label Lists Over a Whopping 70 Side Effects," June 9, 2011.
http://articles.mercola.com/sites/articles/archive/2011/06/09/average-drug-label-lists-over-whopping-70-side-effects.aspx

Mercola, Dr. Joseph, "Drug Company Had Hit List for Doctors Who Criticized Them," April 23, 2009.
http://articles.mercola.com/sites/articles/archive/2009/04/23/Drug-Company-Had-Hit-List-for-Doctors-Who-Criticized-Them.aspx

Mercola, Dr. Joseph, "How Drug Companies Bribe Doctors to Suck You Into Their Web," September 25, 2010.
http://articles.mercola.com/sites/articles/archive/2010/09/25/the-secret-weapon-drug-companies-use-to-manipulate-your-doctor.aspx

Mercola, Dr. Joseph, "New Study Shows Using Statins Actually Worsens Your Heart Function," June 22, 2011.
http://articles.mercola.com/sites/articles/archive/2011/06/22/new-study-show-using-statins-actually-worsens-your-heart-function.aspx

Mitchell, Dr. Roby. http://drfitt.com

National Vaccine Information Center, http://www.nvic.org/reportreaction.aspx

Null, Gary, Ph.D. et al. Death by Medicine, "Introduction," Praktikos Books, 2011.

Null, Gary, Ph.D. et al. "Death by Medicine."
http://www.webdc.com/pdfs/deathbymedicine.pdf.
http://www.wnho.net/deathbymedicine.htm

Olsen, Gwen, "Pharma Doesn't Want to Cure You." Video.
http://www.gwenolsen.com/?page_id=391

Olsen, Gwen, "Rx Companies & the FDA." Video.
http://www.gwenolsen.com/?page_id=391

Olsen, Gwen, "The Mission." Video.
http://www.gwenolsen.com/?page_id=391

Pfizer, Individuals and Grants Payments, 4th Quarter 2009.
http://media.pfizer.com/files/responsibility/grants_payments/pfizer_us_grants_cc_q4_2009. PDF.
http://www.pfizer.com/responsibility/working_with_hcp/payments_report.jsp

PharmedOut, PharmedOut.org. http://pharmedout.org/

Prescription Drug User Fee Act (PDUFA).
http://www.fda.gov/ForIndustry/UserFees/PrescriptionDrugUserFee/default.htm

S.A.N.E. Vax, HPV Vaccine VAERS Reports. Accessed October 2011. http://sanevax.org/

S.A.N.E. Vax, HPV Vaccine VAERS Reports. Accessed February 2013. http://sanevax.org/

S.A.N.E. Vax, Inc., Vaccine Victims – Memorial. http://sanevax.org/victims/memorial.shtml

Scott-Mumby, Keith, M.D., "Jon Rappaport Interviews an Ex-Vaccine Worker." http://www.alternative-doctor.com/vaccination/rappaport.htm

Sinclair, Ian, "Graphical Evidence Shows Vaccines Didn't Save Us," Vaccination Debate, VacLib.org, August 20007. http://www.vaclib.org/sites/debate/web1.html

Statement of The Association Of American Physicians & Surgeons to the Subcommittee On Criminal Justice, Drug Policy, and Human Resources of the Committee on Government Reform U.S. House of Representatives. Submitted by Jane Orient, M.D., June 14, 1999. http://articles.mercola.com/sites/articles/archive/2008/01/02/hepatitis-b-vaccine-part-four.aspx

Sykes, Rev. Lisa Karen, "Glutathione Deactivation," Letter to Congressmen Dan Burton, Dave Weldon, and Senator Chuck Grassley, Coalition for Mercury-Free Drugs (CoMeD), March 15, 2005. http://mercury-freedrugs.org/, http://www.sacredsparkbook.com/HOME%20PAGE.html

Tomljenovic, Lucija and Christopher A. Shaw, "Death after Quadrivalent Human Papillomavirus (HPV) Vaccination: Causal or Coincidental?" Pharmaceutical Regulatory Affairs: Open Access, 2012, S12:001, http://dx.doi.org/10.4172/2167-7689.S12-001

VaccineInjury.Info, "Illnesses in Unvaccinated Children." http://www.vaccineinjury.info/vaccinations-in-general/health-unvaccinated-children/survey-results-illnesses.html

Wysong, Dr. Randy, "Chondroitin," *100 Pet Health Truths*, www.WysongPetHealth.net

Chapter 7
Disease Free

"Your time is limited, so don't waste it living someone else's life. Don't be trapped by dogma - which is living with the results of other people's thinking. Don't let the noise of others' opinions drown out your own inner voice. And most important, have the courage to follow your heart and intuition. They somehow already know what you truly want to become. Everything else is secondary." Steve Jobs

Along with LS, I had myriad minor, "unrelated" problems. Then I began having allergic reactions to dairy products and nuts, which was a new problem. I have come to learn that these symptoms, along with light sensitivity and others are not only symptoms of Lyme disease, but also the signatures of chemical toxicity.

By now, I was anxious to begin the healing program I'd cobbled together, hoping it might be the key to my cure, understanding that it required a leap of faith, and realizing it would be a huge undertaking requiring time, discipline, and money. My husband thought it was foolish and just another example of my desperation.

By that point, I'd already altered our lifestyle in bits and pieces, first by removing toxic products, then by switching to a strictly organic diet, until finally beginning my pieced-together healing protocol in January of 2010. I had gathered a substantial collection of supplements, raw organic ginger root, a closet full of Epsom salts and hydrogen peroxide, and bottles of botanicals, all of which I wanted to use to try to heal myself. I took the plunge on January 18, 2010.

By March, I couldn't see or feel the white spot between my left labia minora and labia majora. I thought I felt and saw changes in my perineum. From what I could see in a mirror, the white spot on my perineum now seemed pinker but still lighter than the rest of my skin. It also felt smoother some days, but then wrinkled again at times. Was I imagining it? There was no denying that it felt more elastic, and was no longer tearing or bleeding. Not only that, but I had no redness or cracking in my bellybutton, the itching rashes under my bra were gone. I began eating nuts and dairy products again without any reactions.

My six-month checkup was scheduled for mid-April, three months after starting the full healing protocol. As the appointment date neared, I felt excited and apprehensive. I was sure the doctor would see my miraculous recovery, but I worried that perhaps I was imagining it; in that case, I'd be extremely disappointed.

To my delight, Dr. Jacobs' examination and test results confirmed what I knew. The white spot on my perineum was smaller and mixed with pink blotches, and the puckering was gone. She described my perineum as "smooth and supple." I actually had to remind her that between my left labias there had been a white spot, which she could no longer find. A body composition analysis showed that I was healing on a cellular level. We were both excited by my recovery, and she didn't scoff at my research or downplay the changes I'd made in my life. Instead, she asked if I would consult with some of her other patients and urged me to write this book.

At my one-year checkup in October 2010, eight months into the full healing protocol, Dr. Jacobs declared that I was completely healed. All of my test result numbers were exactly where they should be, and she changed my medical status from a Lichen

Sclerosis patient back to a regular gynecology patient requiring only annual checkups.

I am totally free of Lichen Sclerosis, and as of 2014, have been free of it for four years. For about two years after completing the year-long healing protocol, my perineum was sensitive, and while pink, I was disappointed it was still paler than the surrounding skin. As more time passed, I came to realize that my body was replacing my LS-affected skin, one cell at a time, with scar tissue. Now, several years after having completed my healing protocol, my skin is completely healed, it is the same color as the surrounding tissue, my perineum is no longer sensitive, and there is no trace that I ever had LS. And while my right labia minora will never regain its former size, what remains is full and healthy looking.

My change in lifestyle is permanent, and I will continue indefinitely to use basic organic products for all personal care and household maintenance, and eat only organic foods at home and as much as possible everywhere else. It is important that we continue chemical detoxification as we are constantly bombarded with toxins in the air we breathe, the water we drink, and the foods we eat out in the real world. I will continue to follow a healthy lifestyle for the remainder of my life, and continue with whole food vitamins, detox tea occasionally, periodic soaks, and perhaps a round or two of botanicals every now and then if I feel they are necessary.

It takes time to heal, but the body can and will heal itself, given the right conditions and help. The rule of thumb is that it takes 3-4 months of healing for every year of illness. I had LS for two years before implementing this program, so I estimated it would take at least a full year of using it to recover completely. However, there were 30 years or longer of dysfunction to get to the point of developing LS, so I estimated that healing would be an ongoing process that could take as long as six years.

Does that sound too long, or not worth the effort? Consider this: in my mid-twenties I complained to a psychologist friend that if I started attending college at the age of 25, I'd be almost 30 by the time I graduated. He said, "But in four years, won't you still be almost 30, even if you don't attend college?" The point is that if total recovery from LS, as well as the problems leading up to Lichen Sclerosis was going to take me six years, those same six years were going to pass whether I chose to follow my healing protocol and continue a healthy lifestyle or not. I might as well pass the time doing what's best for my health.

After eight months, I discontinued a portion of my healing protocol, not only to give my body a rest, but to see if any symptoms reoccurred. Although I stopped taking the botanicals, I continued with the supplements, but scaled them back. Within only one month, I developed the early stages of an eye infection, although it was not as bad as it usually was and never progressed to a full-fledged infection. That was my one and only symptom after stopping the botanical portion of the protocol. I was ecstatic that I did not have any hint of a return of LS, but I was disappointed that an old problem had reared its ugly head again.

Eye infections had started in 1994. I've read that when the body begins to heal itself, it does so in reverse. The most recent problem is the first to go, while the oldest complaints will be the last to be healed. If the protocol is stopped before full healing takes place, some of the symptoms may return. Depending upon what they are, those symptoms are a sign of the stage the body has reached in the healing process. So instead of being disappointed, I saw the eye problem as part of a healing timeline.

It soon became evident to me that although I appeared free of Lichen Sclerosis, the healing program needed to be in place for a *minimum of one year* to allow my body to heal further. It was important to repair the path my body had taken on the road to Lichen Sclerosis. If those pathways were not healed as well, they eventually could lead me to a recurrence of LS.

I have no idea how much longer I would have needed to continue the healing protocol if I'd had Lichen Sclerosis for a longer time, or if my LS symptoms had resurfaced. What I do know is that if I had stopped the protocol and the symptoms of LS had reappeared, I would have finished the protocol and then started the program over and continued for another full year, repeating it until I could stop without a reoccurrence of any symptoms of LS or anything else. Then I'd know I had recovered enough for my body to fully repair itself without further assistance from my healing protocol.

Do I think that my disease was caused by Lyme? No, I do not, because Lyme can mimic the symptoms of toxicity. I now realize the body reacts the same to toxins whether they are chemical, bacterial, or viral in origin. I believe that I suffered toxic overload from numerous sources. The reason I know it isn't from Lyme is because I'd begun to experience escalating health issues long before I'd met my husband, long before he'd contracted Lyme, and long before Lyme was ever identified as a disease.

I also realized that there are very few diseases; those caused by bacteria, viruses, or other pathogens. Instead, "unrelated" chronic and auto-immune conditions such as Lichen Sclerosis are really our body's genetic makeup reacting to toxic overload. It is the only logical common link that explains how these chronic and auto-immune disorders in general and

Lichen Sclerosis in particular affect every gender, age, and race around the world.

Regardless of the source of illness, the healing protocol's design seems to address multiple health issues, which was proven by clearing up *all* of my "unrelated" health problems, as well as those of the case studies.

It was very important that each part of the 3-phase program be integrated simultaneously. Every aspect was chosen to work synergistically. I couldn't try just one or two things and expect to get well. LS sufferers can't just take botanicals or supplements while continuing with a lifestyle that piles on the poisons, and expect to heal. It took years to develop LS, so it would take time, discipline, and a change in mindset to get well. It wasn't cheap, but you can't put a price tag on your health. Everyone has to make that choice for themselves.

As for my husband, this once-doubting critic who had been so angry with me and had accused me of being foolish and desperate now believed that I was really on to something. He went from grudgingly going along with me to being my greatest champion and supporter, telling everyone he talks to that if they follow the healing protocol presented in this book, their diseases and symptoms will heal.

Chapter 8
Preliminary Testing

The following tests are important for establishing a baseline before starting phase three of the healing protocol. They should be repeated periodically to measure progress towards healing:

1. A bio-impedance reading for Intracellular Fluid (ICF) level

2. A blood test for Lyme disease and/or Lyme antibodies

3. A blood test to measure vitamin and mineral levels

4. A blood test measuring cholesterol levels

5. Hs-C-Reactive Protein to measure inflammation

Comparisons to the original, or base-line, numbers will show how the body is healing on a molecular level.

BODY COMPOSITION ANALYSIS

It is important to have a baseline metabolic reading for cellular water levels and electrolytes. To obtain an ICW/ICF reading, a health care provider uses bio-impedance spectroscopy, which requires a small, hand-held, battery-operated device that sends multiple frequencies through the body via leads attached to the wrist and ankle. The meter on the device displays resistance, reactance, impedance, and phase, and calculates fat-free mass, fat mass, total body water, intracellular water, extracellular water, and their percentages. The patient must lie still for approximately 2-3 minutes and feels no sensations during the non-invasive test.

Knowing Intracellular Fluid (ICF) levels is important before starting any therapy because it provides insight into the level at which the cells are functioning and how damaged they are from years of exposure to toxins. Ideally, Intracellular Fluid levels should range between a low of 50% and a high of 60%, with 55% being the target. My initial ICF reading was a low 52.4%. Six months later it was up to 53.6%. Considering I'd only been on my three-phase healing program for four months, it was a significant increase. An ideal measurement is around 55% Intracellular Fluids, and 10 months after starting my healing program, my Intracellular Fluid level was at 55.3%.

LYME DISEASE AND LYME ANTIBODY TESTING

Being tested for Lyme disease and Lyme antibodies is important because Lyme spirochetes are toxic and inflame the immune system. Blood and/or urine testing will determine the presence of Lyme spirochetes (bacteria) or antibodies. Long-term Lyme sufferers frequently test negative. Even though my blood tests showed "inconclusive" for Lyme antibodies, my husband had been treated for Lyme. With the transfer of bodily fluids between husbands and wives, it was possible that microscopic Lyme toxins had entered my body. For this reason I was taking no chances and chose to take Lyme-specific as well as broad-based botanicals for detoxification and healing.

Those testing positive for Lyme disease who are being treated with antibiotics should wait to begin the healing protocol until after stopping the antibiotics. Antibiotics would render the healing protocol less effective as they may interfere with the body's own mechanisms to heal itself.

VITAMIN AND MINERAL TESTING

As a baseline, it's helpful to have a good knowledge of blood serum vitamin and mineral levels, especially Vitamin D, B complex, calcium, and others. If a test shows insufficient vitamin and mineral levels, take supplements. Healing cannot take place without the appropriate nutrients that the body requires to function optimally. More information on vitamin and mineral levels can be found in Chapter 9: Vitamins, Supplements, and Nutraceuticals.

HEAVY METALS TESTING

Many diseases, including auto-immune, Alzheimer's, and other neurological disorders, can be the result of accumulations of heavy metals in our bodies. The heavy metals aluminum, mercury, lead, and iron are known environmental toxins.

We ingest mercury in foods such as fish, aluminums in food ingredients, we absorb aluminum through the use of deodorants, iron from supplements and food sources, lead from very old paints, and lead from solder used to connect copper pipes in homes. We inhale heavy metals that have been released into the environment from automobile exhaust, through manufacturing plants, even if they are hundreds of miles away, and we have heavy metals injected into us if we receive vaccines.

If you have LS or another chronic condition, it's a good idea to be tested for heavy metal poisoning. Blood and urine are tested, along with hair and fingernails, which are the most accurate tests for heavy metal toxicity. If you test positive for heavy metal poisoning, you will need chelation therapy to remove the heavy metals from your body. This can be handled by conventional medical doctors and/or naturopaths.

Infrared sauna is another widely accept[ed method] of removing heavy metals. However, this mu[st be done] under medical supervision to ensure th[at proper] elimination procedures are followed; otherw[ise the] metals may become dislodged and move fro[m one part] of the body to another, creating new health problems.

CHOLESTEROL AND INFLAMMATION

It is important to know your cholesterol numbers, and having a cholesterol baseline helps in monitoring and comparing your level of inflammation over time. Theoretically, if your inflammation goes down, so will your cholesterol level.

In the United States, cholesterol-lowering drug advertisements focus on plaque buildup and platelets. The ads claim that the drugs will reduce "bad" cholesterol but this is an over-simplification. Here are the facts about cholesterol: There are several reasons for elevated cholesterol. One is hereditary, our body chemistry handed down to us through thousands of years of evolution.

Another reason for high cholesterol readings is dehydration. When we don't drink enough water, our cells become dehydrated and the body manufactures more cholesterol to keep the cells hydrated. Before having that morning cup of tea or java, drinking a glass of water first would be more beneficial because not only would it hydrate our cells, but it would aid in flushing toxins out of the kidneys. Most people do not drink enough plain water, as opposed to tea, coffee, or juice, substances that the body must filter to use. What we need is plain, pure water that our body is able to use immediately because it does not first need to be filtered.

The most serious reason the body manufactures high cholesterol is inflammation. Cholesterol lines the uter membrane of every cell, not only acting as a hydrator if not enough water is present, but also as a cell protector or cushion. Unfortunately, inflammation is destructive to cells, so the more inflammation in the cells, the more cholesterol the body manufactures to protect itself. Inflammation usually occurs when the body is burdened by dietary, pathogenic, and environmental toxins, including petrochemicals and heavy metals.

The body manufactures cholesterol because it needs it. A lipid derived from cholesterol lines the outer membrane of every cell. The integrity of every cell requires cholesterol, which is an integral function in building and repairing every cell in our body. In addition, the sterol in chole*sterol* is a necessary precursor for the body's manufacture of all steroid hormones, without which we cannot live.

Cholesterol is a fatty, waxy substance, 75% of which is manufactured in the liver. Because cholesterol is a complex molecule to manufacture and replace, the body efficiently recycles it. Cholesterol's viscous composition doesn't mix well into our watery blood, so it needs a chaperone in the form of LDL (low density lipoprotein) that attaches to and transports cholesterol from the liver to the tissues. In the same way, HDL (high density lipoprotein) attaches to and transports cholesterol from tissues back to the liver for refurbishing. LDL and HDL are not cholesterol at all. They are simply the *protein* shuttles that take cholesterol to and from bodily tissues. The liver is the detoxifier that cleans the blood of cellular debris, "used" cholesterol, toxins, etc. In reality, there is no good or bad cholesterol at all.

Triglycerides, which are large and small fats that we acquire through our diet, are also measured in a cholesterol test. However, testing lumps triglycerides together and doesn't differentiate particle sizes. Particle sizes are modulated by diet, and large triglycerides are synonymous with a diet of whole foods, vegetables, fruits, whole grains, and non-hydrolyzed fats. Small triglycerides develop through a poor diet of white flour, processed, and hydrolyzed fat foods, and it is the elevation of small triglycerides that are linked to heart disease and diabetes.

Our arteries have channels, called gap junctions, between cells, through which nutrients travel. When triglyceride particle size is large, it passes through our arteries and the gap junctions without problem. But when triglyceride particles are tiny, they tend to collect in the channels, and over time, these fats turn rancid and decay. This causes the cells lining our arteries to become damaged, which in turn causes inflammation. To try to heal itself when inflammation is present, the body creates arterial plaque, which is similar to a scab. As inflammation remains or worsens, plaque builds up further, the blood vessels constrict, and blood thickens so it can clot, keeping us from bleeding to death while the body tries to repair and/or replace damaged arterial cells.

When chemical, viral, or bacterial toxins are stored in our cells, it causes inflammation throughout our body and as a result, our body makes more cholesterol to protect itself.

Taking cholesterol-lowering drugs has no impact on plaque buildup because it does not address the body's natural response to cellular damage caused by inflammation. Lipoprotein (a), otherwise known as Lp(a), is composed of a part of low density lipoprotein (LDL), plus a protein called apoprotein a. Testing for an elevation of Lp(a) is the true key in determining if one is at risk for heart disease, not your total cholesterol numbers.

How the reduction of inflammation affects cholesterol is shown in the following charts, using my own test results starting with October 2009, when I was diagnosed with LS.

2009			
Total Cholesterol	238	Low = 111	High = 200
Triglycerides	142	Low = 20	High = 190
HDL	51	Low = 37	High = 92
LDL	158	Low = 0.0	High = 130

LDL interpretations:

Low Risk: Less than 130 mg/dL
Medium Risk: 130 – 139 mg/dL
High Risk: Greater than or equal to 160 mg/dL

But the numbers are only half of the story because it's the ratios that matter most.

- HDL/Cholesterol Ratio: HDL in relationship to overall cholesterol should be above 24%. To calculate the ratio, divide HDL by cholesterol number. In my 2009 chart, HDL was 51 and cholesterol was 238. If we divide 51/238, the ratio is 21%.

- Triglyceride/HDL Ratio: The ideal Triglyceride ratio should be below 2%. To calculate that percentage, divide the Triglyceride number by the HDL number. In my 2009 chart, Triglycerides were 142, and HDL was 51. If we divide 142/51, the ratio is 2.8%.

A year later, before my doctor confirmed that I had cured myself of Lichen Sclerosis, I expected that my test results would prove my body was healing based on the theory that cholesterol levels would drop along with declining inflammation. I was not disappointed and below is my cholesterol test chart for the following year, October 2010:

2010			
Total Chol	195	Low = 111	High = 200
Triglycerides	61	Low = 20	High = 190
HDL	88	L0w = 37	High = 92
LDL	94	L0w = 0.0	High = 130

Total cholesterol level had dropped 43 points, triglycerides had dropped 81 points, HDL had risen by 37 points, and LDL had dropped 64 points.

In terms of ratios, in 2009 my HDL/Cholesterol ratio was 21%. Ideally it should be above 24%. By dividing my 2010 HDL of 88 by the 195 cholesterol number, the ratio was now 45%, well above the 24% minimum.

Likewise, the triglyceride/HDL ratio also improved. The 2009 ratio was 2.8% but should be below 2%. By dividing the 2010 Triglyceride level of 61 by the HDL number of 88, the percentage dropped to 0.69%, or well below the maximum of 2%.

I eat the same food as I always have, except that food is now organic, unprocessed and mostly raw. I stopped using commercial products entirely, switching to very simple, organic-only products, and have allowed my body to recover from years of toxic buildup to the point of overload.

I have never taken cholesterol-lowering medication, which focus on a set of numbers, without addressing whatsoever the underlying cause for the high cholesterol readings.

Keep in mind that cholesterol levels are partially based upon pharmaceutical industry recommendations, which has a profit motive in revamping recommended cholesterol levels. In 2004, the National Cholesterol Education Program, which is part of the U.S. National Institutes of Health, advised patients at risk for heart disease to reduce their LDL cholesterol to specific very low levels. Eight of the nine doctors on the panel making this recommendation were subsidized by the pharmaceutical companies making statin cholesterol-lowering drugs. This probably isn't a coincidence.

In 2013, new cholesterol management guidelines were issued by the American College of Cardiology—American Heart Association Task Force on Practice Guidelines. One of the criteria for placing a patient on cholesterol-lowering medications is "anyone with a greater than 7.5% chance of having a heart attack, stroke, or developing other forms of cardiovascular disease in the next 10 years." In other words, these new guidelines place almost 93%, an estimated 35 million people, into a "risk" category for a condition they don't have and may never develop in a decade. It should come as no surprise that more than half of the 15-member panel making these recommendations have current or recent financial ties to pharmaceutical companies producing statins. Additionally, while the American Heart Association and the American College of Cardiology are non-profit entities, they are heavily subsidized by the pharmaceutical industry.

THE PROBLEM WITH LOW CHOLESTEROL

Very low cholesterol can result in serious consequences, including:

- Depression and suicide: Studies reveal that low cholesterol affects the metabolism of serotonin. Researchers have found that people in the lowest quarter of total cholesterol concentration had more than six times the risk of committing suicide than those with the highest concentrations.

- Aggression and Violence: Dozens of studies show a link between low cholesterol levels and violent behavior.

- Neurological Disorders: Studies show a connection between low cholesterol and Parkinson's disease, while recent studies point out a correlation between low cholesterol levels and an increased risk of ALS, Lou Gehrig's disease.

- Cancer: A recent study showed the correlation between low LDL and a greater risk of cancer in patients with no history of taking cholesterol-lowering drugs.

PROBLEMS RELATED TO USE OF STATINS

- Cancer: One analysis of over 41,000 patient records indicated a higher risk of cancer in those patients on statins. While statins themselves do not cause cancer, forcing the body into dangerously low LDL levels increases the risk of cancer.

- Rhabdomyolysis: Statins can cause this condition of muscle pain and weakness because they deplete the body of CoQ10 (Coenzyme Q10), which is instrumental in building and maintaining muscle tissue. The route by which the body manufactures cholesterol is the same it uses to manufacture CoQ10. Statins block the body's manufacture of cholesterol, and in so doing, block its pathway for CoQ10. The depletion of CoQ10 can lead to fatigue, muscle weakness, soreness, and eventually stroke, heart attack, and heart failure. Statistics show that people on statins are more likely to have strokes and/or heart attacks they are trying to avoid because the heart is a muscle and statins may weaken muscles by depleting CoQ10. Muscle pain and weakness also may be an indicator of tissue breakdown and signal the beginning of kidney damage. For this reason, anyone taking a statin drug must supplement with CoQ10 to avoid depleting the body of this essential enzyme. Note that the body's production of CoQ10 drops off after age 35 so supplementing with ubiquinol is recommended. For people with chronic disease, the body may have a difficult time breaking down CoQ10 into ubiquinol. Ubiquinol is the bio-available, active form of CoQ10 that is readily absorbed and used by the body. Recommended daily dose of ubiquinol is 100-200 mg.

Hs-CRP

Having this test done once a year would be a great way to monitor inflammation due to Lichen Sclerosis, or other health issues. And don't allow a doctor to tell you your cholesterol level is a heart disease indicator without first performing a test for an elevation of Lp(a), and a high sensitivity C-reactive protein test (Hs-CRP), which is an indicator of the level of inflammation in your body. It can indicate inflammation for any number of reasons, including auto-immune diseases, not necessarily heart disease. However, since nearly everyone will have some level of inflammation, the results still do not necessarily indicate heart disease. Having this test done periodically should indicate reduced inflammation readings as healing takes place on a cellular level.

Here are the basic risk levels of Hs-CRP readings:

Low Risk:	Less than 1.0 mg/L
Average Risk:	1.0 to 3.0 mg/L
High Risk:	Above 3.0 mg/L

THICKENED BLOOD

People with chronic illness tend to [have] depleted blood, which makes their blood more sluggish. Thickened blood leads to [low] temperature (less than 98.6°F) and in some cases low blood pressure. Because viruses, bacteria, and other pathogens thrive and proliferate in an oxygen-poor environment, people with this condition are open to additional health problems.

There is a very simple indicator for thickened blood, one that anyone can look for to determine if they fit into this category. Simply touch the tip of the tongue to the roof of the mouth. Underneath the tongue are numerous veins. There are two large dark veins; one on either side of the tongue, which is normal. If there are groups of dark veins that resemble clusters of grapes, it is a sign of thickened blood. A healthy individual will not have them, and the underside of a healthy tongue is pink.

When I was diagnosed with Lichen Sclerosis, my body temperature had been reading 97°F and my blood pressure was below normal. And, not only did I have the grape cluster of veins under my tongue, I had an entire vineyard. But having completed the healing protocol, my temperature is now normal, as is my blood pressure, and the underside of my tongue is a healthy pink.

Sources:

The American Heart Association, "Inflammation, Heart Disease and Stroke: The Role of C-Reactive Protein." http://www.americanheart.org/presenter.jhtml?identifier=4648

Body Composition Analysis Comes of Age, www.impedimed.com. Accessed December 24, 2010

Carey, John, "Do Cholesterol Drugs Do Any Good?" Business Week, January 17, 2008. http://www.businessweek.com/magazine/content/08_04/b4068052092994.htm

Enig, Mary and Sally Fallon, "The Skinny on Fats," The Weston A. ice Foundation, January 1, 2000. http://www.westonaprice.org/know-your-fats/526-skinny-on-fats

Fallon, Sally and Mary Enig, "Dangers of Statin Drugs: What You Haven't Been Told About Popular Cholesterol-Lowering Medicines," The Weston A. Price Foundation, June 14, 2004. http://www.westonaprice.org/modern-diseases/cardiovascular-disease/581-dangers-of-statin-drugs

Gleis, Radhia, CCN and Peter McCarthy, N.D., "Cholesterol Drug Scam – Wake Up America," Cholesterol – The Good, The Bad, The Ugly Truth DVD. http://www.youtube.com/watch?v=y3ubuK57h6Y

Jernigan, David, B.S., *Beating Lyme Disease*, Somerleyton Press, 2008

Mercola, Dr. Joseph, Video Transcript – Interview with Carole Baggerly, Founder Grassroots Health, "Why the New Vitamin D Recommendations Spell Disaster for Your Health," December 11, 2010. http://articles.mercola.com/sites/articles/archive/2010/12/11/vitamin-d-update-carole-baggerly-and-dr-cannell.aspx

Mercola, Dr. Joseph, "The Cholesterol Myth That Is Harming Your Health," August 10, 2010. http://articles.mercola.com/sites/articles/archive/2010/08/10/making-sense-of-your-cholesterol-numbers.aspx

Natural News, "Cardiologists on Big Pharma Kickbacks Release New Statin Drug Guidelines," November 20, 2013. http://www.omsj.org/blogs/cardiologists-double-statin-prescriptions

Rosedale, Ron, M.D., "Cholesterol is NOT the Cause of Heart Disease," May 28, 2005. http://articles.mercola.com/sites/articles/archive/2005/05/28/cholesterol-heart.aspx

Rosedale, Ron, M.D., "Exposing the Cholesterol Myth," March 25, 2008. Cholesterol – The Good, the Bad, the Ugly Truth DVD. http://www.youtube.com/watch?v=y3ubuK57h6Y
http://storesonline.com/site/708446/product/DVD29

Science Daily, "Low LDL Cholesterol Is Related to Cancer Risk," March 25, 2012. http://www.sciencedaily.com/releases/2012/03/120326113713.htm

Chapter 9
Vitamins, Supplements, and Nutraceuticals

"When you actually look at some of the diets experimentally, doing what we call heat maps (DNA or RNA micro-array), you will see the enzymes that are turned on, upregulated, and pro-inflammatory initially in a patient with a particular disease. When you treat them with the appropriate food and functional botanicals as necessary, those activated enzyme profiles will go down and will cleanse. And so the body will be healed." Dr. Jean Dodds and Dr. Karen Becker

Was there one cause for my Lichen Sclerosis? Yes, I believe there was, and is, one cause for Lichen Sclerosis, and that is *toxins* from every conceivable source.

There are far too many factors to try and determine how our bodies interact with toxins that will result in Lichen Sclerosis and it's impossible to pinpoint any one particular toxin when there are so many in multiple combinations. There are also contributing human factors and chemical reactions within the human body that fluctuate by the nano-second. To learn which ones are affected by what toxin or group of toxins at any particular time might take scientists an eternity to figure out. And for anyone with Lichen Sclerosis or another auto-immune disorder, there just isn't that much time to wait for an answer.

For anyone, sick or not, it is in our best interests to limit our exposure to as many toxins as practicable. The complete protocol spelled out in this book calls for the elimination of as many daily toxins as possible and provides the reader with a multi-layered framework for healing from the multitude of possibilities that have contributed to disease in general and Lichen Sclerosis in particular.

As described in Chapter 8, it's important to have readings of blood serum levels for important nutrients such as vitamins and minerals and to discuss the test results with a healthcare professional to get a clear picture of the state of a person's health on all levels. If, for instance, someone already has sufficient levels of vitamin D_3 without supplementation, then there would be no advantage in taking more.

Because most conventional doctors are not amenable to alternative medicine, I presented the list of ingredients I compiled for the LS healing protocol described in this book to my homeopathic practitioner for his consideration. He reviewed the list and checked product websites for further clarification, and I was relieved when he said *"If you want to go ahead with this, there's nothing in it that can hurt you."*

In this healing protocol, each vitamin, supplement, and nutraceutical has been chosen because they work together to optimize not only healing, but to bring all systems back into harmony to restore the body so it functions at the highest level.

When I was diagnosed with LS, I was not on any type of over-the-counter or prescription medication. This was fortunate because, as discussed previously, medications inhibit the body's normal functions. Coupled with the suppressive and mutative qualities of environmental toxins, the body must struggle to function as designed.

While natural supplements work with the body by providing key elements it needs, many prescription drugs either inhibit the body's natural production of important molecules, proteins, enzymes, and other chemicals, or else they interfere with the ability to assimilate nutrients.

An example of medication interfering with the body's assimilation of nutrients is found in the group known as corticosteroids, of which Clobetasol, a treatment for LS, is one. Corticosteroids suppress the immune system, impair vitamin D metabolization, and reduce calcium absorption, none of which is beneficial to the health of the patient using it.

Although some vitamins and supplements might be safer than prescription medications to accomplish the same results, there can be problems mixing them with prescription drugs. For example, Vitamin E, which the immune system needs in order to fight off viruses and bacteria, also acts as an antioxidant as well as the body's own natural blood anticoagulant. It also helps widen our blood vessels. It would seem logical then, that increased intake of Vitamin E would be more beneficial to heart health than taking anticoagulants or antiplatelet medications like Warfarin (Coumadin®).

But when Vitamin E intake is increased while taking drugs such as Warfarin, there is an increased risk of bleeding. According to the government's Vitamin E Fact Sheet:

"Vitamin E, plus other antioxidants (such as Vitamin C, selenium, and beta-carotene) reduced the heart-protective effects of two drugs taken in combination..."

Let me see if I got that right. According to the medical establishment, the government, and the pharmaceutical industry, *natural whole vitamins and minerals*, which the body can use immediately because they are bioavailable, and which offer all of the natural protection our body requires, *interfere with prescription medications*. Shouldn't it be the other way around? Shouldn't it be that these *drugs interfere* with the body's natural metabolism?

The human body is dependent upon many micronutrients, molecules, proteins, enzymes, amino acids, etc., that all work in combination and actually need each other in order to complete a process. Just as production lags when a worker is out sick or is underperforming, the body is the same way. If it is low or missing key elements, it cannot function optimally.

Some drugs have addictive or other dependent properties that can cause great harm when they are stopped without being tapered off under medical supervision. Anyone taking prescription medications must not stop taking them or begin any type of therapy without first consulting a physician. Doing so without proper medical supervision could have dire consequences. It is best never to step onto that allopathic drug treadmill in the first place, and this is why I am extremely thankful that my only "drugs" at the time of my Lichen Sclerosis diagnosis, were, and continue to be, natural whole vitamins.

HERXHEIMER REACTION

Adolf Jarisch, an Austrian dermatologist, and Karl Herxheimer, a German dermatologist, are credited with the discovery of the Herx reaction. Both doctors observed reactions in patients with various stages of syphilis when they were treated with Salvarsan, mercury, or antibiotics. Patients with early stage syphilis had a 50% reaction to treatment, while patients in the late stage of the disease had a 90% reaction to treatment.

Although you may not have heard of the Herxheimer reaction, you've probably experienced it at least once. The way it works is that when starting a course of treatment, especially an allopathic therapy, the patient often feels worse before feeling better, which is considered a positive sign that the drugs are working. Homeopathic medicine also considers a worsening of symptoms as a sign of being on the correct path to healing.

A Herxheimer reaction typically occurs during, but is not limited to, antibiotic therapy, when there is massive die-off of bacteria. These bacteria give off a toxin and inflame the immune system. It is our body's reaction to viral and bacterial toxins that make us feel sick in the first place, and, as bacteria and/or viruses die, they produce a secondary toxin. The body's reaction to this massive toxic die-off can take the form of a yeast infection, chills, fever, muscle pain, and rash. The intensity of the reaction is an indicator of the amount of die-off, which also indicates the level of inflammation.

Quite often, in addition to medical intervention for the initial illness, mainstream medicine focuses on treating symptoms of disease, dispensing more prescriptions for side effects, and ignoring and usurping the body's own mechanisms for self-healing.

Unlike many approaches, the alternative medicine route I took views a Herxheimer reaction as an indication of poor protocol management, so my protocol takes steps to ensure that no Herxheimer reaction occurs. This healing protocol for LS does not treat disease or its symptoms. The goal is not to blast any bacteria, virus, or disease into oblivion. Instead, through a change in mindset and lifestyle that uses organic, whole food nutrition, and carefully chosen non-toxic products, vitamins, supplements and nutraceuticals, the protocol focuses on providing diseased bodies with the building blocks needed to work its way back to health.

The human body was designed so that a healthy human being with a strong and vital immune system is not a viable host for disease. Only when the body is deficient, dysfunctional, or compromised can disease get a foothold and proliferate.

Toxins from the non-organic chemicals we ingest from all sources, and the chemical-laced products we use externally have wreaked havoc on our bodies. Fluoride in water has slowed down our thyroid, parabens have promoted the proliferation of cancer cells, and chemicals such as sodium lauryl sulfate have modulated our cells by destroying their protein structure.

I'm sure you've heard how exercise boosts the immune system and how it is important to get more oxygen into our system, but no one ever really explains why. It's important because viruses and bacteria thrive in an oxygen-poor atmosphere, so the converse is true. They can't survive in an oxygen-rich environment.

Think about it. What is a Petri dish if it isn't a closed, oxygen poor environment? Chemicals have turned our bodies into Petri dishes where bacteria and viruses can now harbor and thrive. As they proliferate, the body becomes even more sluggish, inviting in similar organisms to inhabit us as well. These other organisms are sometimes referred to as co-infections. One example of a virus and its co-infection is Hepatitis B. People with Hepatitis B will often contract Hepatitis C, Hepatitis D, and HIV.

Viruses and bacteria are living organisms, and all living organisms communicate. The viruses and bacteria in the human body also communicate with each other. They take many forms and change shape, and this is how "superbugs" and "drug resistant" organisms survive. When the same drugs are prescribed repeatedly, there are always surviving organisms and they alter their form. This makes them resistant to specific drugs because that drug is focusing only on a specific form of virus or bacteria. The scenario continues with every new drug that comes along, resulting in multi-resistant strains.

As described in Chapter 5, I found a group of nutraceuticals (botanicals), some of which had been developed to address the toxins of Lyme disease and its co-infections. While the original intent was to help the human body overcome and heal from Lyme disease toxins and those of its co-infections, the botanicals are broad spectrum enough to address *any* bacteria, virus, or co-infection, regardless of the origins.

Why would these botanicals be important, especially if we have never had Lyme disease? It's because we've all got pathogenic bacteria, as well as dormant viruses, inside us, clogging our body's streamlined systems, and adding another kink to the machinery. We harbor dormant viruses such as Herpes Varicella-Zoster, which takes the form of chicken pox as children and shingles as adults. Anyone with warts harbors a strain of the Human Papilloma Virus (HPV), and anyone who has had, or still gets cold sores has yet another strain of the Herpes virus. The Centers for Disease Control estimate that 92% of Americans have one or more strains of the Herpes virus, even if they've never had any symptoms.

Why does this matter to a person with Lichen Sclerosis? It's because Lichen Sclerosis is merely the tip of the illness iceberg. When I examined my life closely, even though I thought I was healthy, I realized that for years a number of little, seemingly unrelated things had been going wrong, well before getting the diagnosis of Lichen Sclerosis.

If I were going to get well, I needed a plan of attack that would address every conceivable way in which Lichen Sclerosis could have evolved, and to do so I would leave no stone unturned. I refused to allow this disease to become a permanent part of my life.

VITAMIN AND SUPPLEMENT FORMAT

Vitamins and supplements come in capsule, soft gel, or liquid, which are the preferred formats. Hard tablets will suffice if no other form is available. Capsules can be easily pulled apart and contents added to food or liquids. This is also important when contents must be divided over the course of a day, or an adult-size portion reduced due to child's age or weight. Soft gels can be pierced and contents added to food or liquids. Liquid vitamins and supplements can be taken orally or mixed with food or drink. All vitamins and supplements (except TPP Protease) should be taken with meals.

In the healing protocol for very young children, some vitamins are not essential and are indicated as such. However, if the reader wishes to include them for their child, the Homeopathic Rule of Thumb should be followed. As I began learning more about vitamins, I began taking not only a multi-vitamin, but individual supplemental vitamins as well.

VITAMINS

This section covers the vitamins that I and others have used during the healing protocol. It wasn't until I was nearly 50 that I began taking vitamins on a regular basis, and those consisted of your typical once or twice a day multi-vitamin.

I thought I was doing right by my body by using these items, but actually it was not only a hodgepodge of individual vitamins and minerals, but I found out that they were mostly synthetic vitamins. Synthetic vitamins may be better than no vitamins at all, but not only are they isolates, they are not bio-available, meaning they are not readily assimilated. Isolates means they are only part of a vitamin family, not the entire vitamin family that makes them a whole vitamin. They contain fillers and other ingredients that the human body does not need.

As I learned more about vitamins, the quality of the ones I was taking improved, but it wasn't until I was nearly finished with my healing protocol that I settled on organic whole food vitamins. Whole food vitamins are more expensive than the cheaper synthetic isolates. There are several whole food vitamins on the market, and they are available powdered and scoopable, or as capsules.

In nature, whole foods contain not only the vitamins and minerals we need, but contain the co-factors and transporters that synthetic, isolated vitamins do not contain. If they aren't derived from natural sources, they are synthetically made.

Vitamin manufacturers don't usually state the sources from which their vitamins are derived. Most of the isolates are imported from China. By isolates, as an example, Vitamin A (beta-carotene) will be marketed as an isolated beta-carotene, whereas in nature, beta-carotene is part of a complete family of carotenoids that includes alpha-carotene, canto-zantheen, gamma-carotene, omega-carotene, and others. Beta-carotene by itself is not a whole vitamin, but a partial vitamin that is combined with other chemical ingredients.

Are *Your* Vitamins Synthetic?

How can you tell if the vitamin/mineral supplements you are taking are synthetic or not? Actually, it's pretty simple. If the vitamins are from blends of whole fruits, vegetables, and/or their juices, then they are whole food vitamins. For instance, the Vitamin E that I currently take is made up of organic strawberry, cherry, blackberry, blueberry, raspberry, beet, carrot, spinach, broccoli, tomato, kale, red cabbage, Brussels sprout, bell pepper, cucumber, celery, garlic, ginger, green onion, cauliflower, and asparagus.

There are definite clues to whether your vitamins are natural or synthetic. If their names include or end in any of the following, they are synthetic:

- **ate** – Typically anything that ends in "ate" is synthetic. That includes, but is not limited to acetate, palmitate, monitrate, mononitrate, pantothenate, bitrate, bitartrate, picolinate, etc.

- **ide** – Anything ending in "ide" is another indicator that it is synthetic, including, but not limited to chloride, hydrochloride, niacinamide, etc.

- **in** – d-Biotin, riboflavin, cobalamin, etc. are synthetics.

- **ic** - Ascorbic, pteroylglutamic, aminobenzoic are all examples of synthetic vitamins.

- **dl** – Any vitamin that includes the letters dl is synthetic. An example is dl-alpha-tocopherol (synthetic Vitamin E).

The same rule of thumb used for the ingredients in personal or home care products can be applied to vitamins and supplements. If it didn't grow in nature on a tree, bush, flower, or contains a name you cannot pronounce or have no idea what it is, then do not swallow it.

Vitamin C is often marketed as ascorbic acid and I believed it was natural Vitamin C. But Vitamin C must be derived from citrus, or rose hips, which contain higher concentrations of Vitamin C than any other source including citrus fruits. Synthetic ascorbic acid is tart and can be added to beverages or foods. Rose hip powder is naturally sweet and can be added to food or liquids, or simply taken alone.

Listed below are the vitamins to use during the year-long healing protocol unless preliminary testing shows optimal levels. *If there is a medical reason why a particular vitamin or supplement cannot be taken, then omit it from the healing protocol.*

All vitamins are to be taken 7 days a week for the entire duration of the healing protocol.

As previously discussed, it is a good idea to have your blood analyzed to determine vitamin and mineral levels before adding vitamins. I prefer to take vitamins as capsules with powder contents. This makes it easy to travel with, open the capsule and mix the contents into food, or taken in smaller doses as needed. Some vitamins are available as soft gels and can be pierced to mix contents into food or liquid, or taken in smaller doses as needed. When giving vitamins to children, follow manufacturer's directions, or follow the Homeopathic Rule of Thumb.

HOMEOPATHIC RULE OF THUMB FOR CHILDREN

To calculate herbal formulas for children younger than 6: Divide child's weight into 150

Examples:

10 lbs/150 = 0.06, or 6-10 drops per day
30 lbs/150 = 0.20, or ¼ of adult dose
75 lbs/150 = 0.5, or ½ of adult dose

(Homeopathic Rule of Thumb for Children provided by Dr. Steven Coward, Asheville Health & Homeopathy, Asheville, North Carolina)

Where a dosage range is given, such as 2-3 times per day, always begin with the lowest dosage. For small children under the age of 6, always test using a drop or two to be certain there is no adverse reaction. Capsules and soft gels can be opened or pierced and contents can be added to food or liquids.

MULTIVITAMINS

Multivitamins are helpful in providing a little bit of everything. Because the body requires many nutrients, a one-a-day vitamin providing the maximum amounts of optimum nutrition would be the size of a golf ball. Any multivitamin that provides the best nutrition will most likely be taken in divided doses over the course of a day. For instance, I took six multivitamins per day without iron for menopausal women that my physician had recommended: two with breakfast, two with lunch, and two with dinner. However, they were hard tablets I will no longer take because not only were they synthetic vitamins, they included ingredients such as titanium dioxide. Now I take only organic whole food vitamins, even though they can be pricey. Whichever multi-vitamins you select, take the full dose the manufacturer recommends, unless they are to be given to children, in which case follow the "Homeopathic Rule of Thumb.

How to Take Multivitamin Capsules or Tablets:

- Children Under 6: Children's formula, follow manufacturer's directions or follow "Homeopathic Rule of Thumb." Always give children vitamins with meals. Note that whole food multivitamin capsules are preferable over children's chewables which are usually mostly sugar and artificial color.

- Children Ages 6-12: Children's formula (same as for Under 6 above)

- Teens to adult: Use the adult formula and dose, per the manufacturer's directions and always take vitamins with meals.

- Menopausal women should take a no-iron formula and always with meals.

All vitamins are to be taken 7 days a week for the duration of the healing protocol.

B-COMPLEX and B12 VITAMINS

B Vitamins are required for production of DNA in all cells, as well as metabolizing fat and carbohydrates. B vitamins are abundant in whole, unprocessed foods, and are concentrated in meats such as liver, as well as in poultry, dairy products, eggs, and seafood. They are also found in nutritional yeast, whole grains, bananas, potatoes, lentils, and beans. Together they play a major role in:

- Promoting normal immune function
- Promoting cell metabolism (growth and division)
- Maintaining healthy skin and muscle tone
- Enhancing immune and nervous system function
- Preventing anemia

People on restrictive diets or who have digestive issues can easily become deficient in B-complex and Vitamin B12. Symptoms of deficiency include:

- Chest pain and/or shortness of breath
- Fatigue/weakness
- Dizziness, fainting, or balance issues

- Cognitive impairment (confusion, memory loss, or dementia)
- Neurological issues including coldness, numbness, or tingling of hands or feet
- Diminished nervous system function or slow reflexes
- Pale or yellowing skin
- Sore mouth and tongue

Toxicity

Since the body excretes excess B vitamins, toxicity is not an issue.

How to Take Vitamin B Supplements:

B-complex capsule, 50 mg

- Children under the age of 6: Follow the Homeopathic Rule of Thumb.
- Children ages 6-12: 1 capsule per day with food or drink.
- Teens to adult: 1 capsule per day with food or drink.

B-12 capsule, 1000 mcg

- Children under age 6: Not essential for very young children, but if included, use Homeopathic Rule of Thumb and give with meals.
- Children ages 6-12: 1/2 capsule twice per day with meals.
- Teens to adults: 1 capsule per day with meals.

Vitamin B12 is also available in sublingual liquid form.

All vitamins are to be taken 7 days a week for the entire duration of the healing protocol.

VITAMIN C

Vitamin C acts as an antioxidant and is integral to the growth and repair of tissues throughout the body, as well as in wound healing, collagen production, and the repair and maintenance of teeth and bones.

Vitamin C deficiency includes:

- Dry, splitting hair
- Gingivitis and bleeding gums
- Rough, dry, or scaly skin
- Slow wound healing
- Bruising easily
- Nosebleeds
- Frequent infections

Optimal Vitamin C intake has been shown to be effective in protecting against or reducing the symptoms of:

- Common cold
- Cardiovascular disease
- Hypertension
- Cancer
- Osteoarthritis
- Macular degeneration
- Cataracts
- Asthma
- Auto-immune response

Drug Interactions

- Aspirin and over-the-counter anti-inflammatory drugs can deplete Vitamin C levels.

- Vitamin C supplementation can inhibit the release of Acetaminophen, Tetracycline, Doxycycline, and Minocycline, thereby increasing the levels of the drug in the bloodstream.

- Barbiturates may decrease the effectiveness of Vitamin C.

- Vitamin C may decrease the effectiveness of some chemotherapy drugs.

- Vitamin C may increase the body's absorption rate of aluminum from antacids, deodorants, from cooking ingredients containing aluminum, aluminum cookware, as well as the aluminum adjuvants in vaccines.

Raw, whole food Vitamin C is preferable to any other form. Studies show that natural Vitamin C with flavonoids is more slowly absorbed and is 35% more bio-available than its synthetic counterpart.

Unfortunately, most Vitamin C supplements are a synthetic isolate derived from corn, which may be GMO.

The most highly concentrated and naturally bio-available form of Vitamin C is rose hip powder. In addition to containing Vitamin C, rose hip powder includes Vitamins A, D, E, flavonoids, lycopene, and iron. Pure rose hip powder, with no additives is sweet but very sticky when moistened in the mouth. Rose hips are often added to powdered synthesized Vitamin C, which can taste very sour. Rose hip powder is also available in capsule form, which is the way I prefer to take rose hips. Read labels carefully before selecting rose hip capsules to ensure that they include only pure rose hip powder, without anti-caking agents or other additives.

Toxicity

Vitamin C is considered safe because the body excretes excess Vitamin C. However, people having too much iron in their blood should be cautious about raising their intake of Vitamin C because it will increase their iron absorption.

Taking more than 2000 mg of Vitamin C per day may cause diarrhea, gas, or stomach upset.

Always consult with a health care professional before taking large quantities of Vitamin C, especially before giving it or any vitamin to children.

How to Take Vitamin C Supplements:

150 mg capsule

- Children under age 6: Not essential for very young children, but if included, use the Rule of Thumb and always give with meals.
- Children ages 6-12: 1 capsule per day, always with meals.
- Teens to Adults: 1 capsule 2x per day, always with meals.

All vitamins are to be taken 7 days a week for the entire healing protocol.

VITAMIN D_3

Vitamin D_3, also known as Cholecalciferol, is a fat-soluble vitamin not normally present in most foods unless added, and which humans naturally obtain via exposure to sunshine. It must be processed in the liver and the kidneys to be activated. While all vitamins are important, Vitamin D is the cornerstone, a precursor vitamin without which all other vitamins and bodily processes could not function. It is essential for calcium absorption, the modulation of neuromuscular and immune function, reducing inflammation, and encoding genetic proteins that regulate cell proliferation, differentiation, and apoptosis, or cell death.

Vitamin D_3 isn't really a vitamin at all. Cholecalcipherol (D_3), is actually a secosteroid, which is a molecule that is similar to a steroid. In Vitamin D_3 whole food supplements, only about 60% is able to adhere to a binding protein, allowing it to be used. Even less is usable from synthetic vitamins.

Many diseases are attributed to a Vitamin D_3 deficiency, including:

- Alzheimer's
- Autoimmune disorders
- Chrohn's
- Chronic pain
- Dementia
- Depression
- Diabetes
- Heart conditions
- Hypertension
- Macular degeneration
- Muscle weakness and wasting
- Multiple Sclerosis
- Soft Bones in children
- Osteoarthritis
- Osteoporosis
- Periodontal problems
- Respiratory infections
- Rheumatoid arthritis

- Rickets
- Cancer

The best source for Vitamin D_3, and the only kind that is completely metabolized, comes from the sun's ultra-violet B (UVB) rays, which stimulate the skin to produce Vitamin D_3. Sun UVB exposure will stimulate excessive production of Vitamin D_3 by the skin. What prevents us from overdosing on sun-produced Vitamin D_3 is our body's production of the enzyme 24-hydroxylase, which reduces excess amounts of Vitamin D_3.

Geographic latitude, time of day, cloud cover, smog, skin melanin content, and whether or not an individual uses sunscreen all play a role in Vitamin D_3 deficiency. Anyone living in the northern United States, above 42° north latitude (the northernmost states, New England, and northern California) will have insufficient sun exposure from November through February.

Sunscreen use, encouraged because of the fear of melanoma, coupled with sedentary lifestyles, foster Vitamin D_3 deficiency in most people in the U.S. Only a blood test can determine the serum levels of Vitamin D_3 and whether supplementation is required. I prefer the 25(OH)D test because it screens for serum concentrations of Vitamin D_3 obtained through the skin from sunshine, from food, and from supplementation. It has a circulating half-life of 15 days.

Keep in mind that the Recommended Daily Allowance (RDA) established by the FDA is based on an *average* 2,000 calorie diet and are the *minimum* daily requirements only. The FDA's Vitamin D_3 serum concentration recommendations are for an adequate amount that is just enough to get by without getting rickets or other severe conditions. But adequate does not mean optimal, not by a long shot.

In fact, Vitamin D_3 may be our greatest antioxidant. Breast and colorectal cancer statistics from 175 countries were mapped according to a country's distance from the equator and sunlight measurements. The graphs show increasingly higher rates for both cancers the further a country is from the equator. For example, breast cancer rates in the US, Canada, and Australia were 75.8-101.1 per 100,000, while breast cancer rates in Africa, China, and the Middle East countries were 0.1-28.0 per 100,000.

The National Institutes of Health, Office of Dietary Supplements suggests the following sun exposure for obtaining a *minimum* of Vitamin D_3 synthesis:

- 5-30 minutes of sun exposure at least twice a week
- Best time of day is between 10 AM and 3 PM
- Exposure on face, chest, arms, legs, and back
- Do not use sunscreen during that time

The chart below shows various levels of Vitamin D in the blood.

OPTIMUM SERUM 25(OH)D LEVELS	
Deficient	Less than 50 ng/ml
Optimal	50-70 ng/ml
Cancer or Heart Disease Treatment	70-100 ng/ml
Excessive	Greater than 100 ng/ml

*Serum concentrations are indicated as nanograms per milliliter (ng/ml)

When I was diagnosed with Lichen Sclerosis, although my Vitamin D_3 serum concentration was at the bottom of the optimal range, at 50 ng/ml, my doctor recommended supplementation. A year later, with more sun exposure coupled with supplementation, my serum Vitamin D_3 level was well into the optimal level of 63 ng/mL.

Now, my doctor-recommended winter intake of supplemental Vitamin D_3 is 5,000 IU twice a day in capsule form because I live in a northern climate with minimal sunlight in winter. In the summer I spend a lot of time in the sun and take no Vitamin D_3 supplement. I also do not use any kind of sunscreen.

The Vitamin D Council recommends Vitamin D_3 supplementation as shown in the chart below. Note that the Council *requires Vitamin D_3 blood serum 25 (OH) D testing and a doctor's approval before implementing these guidelines*:

Recommended Daily Vitamin D_3 Dosage Guidelines	
Children Below the Age of 1	25 IU per pound of body weight
Children Age 1 – 4	25 IU per pound of body weight
Adolescents Ages 5-18	2500 IU
Adults	4000 IU - 5000 IU
Chronically Ill	Dosages may be as much as 10,000 IU, but only under physician's care

The rule of thumb for Vitamin D_3 supplementation is 25 IU's per pound of body weight. This means that for a child weighing 40 pounds, the *average* dose would be 960 IU per day. An adult weighing 170 would require over 4000 IU per day.

Drug Interactions

People with the following conditions should use Vitamin D_3 supplementation only under the direction of a knowledgeable physician or endocrinologist:

- Primary hyperparathyroidism
- Sarcoidosis
- Granulomatous TB
- Some Cancers

Anyone taking thyroid medications and/or statins should always consult with their physician before taking Vitamin D₃ supplements. These supplements may interact with some medications and could cause Hypercalcemia, a condition in which calcium levels are elevated, and which can be devastating to health.

And finally, do not fall victim to any "pharmaceutical grade" Vitamin D or any other vitamin prescription supplement. You only need the real deal. But be tested for Vitamin D serum levels before taking any supplements.

How to Use Vitamin D₃ Supplements:

1000 IU capsule

- Children under 6: Use Rule of Thumb (taken with meals)
- Children ages 6-12: 2000 IU per day in divided doses throughout the day, always with meals.
- Teen to Adult: 3000 IU per day in divided doses throughout the day, always with meals.

All vitamins are to be taken 7 days a week for the duration of the healing protocol.

VITAMIN E

Vitamin E acts as an antioxidant in protecting the skin's cell membranes from free radicals. It also is involved in the flow of genetic information from cells to the proteins they produce that determine structures such as hair or eye color (gene expression), as well as activities of molecules and enzymes in immune and inflammatory cells. It has also been shown to inhibit blood clots and opens the blood vessels. Vitamin E inhibits the activity of enzymes involved in cancer cell proliferation.

While outright deficiency of Vitamin E is rare, people with fat-malabsorption or on low-fat diets may be deficient in this valuable nutrient. Fat is required in the digestive tract in order to absorb Vitamin E. Deficiency symptoms include:

- Severe muscle weakness (Ataxia)
- Poor memory or cognitive function (Alzheimer's Disease)
- Impaired immune response
- Prickling or numbness of the fingers or toes (Peripheral neuropathy)
- Cataracts and macular degeneration (Retinopathy)
- Weak or diseased skeletal muscles (Skeletal myopathy)

Drug Interactions

Drug interactions may occur with Vitamin E supplementation beyond 400 IU per day. Anyone using the following prescription medications or treatments should check with a physician before taking Vitamin E:

- Anticoagulant and antiplatelet medications Warfarin (Coumadin®)
- Simvastatin (Zocor®) and niacin
- Chemotherapy and radiation

Always consult with a health care professional, especially before giving children vitamins.

How to Use Vitamin E Supplements:

400 mg soft gel

- Children under 6: Not essential for very young children, but if included, use the Homeopathic Rule of Thumb and give with meals.
- Children ages 6-12: 1/2 soft gel 2x per day with meals.
- Teens to Adults: 1 soft gel per day with meals

All vitamins are to be taken 7 days a week for the duration of the healing protocol.

CALCIUM

We think of calcium as merely the factor for building strong teeth and bones. However, calcium is integral for a multitude of other bodily functions including:

- Cell signaling
- Stabilizing and optimizing proteins and enzymes
- Blood clotting
- Protects against lead toxicity

Calcium also reduces the risk of the following diseases:

- Colorectal cancer
- Osteoporosis
- Kidney stones
- Hypertension

- Preeclampsia (pregnancy-induced hypertension)

Recommended Dietary Allowances (RDAs) for Calcium

Age	Male	Female	Pregnant	Lactating
0–6 months	200 mg	200 mg		
7–12 months	260 mg	260 mg		
1–3 years	700 mg	700 mg		
4–8 years	1,000 mg	1,000 mg		
9–13 years	1,300 mg	1,300 mg		
14–18 years	1,300 mg	1,300 mg	1,300 mg	1,300 mg
19–50 years	1,000 mg	1,000 mg	1,000 mg	1,000 mg
51–70 years	1,000 mg	1,200 mg		
71+ years	1,200 mg	1,200 mg		

Remember that these numbers are the *minimum* allowances.

Toxicity

Elevated blood calcium levels (hypercalcemia) can occur if supplementation is twice the level of the recommended daily allowances listed in the previous table (as opposed to drinking milk or eating calcium-rich food).

A blood test can easily determine if calcium supplementation is required, especially for mature women, and may be obtained before taking calcium supplements, but it is not a prerequisite.

How to Take Calcium Supplements:

1200 mg capsule or soft gel

- Children under 6: Not essential for very young children, but if included, Use Rule of Thumb. Always give calcium with meals.

- Children ages 6-12: 300 mg 3x per day, with meals.

- Teens to Adults: 600 mg 2x per day, with meals.

All vitamins are to be taken 7 days a week for the duration of the healing protocol.

SUPPLEMENTS

As with vitamins, all supplements are to be taken 7 days a week for the duration of the healing protocol.

TPP™ PROTEASE

In Chapter 2: Toxic Topicals, we discussed the havoc wreaked on cells by sodium lauryl and sodium laureth sulfates (SLS) when they form chemical bridges that disrupt the hydrophobic (water) process needed to maintain protein structure in the cells. As previously noted, this damage is usually irreversible because by depriving our cells of the water needed to maintain their structure, these chemical bridges lead to a protein buildup in our cells.

TPP™ Protease's proteolytic enzyme ability to break down excess proteins was exactly what I needed to undo the damage caused by sodium lauryl and laureth sulfates in my body. Once I eliminated the chemicals from my life, no new cell damaging bridges would be built, and, with the help of TPP™ Protease, existing unwanted bridges would be destroyed.

Most people know that proteolytic enzymes act as digestive enzymes and when taken with meals, aid in the digestion of proteins in our food. However, I believe that when taken on an empty stomach, these protein digesting enzymes go on a search and destroy mission throughout the body to eliminate protein buildup anywhere they find it, including those toxin-created chemical bridges in our cells.

According to the manufacturer of TTP™ Protease, *"As An Immune Modular: The formation and persistence of immune complexes in the system may in the long-term lead to autoimmune conditions and other complications. It is thought that immune complexes end up depositing themselves along the lining of blood vessels and on the surfaces of organs as they circulate in the blood stream, creating areas of inflammation or impeding the normal functioning of the body. Orally administered proteolytic enzymes break down the immune complexes and the antigens, thus alleviating any potential problems that may be created by an overacting immune system. It has also been shown that proteolytic enzymes control the over expression of some of the cytokines, thus modulating the adverse impact of their higher concentrations in the body (Buford et al, 2008)."*

While there are many proteases on the market, for the healing protocol ***only*** TPP™ Protease by Transformation Enzymes is acceptable and comes as a powder in large capsules. For anyone who can't or doesn't want to swallow a capsule they can be opened and the contents emptied into water and the taste is bland. These are to be taken without food, 1 hour before or after eating so as not to waste the proteolytic enzymes by digesting food.

How to Take TPP™ Protease Supplements:

- Children under 6: 1/2 capsule 2x per day *OR* use the Homeopathic Rule of Thumb. Take with water, *1 hour before or after eating.*

- Children 6-12: 1 capsule 2x per day, with water, *1 hour before or after eating.*

- Teen to Adult: 1 capsule 3x per day, with water, *1 hour before or after eating.*

Ingredients: Tzyme™ Protease Blend (638 mg), peptidases, bromelain, papain

All supplements are to be taken 7 days a week for the duration of the healing protocol.

PROBIOTICS

The human body is literally covered with bacteria. It is estimated that we carry 5 pounds of bacteria in our intestinal tract and 25 pounds overall. You might say that our bacteria are our first line of defense. People are now so worried about "germs" they constantly use chemical sprays, cleaners, wipes, and hand sanitizers, the latter of which contain chemicals such as the hormone-disrupting triclosan. By using these products, we are, in fact, weakening our body's defenses rather than keeping them strong and healthy by exercising them to fight germs and infections.

Our external bacteria are our first line of external defense. They protect the skin from pathogenic germs that might otherwise enter through the pores. Internal bacteria begin at the nose, eyes, and mouth, lines the entire digestive tract, and end at the anus.

Bacteria are voracious eaters designed to consume everything that poses a threat to our health, both inside and outside of the body.

One of the main suppressors of our beneficial internal bacteria, or flora, is processed foods. Processed foods contain simple processed sugars that inhibit our beneficial bacteria, allowing disease-causing, or pathogenic, bacteria to proliferate and overwhelm the good kind.

Other things that inhibit beneficial bacteria are medications, especially antibiotics.

Anyone who is chronically ill most likely has impaired beneficial flora. That means it's imperative to reintroduce and promote "good" bacteria.

The first step is to eliminate processed food from your diet, especially processed sugars and artificial sweeteners.

Next, stop using antibacterial soaps for bathing, and stop using hand sanitizers. Washing hands with ordinary soap, preferably organic, which I believe is a must, will reduce "germs" by 99%. It is not necessary to use chemical cleaners, wipes, or any other commercial antibacterial product.

Another great way to enhance internal beneficial flora is to take a good probiotic. The best is one that contains millions of different types of living beneficial bacteria. Raw milk is a healthy, bacteria-rich probiotic, but sadly it's not always available in all areas.

Yogurt is often recommended as a source of probiotics, but all commercial yogurts are pasteurized, which means that no live beneficial natural bacteria remain and only a handful of bacterial "cultures" have been added. Flavored yogurts also contain sugar. Only plain, unflavored, unpasteurized yogurt contains live beneficial probiotics.

Probiotics in capsule form are preferable, especially when adjusting children's dosages, but they are also available as tablets. Note that some probiotics must be refrigerated before opening, whereas others only require refrigeration once they have been opened to keep the beneficial bacteria alive.

For older children and adults, one full probiotic capsule or tablet per day should be all that is needed. For very young children, the capsules can be opened to provide the appropriate amount, which may be mixed with cold food or drinks (hot food or liquids will kill the bacteria).

How to Take Probiotics:

- Children under 6: 1/2 capsule per day with meal, OR use the Homeopathic Rule of Thumb.

- Children ages 6-12: 1 capsule per day with meal.

- Teen to Adult: 1 capsule per day with meal.

All supplements are to be taken 7 days a week for the duration of the healing protocol.

MOLYBDENUM

Molybdenum is an essential trace element necessary for every life form. It acts as a co-factor for numerous enzymes that are catalysts for the metabolism of sulfur-containing amino acids, the antioxidant capacity of blood plasma, and the body's ability to metabolize drugs and toxins. Increased molybdenum helps the liver to detoxify itself, and slows the degeneration of tissues, along with other symptoms of toxic overload.

Tolerable Upper Intake Level (UL) for Molybdenum	
Age Group	UL (mcg/day)
Infants 0-12 months	Not possible to establish
Children 1-3 years	300
Children 4-8 years	600

Tolerable Upper Intake Level (UL) for Molybdenum	
Age Group	UL (mcg/day)
Children 9-13 years	1,100
Adolescents 14-18 years	1,700
Adults 19 years and older	2,000

There have been no reports of adverse reactions to Molybdenum supplementation.

How to Take Molybdenum:

- Children under 6: 1/2 of a 300 mcg capsule 2x per day OR use the Homeopathic Rule of Thumb. Give with meals.

- Children ages 6-12: 1 300 mcg capsule 2x per day with meals.

- Teen to Adult: 1 300 mcg capsule 3x per day with meals.

All supplements are to be taken 7 days a week for the entire duration of the healing protocol.

L-LYSINE

We live in a world filled with viruses. For example, the Centers for Disease Control and Prevention estimate that 92% of the population, if tested, would show positive results for six different strains of the Herpes virus alone. Viruses are living organisms that need to eat in order to survive and multiply. And their sole form of nutrition is the amino acid arginine.

There are two types of arginine: one is a free-form amino acid that the body produces. The other type comes from food, and all foods contain arginine, some more than others. Food-derived arginine is the type that viruses thrive on.

L-Lysine is also an amino acid, and its key function is to speed up the breakdown of dietary arginine, which limits its absorption into the intestines. This means that L-Lysine acts to starve viruses of the food they need to survive and proliferate. When I began my LS protocol, I took L-Lysine by capsule, then later switched to L-Lysine Amino Acid Powder.

How to Take L-Lysine:

L-Lysine 500 mg capsules:

- Children under 6: 1/2 capsule per day with meals; OR use the Homeopathic Rule of Thumb for dosage.

- Children 6-12: 1 capsule per day with meals.

- Teen to Adult: 1 capsule per day with meals.

L-Lysine crystals: 1/4 teaspoon = 600 mg
(The crystals taste similar to salt and can be sprinkled on or mixed into food.)

- Children under 6: 1/8 teaspoon per day with meals OR use the Homeopathic Rule of Thumb for dosage.

- Children ages 6-12: 1 scoop per day with meals. (The scoop is provided with the container)

- Teen to Adult: 1 scoop per day with meals. (The scoop is provided with the container)

All supplements are to be taken 7 days a week for the duration of the healing protocol.

Note: Because L-Lysine starves viruses, instead of getting vaccines such as flu shots, adults may take 1/2 teaspoon (1200 mg), children 6 and older may take 1/4 teaspoon (600 mg), and children under age 6 may take 1/8 teaspoon (300 mg) of L-Lysine crystals per day with meals as a precaution.

EVENING PRIMROSE OIL (EPO)

Evening primrose oil is derived from the seeds of the wildflower that grows throughout the United States. The EPO seeds contain Linoleic Acid (LA), as well as *gamma*-Linolenic Acid (GLA). These essential fatty acids are part of the Omega-6 family of fatty acids.

In order for the body to function optimally, it needs a healthy balance of Omega-3 and Omega-6 fatty acids. Evening primrose oil is one of the richest sources of Omega-6 fatty acids. Essential fatty acids are called *essential* because they are not produced in the body and must be obtained from food, and they are integral for our overall health and for the health of our organs. Evening primrose oil's rich *gamma*-linoleic acid supports our cardiovascular, immune, nervous, and reproductive systems, and helps to maintain cell health. EPO also has an anti-inflammatory and antioxidant effect on blood thinning and blood vessel dilation.

Whole foods that are high in omega-6 fatty acids include meats, liver, and whole grains. Unfortunately, our Western diet is high in the wrong *type* of omega-6 fatty acids, trans-fats, which mainly come from grain-fed meats, processed vegetable oils, and processed cereals.

Evening primrose oil has been used by native cultures and early American settlers for the treatment of ailments such as bruises and hemorrhoids. It is currently being used to reduce the symptoms of:

- ADHD
- Alzheimer's Disease
- Arthritis
- Asthma
- Chronic fatigue syndrome
- Fibrocystic breast disease
- Heart disease
- Hives
- Hot flashes
- Inflammation from Lupus
- Irritable bowel syndrome
- Itching from skin conditions
- Breast tenderness
- Mood swings
- Multiple sclerosis
- Peripheral Neuropathy (numbness, tingling, pain, burning, or lack of sensation in hands, feet and legs)
- Osteoporosis
- Preeclampsia (pregnancy-induced hypertension)
- Rashes
- Raynaud's disease
- Redness and scaling caused by eczema and dermatitis
- Rosacea

- Skin ulcers

It is important to take an Omega-3 fatty acid such as fish oil when taking evening primrose oil. The Omegas work synergistically and provide more bang for the health buck than if either is taken alone.

Toxicity

While evening primrose oil is generally safe when used in recommended dosages, it's best to first consult a health professional, especially one well versed in botanical medicine. Children especially should be medically supervised when taking supplements.

Side Effects

Possible side effects from taking EPO are:

- Loose stools and stomach pain, which occur if the dosage is too high
- Do not take if one has bleeding disorders
- Interactions with schizophrenia medications including chlorpromazine, fluphenazine, perphenazine, promazine, and thioridazine
- Interactions with nonsteroidal anti-inflammatory drugs
- Interactions with anticoagulant and antiplatelet medications and herbs
- Interactions with seizure medications, including the onset of seizures.

The best EPO is obtained by cold pressing. Evening primrose oils that are not cold-pressed are obtained via hexane baths, the petrochemical that is a known carcinogen. This hexane process contaminates the oil and must be avoided.

Certified organic evening primrose oil is available in liquid oil form (which must be refrigerated), or in soft gel form. As with all Omega essential fatty acids, EPO has a short shelf life of only 6 months. Refrigerate for best results.

How to Take Evening Primrose Oil:

Evening Primrose Oil 500 mg soft gel

- Children under 6: Use Homeopathic Rule of Thumb and give with meals.
- Ages 6-12: 1 capsule 2 times per day with meals.
- Teen to Adult: 1 capsule 2 times per day with meals.

Evening Primrose Oil Liquid: 1/8 teaspoon = 500 mg

- Children under 6: Use Homeopathic Rule of Thumb and mix with food or in a drink.
- Ages 6-12: 1/8 teaspoon 2 times per day mixed with food or in a drink.
- Teen to Adult: 1/8 teaspoon 2 times per day mixed with food or in drink.

All supplements are to be taken 7 days a week for the duration of the healing protocol.

OMEGA-3 FISH OIL/KRILL OIL

Fish oil contains essential omega-3 fatty acids that are essential for optimum health. As with Omega-6s, they are essential because the body cannot manufacture them and Omega-3 fatty acids are integral to the structure of every cell membrane, as well as in the formation of compounds that control metabolism. Omega-3s play an important role in maintaining brain health and immunity, and they are anti-inflammatory. Signs of a deficiency in essential fatty acids include dry, flaky skin, dull hair, brittle nails, and skin conditions such as eczema, psoriasis, and acne.

Foods that are rich in healthy Omega-3 fatty acids are free-range eggs, flax seed oil (cold pressed), grass-fed meats, and fish such as wild caught Alaskan salmon, halibut, cod, rainbow trout, sardines, and shrimp, all of which, unfortunately, are missing from most Americans' diets.

Only fish oils contain the major dietary source of EPA and DHA:

- **EPA** - Eicosapentaenoic acid are potent chemical messengers that play critical roles in immune and inflammatory responses by regulating the activity of multiple genes involved in inflammation.

- **DHA** – High concentrations of docosahexaenoic acid are found in the cell membranes of the retina and are required for the normal development and function of the retina.

Combined, EPA and DHA play a role in suppressing inflammatory immune response. Because some people cannot tolerate fish oil, which can produce gastrointestinal discomfort, krill oil, derived from miniscule shrimp-like crustaceans, may be used instead. However, krill oil may not be suitable for people who have shellfish allergies. Krill Oil contains EPA and DHA, along with:

- **Phospholipids** – These lipids are fat derivatives and affect cell membrane properties of fluidity, flexibility, and permeability. Phospholipids in the brain contain high levels of DHA, which plays an integral role in the central nervous system's function. Phospholipids are easily and fully absorbed because the body needs fewer metabolic steps and less energy to digest and distribute them.

- **Astaxanthin** – This molecule is part of the carotene family and is a potent antioxidant that displays powerful anti-inflammatory properties.

Both Omega-3 fish oil and krill oil support optimal health for:

- Aging
- Vision
- Metabolism
- Inflammation
- Cardiovascular system
- Fetal development
- Skin, hair, nails
- Arthritic conditions
- Cognitive function

How to Take Fish Oil or Krill Oil:

1000 mg Fish Oil or Krill Oil

- Children under age 6: 1/2 capsule per day with meals, or use the Homeopathic Rule of Thumb.

- Children 6-12: 1 capsule 2 times per day with meals.

- Teen to Adult: 1 capsule 3 times per day with meals.

All supplements are to be taken 7 days a week for the duration of the healing protocol.

COENZYME Q10

Coenzyme Q_{10} (CoQ10) is a member of the ubiquinone family of compounds found in all mammals. But only the fully oxidized ubiquinone, Coenzyme Q_{10}, is found in humans. Ubiquinones are lipid-soluble molecules found in all cell membranes, as well as lipoproteins and are integral to a variety of functions in the body:

- Mitochondrial Function – The conversion of energy from carbohydrates and fats to the form of energy used by cells requires CoQ_{10} to be present in the inner mitochondrial membrane.

- Lysosomal Function – Lysosomes are specialized "organelles" that digest cellular debris, which is important in controlling auto-immune and inflammatory disorders.

- Antioxidant Functions – Coenzyme Q_{10} acts as an effective fat-soluble antioxidant that protects cell membranes and neutralizes free radicals.

- Vitamin E Interaction – When combined, Vitamin E and Coenzyme Q_{10} work as the principal fat-soluble antioxidants in membranes and lipoproteins.

- Biosynthesis – Coenzyme Q_{10} is synthesized in most human tissues and requires Vitamin B_6, a B-complex vitamin, to form. Since the two go hand-in-hand, an appropriate nutritional level for vitamin B_6 is also a nutritional indicator for Coenzyme Q_{10}, and vice versa.

Coenzyme Q_{10} is an important factor in health, not only in preventing disease, but also in mitigating illnesses. CoQ_{10} has been shown to have a positive influence on:

- Energy metabolism in the tissues of the liver, heart, and skeletal muscle
- Inhibiting atherosclerosis
- Mitochondrial encephalomyopathies
- Cardiovascular diseases
- Angina pectoris
- Hypertension
- Vascular endothelial function (blood vessel dilation)
- Diabetes mellitus
- Parkinson's Disease
- Huntington's Disease
- Friedreich's Ataxia – a central nervous system disorder that damages muscles, including the heart
- Cancer

Coenzyme Q_{10} Deficiency

Coenzyme Q_{10} is key in the manufacture and sustainability of tissue cells and is an integral part of lipoproteins. Since statins, the cholesterol lowering drugs, reduce low density lipoproteins, they cause muscle pain and weakness in many people on statins who do not take CoQ_{10} supplements. This happens because the statins cause a deficiency of CoQ_{10}.

Toxicity

In some cases, supplementation of 1200 mg per day of CoQ_{10} has produced nausea, diarrhea, heartburn, loss of appetite, and abdominal discomfort.

Drug Interactions

- Warfarin (Coumadin®) – Supplementation of CoQ_{10} can decrease the anti-coagulant's effectiveness

- Statins – Statins inhibit cholesterol production, and as a result, inhibit Coenzyme Q_{10} synthesis as well. Examples of statins include:
    - Altocor
    - Crestor
    - Lipitor
    - Mevacor
    - Pravachol
    - Zetia
    - Zocor

How to Take CoQ_{10}:

CoQ_{10} 200 mg capsule:

- Children under 6: Give with meals and use Homeopathic Rule of Thumb for dosage.

- Children ages 6-12: 1/2 capsule twice a day, taken with meals.

- Teen to Adult: 1 capsule per day taken with meals.

All supplements are to be taken 7 days a week for the duration of the healing protocol.

DETOX TEA

Detox tea does exactly what it says. Specific herbs are used to aid the body in eliminating toxins from organs, tissues, blood, and the lymphatic system. It doesn't matter which brand you select as long as they contain the right ingredients, which should include most or all of the following:

- Alfalfa
- Burdock Root
- Cascara Sagrada
- Chamomile Flower
- Chicory Root
- Corn Silk
- Dandelion Root
- Echinacea Augustifolia Root
- Ginger
- Hibiscus Flower
- Licorice Root
- Milk Thistle
- Red Clover Flower
- Rose Hip
- Sarsaparilla
- Shavegrass
- Siberian Ginseng
- Slippery Elm Bark
- Yellow Dock

Because no commercial detox tea included all the required herbs, I combined one teabag of Yogi Detox Tea and one teabag of Triple Leaf Detox Tea in 10 oz of boiling water, then steeped for 15 minutes. I found adding a sliver or two of raw organic ginger root made the tea taste better. Then I drank it all as soon as it was cool enough. I drank 1 cup of this detox tea each day and also drank another cup during the 30-minute healing soak (see next page for this soak). Drinking the tea while soaking induced intense sweating, one of the main ways in which the body eliminates toxins. Having completed the healing protocol and continuing to live an organic lifestyle, I no longer sweat profusely when drinking detox tea during a healing soak. I assume this means that I have now eliminated the massive amount of toxins in my system.

How to Use Detox Tea:

In young children, always start with just a few drops to test for tolerance. Even though detox teas are made up of natural herbs, some children may react to some of the ingredients in herbal teas.

- Children under 6: One half cup detox tea per day, especially during healing soak.
- Children ages 6-12: One cup detox tea per day, especially during the healing soak.
- Teen to Adult: One to two cups detox tea per day, especially during healing soak.

Detox tea should be consumed 7 days a week for the duration of the healing protocol.

HEALING SOAKS

Healing soaks can be taken every day if necessary, but take at least three soaks per week. There are six components to healing soaks: hot water, Epsom Salts, Hydrogen Peroxide, freshly ground ginger root, and dry skin brushing.

- **Hot water** – The water does not need to be much hotter than body temperature, and certainly should not be more than 100° degrees. Fill a bathtub with 99°-100° water that is deep enough to cover the entire body up to the neck.

- **Epsom salts (unscented only)** – The main components of Epsom salts are magnesium and sulfates. Magnesium reduces inflammation, improves oxygen use, and helps in the regulation of over 300 enzymes. The sulfates pull out toxins and improve the absorption of nutrients; they also aid in the formation of joint and mucin proteins, as well as in the growth of brain tissue. Caution: DO NOT use agricultural-grade Epsom salts as they may contain impurities. Epsom salts are available in supermarkets and pharmacies. For a standard sized bathtub, use 4 cups of Epsom salts. For an extra-large tub, use 8 cups of Epsom salts.

- **Hydrogen Peroxide** – Hydrogen Peroxide (H_2O_2) super oxygenates bathwater; it breaks down toxins and detoxifies pesticides and petroleum-based toxins; it oxidizes heavy metals, and it kills anaerobic microbes. Friendly microbes are aerobic and thrive on oxygen, so by soaking in the super oxygenated water, we absorb the oxygen molecule, thereby oxygenating the bloodstream. As discussed in a previous chapter, people with chronic illnesses may have thickened, oxygen-poor blood and it acts as a host for pathogens. For the Healing Soak, use ordinary 3% Hydrogen Peroxide solution typically found in supermarkets and pharmacies. It is not necessary to use purified Hydrogen Peroxide designed for internal use. For standard tubs, add 32 oz of Hydrogen peroxide. For extra-large tubs, add 64 oz of Hydrogen peroxide.

- **Ginger Root** – Ginger root has both dilating and anti-inflammatory properties that enhance cardiovascular health and circulation. Used externally, ginger root will help dilate pores to better accept the detoxification and healing properties of the other ingredients used in the soak, and will increase surface blood flow. Use fresh ginger root (organic if possible) that is smooth and without wrinkles. It should be unpeeled, and crisp and moist when sliced. Grate the ginger root by hand or use a hand-held blender. Store ginger root in an uncovered container in the refrigerator and note that it will form a scab where it was cut. This is normal. For the healing soak, wrap the freshly grated ginger root in loose-tea tea balls or use cheesecloth, but I found that the toe section of a clean pair of pantyhose worked best. Fill with freshly grated ginger, then knot the cut end of the pantyhose and place the entire container holding the grated ginger into the hot water; this will disperse plumes of yellow ginger root oil into the water. For standard tubs, use 2 tablespoons of freshly grated ginger root. For extra-large tubs, use 4 tablespoons of freshly grated ginger root.

- **Dry skin brushing** – Before stepping into the healing soak and to help open the pores, dry brush the entire body. The face and genital areas do not need to be dry brushed. Start with the extremities and work toward the heart, and be sure to brush the palms and soles of the feet. Think of it as pushing toxins along the lymphatic pathways to help clear them out of the body. Use a soft brush, and gentle strokes. Be careful not to brush so hard as to make the skin raw. Dry skin brushing should take no longer than 5 minutes.

- **Drink a Cup of Detox tea** - Drinking a cup of detox tea during soaks will induce sweating, which will further assist in eliminating toxins.

- **Duration** – Immerse the entire body up to the neck in the healing soak and remain in the preparation for 30 minutes. If the water begins to cool, add more hot water. Once time is up, shower to remove the residual Epsom salts that may remain on the skin.

Take healing soaks 3-4 times per week.

Warning: After the soaking period is up, it is possible to become dizzy when standing up to get out of the tub. Take your time and wait until the sensation passes. This may not happen to everyone, but it is not unusual and no cause for alarm.

Now that I have healed, in addition to not sweating when I drink detox tea during a healing soak, I also no longer become dizzy when getting up from the tub.

NUTRACEUTICALS

Previous chapters covered the many different toxins that impede our health, including environmental toxins which cause most of the damage, viruses, co-infections, and pathogenic bacteria that have been chemically enabled to get a foothold. The whole point of the healing protocol is to address our physical dysfunction and the resulting illnesses and disorders.

Much in the same way that allopathic medicine treats the body part by part, so do many who dabble in alternative methods, patching together a hodgepodge of the most publicized diets, vitamins, cleanses, or lifestyles. When they hear that Vitamin D_3 is beneficial, they take supplements without knowing whether they're synthetic or natural, and have no idea what their Vitamin D_3 serum level is or if they even need supplementation, let alone knowing the correct dosage if they need it. Likewise, people stop eating specific food groups, not because they have reactions to those food groups, but because they've heard they are "bad" for us, but totally miss the point that they brush their teeth with poison.

The downfall of all of these attempts to be healthy is that they are one dimensional whereas our body is complex. Unfortunately, most people focus on just one aspect of health, such as food elimination or a topical application, while missing the big picture. And what is typically overlooked are the toxins that viruses, co-infections, and pathogenic bacteria create, and how to address them. They make us sick, too. They are toxic and cause both inflammation and auto-immune reactions, and we are deluding ourselves if we think we can be healthy without addressing every conceivable angle of toxicity.

When I was healing myself of LS, I used nutraceuticals developed by Dr. David Jernigan, who spent two decades developing and improving his unique nutraceuticals. He became interested in developing botanical formulas, which are based on Chinese medicine and made from organically grown herbs, in his efforts to cure his own Lyme disease and its accompanying co-infections. He succeeded and his botanical formulas later cured his daughter of the dangerous West Nile Virus. Dr. Jernigan has treated thousands of patients successfully with his nutraceuticals at his clinic in Wichita, Kansas and they have been proven non-toxic in independent laboratory testing, even at 150 times their prescribed dosage.

When I first learned of these nutraceuticals, I didn't understand what they were or how they worked, and thought they sounded like hocus pocus, which made me skeptical. For instance, I read that one nutraceutical that focuses on healing the brain uses potencies of cerebellum, temporal lobe, and the like and wondered where the tissues came from and how pure they were.

As I considered using the Jernigan nutraceuticals, knowing that they are successfully used in treating various conditions, I read everything I could about them, trying to grasp exactly how they worked. I was concerned, knowing the dangers of pharmaceutical vaccines and worried about putting anything foreign into my body that could cause problems. But my assumptions about the tissues used in the botanicals were *incorrect* because only the *imprints* of healthy tissues are used to stimulate the healing response, *not the actual tissue itself.* This is also how homeopathy works.

An example of how this works is the photograph, which captures an *image* of a person or thing, not the actual person or thing in the real physical sense. When our brain sees that image, *it recognizes that image as the person or thing,* even though it's only the image, and an emotional response is elicited.

Nutraceuticals work the same way. They do not contain any physical tissue; only the biochemical imprints of healthy animal tissues that most closely match ours. When the nutraceuticals are used, the body recognizes these imprints, or images, and is then stimulated to respond and heal because of that impulse from the image of the healthy tissues. This is the driving force that enabled all botanical ingredients to work on all the affected areas of my body.

These imprints are akin to jumper cables used to start a dead battery. By themselves, they will not keep us going but will give us a start. Once that happens, we must provide our body with the nutrients it needs to recharge itself in the form of non-toxic products, organic whole food, whole vitamins, enzyme supplements, and any necessary herbal nutraceutical formulas that will further aid our ability to recharge and heal ourselves.

Another aspect of the nutraceuticals is based upon frequencies. Everything in nature has its own frequency and the herbs used in the nutraceuticals are frequency matched.

How this works is like a mathematical equation. In algebra, two negatives create a positive. In the nutraceutical formulas, herbal frequencies are matched to address discordance frequencies in our bodies. When the two frequencies combine, the discordant frequencies are neutralized.

Even though I was skeptical about whether the nutraceuticals would do anything to help, I also knew I'd made up my mind to leave no stone unturned to rid myself of LS and I'm grateful I did.

In this healing protocol, the combination of vitamins and supplements, coupled with quick sequencing of botanical rotations, do not allow any organism in our body to become resistant or able to hide. It is the opposite of conventional medicine, where the same formulas are used repeatedly, which encourages drug-resistant "super" organisms.

This healing protocol does not treat any particular disease. Instead, it enables the body to fight against toxic invaders, no matter what form they may take or where they occur, and in doing so, allow the body to heal itself.

In using this healing protocol, *all* nutraceuticals must be taken in the *exact order* described later in this chapter. And unless there is a medical issue, do not pick and choose vitamins, supplements, or nutraceuticals, or cavalierly mix and match them. The protocol has been developed so that the components work synergistically; this means that the order in which they are taken delivers a one-two punch, followed by the final knockout. Also, note that the protocol *must be completed* in the order outlir   even when it's obvious that healing is taking place

NEURO-ANTITOX II™ FORMULAS

These formulas were designed specifically to bind with toxins of all types and help the body eliminate them, including bacterial or viral die-off, environmental heavy metals, and chemicals such as benzene. Since toxins are found in every part of the human body, every part of the body is targeted by these nutraceutical formulas.

To prepare the body for Phase 3 of the healing protocol, take the Neuro-Antitox II™ nutraceutical formulas for two weeks before starting the healing protocol and continue taking them for the 12 months of the protocol. Take all the nutraceutical formulas 6 days per week; you decide which day to skip.

- **Neuro-Antitox II™ CNS/PNS** – Take for two weeks before starting and throughout the entire healing protocol. This formula targets the Central Nervous System and Peripheral Nervous System and symptoms of neuro-toxicity, which include brain fog, headaches, ear aches, visual disturbances, neuritis (nerve inflammation), or neuralgia (nerve pain). This is one of three Neuro-Antitox II™ formulas to be taken simultaneously during the duration of the healing protocol.

- **Neuro-Antitox II™ Musculo-Skeletal** – Take for two weeks before starting and throughout the entire healing protocol. This is one of three Neuro-Antitox II™ formulas to be taken simultaneously during the duration of the healing protocol.

  This formula benefits people having symptoms of rheumatic and arthritic conditions, muscle and joint pain and/or weakness, burning, tingling, radiating pain, or swelling of extremities.

- **Neuro-Antitox II™ Cardio** – Take for two weeks before starting as well as throughout the entire healing protocol. It is taken with the previous two formulas on the list.

  This formula targets heart problems, including angina, palpitations, hypertension, arrhythmia, valve problems, related shoulder and arm pain, shortness of breath, and chronic fatigue.

- **Yeast Ease**™ - Take for two weeks before starting the healing protocol and continue taking throughout the 12-month duration.

  The body tries to cleanse itself of toxic invaders by killing them off; this process results in inflammation and the massive die-off of pathogenic organisms and cells, which in turn leads to a secondary release of toxins. This process is one cause of degenerative disease. When this happens at the start of and during the healing protocol, there is massive toxin die-off and release that initially overloads the body's normal channels of elimination, including the liver, kidneys, and lymphatic system. While the Neuro-Antitox II™ formulas are designed to bind with and aid the body in eliminating these toxins, the body isn't fully prepared for this onslaught, which can cause a yeast overgrowth or infection. Although I did not have a yeast infection during the healing protocol, within a month or two of starting the healing protocol I started to feel itchy all over and decided to add Yeast Ease™ to the regimen. It worked so well that I continued to take it for the remainder of the protocol, and people in the case studies who took Yeast Ease™ at the beginning and throughout the healing protocol did not experience itchiness at all.

The following three nutraceuticals will be <u>alternated every three months</u> during the healing protocol, and taken with Neuro-Antitox II™ and Yeast Ease™ formulas.

- **Borrelogen**™ - This nutraceutical was developed to facilitate the body's antimicrobial control mechanisms. It addresses co-infections, including those of Lyme disease. This formula also contains Virogen™, which was developed to combat viruses in general, and specifically genetically engineered microbes that contain the DNA of viruses, parasites, and bacteria. I consider it the antidote to the toxins contained in genetically modified foods and vaccines. It enables the body to register the first punch against toxic overload.

- **Lymogen**™ - This formula helps the body to attack bacterial infections and co-infections. The broad-spectrum herbal combinations used in Lymogen have their own unique antibiotic-like properties and help deliver the second punch.

- **Microbojen**™ - This powerful, broad-based nutraceutical was formulated for the worst-case scenario to help someone who has contracted a combination of eleven different fatal or extremely debilitating diseases, including Lyme, Smallpox, Anthrax, HIV, Hepatitis B, Hepatitis C, West Nile Virus, Epstein-Barr Virus (EBV), Mycoplasma fermentans incognitos, Cytomegalovirus (CMV), and Bubonic Plague. Microbojen helps the body deliver a full knock down punch to these illnesses.

The final knockout punch will be delivered during the fourth quarter and final three months of the healing protocol, when **all** the nutraceuticals are taken.

Nutraceutical Toxicity:

Always test nutraceutical formulas before beginning any regimen. Start with a few drops. If tolerance is a problem, discontinue use. Note that nutraceutical dosages are the recommendations of the manufacturer.

The contents of the nutraceutical formulations are certified by the manufacturer and have been independently tested at 150 times the recommended dosages and proven to be safe and non-toxic.

How to Take Nutraceuticals

All nutraceutical formulas must be taken <u>6 days per week</u> throughout the healing protocol; you decide which day to skip.

Nutraceuticals are taken sublingually, meaning they are held under the tongue, to enhance absorption of the formulas through under-tongue receptors that bypass the digestive system and help deliver the nutraceuticals directly into the bloodstream and throughout the body. Swallowing reduces the effectiveness of the nutraceuticals as digestive fluids interfere and delay it from entering the bloodstream. Note: Although the eyedropper will appear only half full, one squeeze equals a full eyedropper dose.

All of the 4-ounce size nutraceuticals contain alcohol. The 2-ounce size contain apple cider vinegar and may be more suitable for children. Either choice protects the contents of the bottle from contamination after opening and use. To reduce the alcohol taste, add nutraceuticals to a glass and let sit for up to 30 minutes before putting them under the tongue. The longer the nutraceuticals remain under the tongue, the more the saliva will break down the alcohol and render it nearly tasteless. Because as many as 7 nutraceuticals may be taken at one time, I found it convenient to empty the eyedropper contents for each botanical into a glass and take them sublingually all at once.

All formulas are liquid and should be taken 15 minutes before or after food or drink (other than water), and 15 minutes before or after brushing teeth, using mouthwash, or other oral preparations.

Always pre-test by taking a few drops to determine tolerance. Although these nutraceuticals are derived from organic herbs used on thousands of patients and have been tested for toxicity, there is always the possibility of sensitivity in any given individual. If you detect or develop sensitivity to any of the nutraceuticals, discontinue further use.

For children under 6, always start with the minimum dosage and increase to maximum dosage if necessary.

- Children under age 6: Combine 10 drops of each nutraceutical in 1-2 oz water. Administer 1 to 2 times per day, 6 days per week.

- Children ages 6-12: Combine in a glass 1 eyedropper of each nutraceutical, then have the child hold the liquid *under* the tongue for a minimum of 15 seconds, then swish it around the mouth and gums and swallow. Repeat twice per day, 6 days a week.

- Teen to Adult: Combine in a glass 1 eyedropper of each nutraceutical, then hold contents *under* the tongue for a minimum of 15 seconds, swish around the mouth and gums and swallow. Repeat 3 times per day, 6 days per week.

REPLACING CLOBETASOL WITH ORGANIC EXTRA VIRGIN OLIVE OIL

The health benefits of first pressed, cold pressed, organic extra virgin olive oil as a moisturizer replacement was discussed in Chapter 2, and in Chapter 3, the benefits of this Omega-3 oil in our diet was examined; but as part of the healing protocol, it is used topically as an LS healing agent. You may still be hesitant to replace Clobetasol, or other LS prescription ointment with something as simple and healthy as organic extra virgin olive oil, but why is that?

When we are prescribed Clobetasol, we are advised of the dire consequences we'll face if we don't use it. The threat of cancer that may evolve from the untreated disease scares us into believing that if we don't use it, we'll be worse off than we already are. We think we have no other options. But in the healing protocol we have choices.

Even the best educated, most health conscious, savvy readers may agree with what I've presented in this book but will continue using Clobetasol out of fear. I know that fear, but if we continue to use Clobetasol, it will contribute to our slow but steady decline because it is a concoction of toxic chemicals that not only burn when we apply it, but it is absorbed into the body through the skin. Clobetasol's immuno-suppressive properties further weaken our immune system, making us sitting ducks for worsening symptoms, new diseases, and more drugs to treat new symptoms. This is a vicious cycle. *Break it now!*

If Clobetasol really made a difference, you wouldn't be reading this book. Ask yourself these questions:

- Has Clobetasol, or any other prescription cream stopped the progression of my disease?
- Has it eliminated my symptoms?

- Is Clobetasol, or any other prescription topical ointment strengthening my immune system?
- Does it soothe and heal my skin?
- Will Clobetasol, or any other prescription ointments help my body recover from disease?

If the answer is "NO" to any of these questions, then why use it?

I used Clobetasol once. It burned my skin so badly that I decided then and there that not only did I need my immune system functioning optimally, but there had to be something that would have soothing, healing properties for my LS-affected skin.

Any organic extra virgin olive oil will suffice, but my preference is for Olio Beato organic brand because it has the lowest acidity of all organic extra virgin olive oils on the market and is hexane-free. This is important because no one with LS needs high acid or a chemical solvent residue on their most sensitive area.

During the healing protocol, I bought a new bottle of organic extra virgin olive oil every six months and filled as many eyedropper bottles as needed, keeping one in the bathroom, one next to my bed, and one to bring along when I traveled. (Note: empty nutraceutical bottles are easily washed and are perfect for storing personal size organic extra virgin olive oil). Because olive oil has a 6-month shelf life, the remaining bottle of olive oil was used for cooking.

Application

- Gently cleanse affected area after urinating or defecating and after every bath or shower.
- Wash hands with organic soap.

- Use a generous amount of olive oil on fingertips (anywhere from 3-10 drops or more depending upon the extent of affected skin), rubbing fingertips together and gently applying a generous film of oil to the entire affected area.

- Use 7 days per week, as often as necessary.

For those with ultra-sensitive skin, a small spray bottle of pre-filtered water is helpful in cleansing the area before re-applying a generous film of olive oil.

When traveling, to cleanse myself I took a small pre-moistened piece of soft cotton cloth in a small, purse-size container. I used my own filtered water that I was certain contained no chlorine or fluoride to pre-moisten.

Organic extra virgin olive oil will soothe and heal our skin as the healing protocol restores our health. Can you say the same thing for Clobetasol, or any other LS prescription ointment? I didn't think so.

Sources:

National Institutes of Health, Office of Dietary Supplements, "Vitamin E Fact Sheet." http://ods.od.nih.gov/factsheets/vitamine

National Institutes of Health, Office of Dietary Supplements, "Vitamin E Quick Facts." http://ods.od.nih.gov/factsheets/VitaminE-QuickFacts/

National Institute of Health, Office of Dietary Supplements, "Vitamin D Fact Sheet." http://www.ods.od.nigh.gov/factsheets/vitamind.asp

National Institutes of Health, Office of Dietary Supplements, "Vitamin B12 Quick Facts." http://ods.od.nih.gov/factsheets/VitaminB12-QuickFacts

National Institutes of Health, Office of Dietary Supplements, "Vitamin B12 Dietary Supplement Fact Sheet." http://ods.od.nih.gov/factsheets/VitaminB12-HealthProfessional

National Institutes of Health, Office of Dietary Supplements, "Calcium- Recommended Daily Allowances."
http://ods.od.nih.gov/factsheets/calcium

Dr. Karen Becker, "Is Your Vet a Cautious or Casual Vaccinator?" March 13, 2013.
http://healthypets.mercola.com/sites/healthypets/archive/2013/03/13/pet-vaccine-dangers.aspx?e_cid=20130313_PetsNL_art_1&utm_source=petnl&utm_medium=email&utm_content=art1&utm_campaign=20130313

Cannell, John, MD, "Betrayal of a Nation: Why U.S. health authorities are keeping you vitamin D deficient and who stands to gain," Natural News, April 27, 2011.
http://www.naturalnews.com:80/032202_vitamin_D_deficiency_disease.html

Dodds, Dr. W. Jean, "Nutrigenomics and Customized Functional Nutrition for Pets," March 13, 2013.
http://healthypets.mercola.com/sites/healthypets/archive/2013/03/13/pet-vaccine-dangers.aspx?e_cid=20130313_PetsNL_art_1&utm_source=petnl&utm_medium=email&utm_content=art1&utm_campaign=20130313

Drake, Victoria J., Ph.D., "Vitamin C," Linus Pauling Institute, Micronutrient Center, Oregon State University, November 2009.
http://lpi.oregonstate.edu/infocenter/vitamins/vitaminC/

Drake, Victoria J., Ph.D., "Molybdenum," Linus Pauling Institute, Oregon State University, April 2007.
http://lpi.oregonstate.edu/infocenter/minerals/molybdenum/

Drake, Victoria J., Ph.D., "Essential Fatty Acids," Linus Pauling Institute, Oregon State University, April 2009.
http://lpi.oregonestate.edu/infocenter/othernuts/omega3fa/

Drake, Victoria J., Ph.D., "Coenzyme Q$_{10}$", Linus Pauling Insistute, Oregon State University, March 2012.
http://lpi.oregonsate.edu/infocenter/othernuts/coq10

Hepatitis B Foundation, "Hepatitis B Co-Infections."
http://www.hepb.org/hepb/co-infections.htm

Mohr, Sharif B. et al, "Mapping Vitamin D Deficiency, Breast Cancer, and Colorectal Cancer," September 19, 2008. Abstract.
Ucsdnews.ucsd.edu/newsreel/health/moorescancer06.asp

Mountain Rose Herbs, "Organic Evening Primrose Oil Profile."
www.mountainroseherbs.com/learn/oilprofile/eveningprimrose.php)

Perry, Dr. Leonard, University of Vermont Extension, Department of Plant and Soil Science, "Rose Hips," September 2011. http://www.uvm.edu/pss/ppp/articles/rosehips.html

The Professional Supplement Center, "Cholecalciferol? Oh! You Mean Vitamin D." http:://www.professionalsupplementcenter.com)

The Vitamin D Council, "Vitamin D Supplementation." http://www.vitamindcouncil.org/about-vitamin-d/how-to-get-your-vitamin-d/vitamin-d-supplementation/

Chapter 10
The Healing Protocol

There are three important steps that I undertook in healing myself of LS, and believe that the combination of these three actions or phases, none of which can be eliminated, resulted in my body's ability to eliminate Lichen Sclerosis.

Phase 1 focused on removing all toxic products in favor of only organic ones. Phase 2 eliminated all non-organic foods. Phase 3 is the healing protocol. The first two phases should be implemented as quickly as possible. For maximum healing benefit, all three phases need to be combined simultaneously.

PHASE 1: ELIMINATION OF TOXIC TOPICALS

This phase recommends the removal of all toxic products from the home. This includes shampoo, deodorant, toothpaste, powder, skin care products, beauty products, dish and laundry detergents (including those touted as "natural"), household cleaning agents, pharmaceutical topical creams and ointments, and anything else that includes ingredients that are chemically derived. It is best to eliminate these products as quickly as possible since they tend to be absorbed through the skin.

All should be replaced with organic non-toxic products. It is imperative that the replacement products be organic and contain no hazardous ingredients. If you're unsure of ingredients, query the Environmental Working Group's "Skin Deep" database.

I cannot stress enough that Clobetasol, or other prescription topical ointment be eliminated at this time or it will continue to inhibit the body's ability to heal and reestablish full immune system functionality.

PHASE 2: ELIMINATION OF CHEMICAL CONSUMPTION

I recommend that all non-organic food be phased out as quickly as possible and replaced with organic versions. This includes pre-packaged foods, items with blanket ingredients such as "spices" or "seasoning," as well as every ingredient used for home cooking. Choose organic meats, poultry and wild caught seafood with the least amount of contaminants (listed on the Monterey Bay Aquarium Seafood Watch website). Bison is an excellent substitute for beef.

Many large supermarkets now carry a wide selection of organic foods, as do health food stores and food co-ops. What you can't find in stores is usually available on-line. There are now organic substitutes for everything, including every herb, spice, and even Bisquick.

Avoid food items in cans or plastic because of possible BPA contamination, and specifically look for items sold in glass containers.

Get an under-counter water filtration system as well as a shower head, or if possible a whole house water filtration system.

Instead of using chemical cleansers, use plain organic soap. White vinegar, water, and a sponge mop do a better, non-toxic job of cleaning than toxic liquid floor cleaning systems. White vinegar also works fabulously as a dishwasher rinse aid. For surfaces that need an abrasive cleanser, combine water, white vinegar (or hydrogen peroxide), and a little baking soda. By using nothing more than various combinations of water, soap, vinegar, hydrogen peroxide, and baking soda, you will get everything clean without toxic fumes or toxic buildup. You'll also replace a multitude of expensive manufactured items with a few cheap, healthy ones.

Phase out and avoid non-prescription, over-the-counter medications if possible, but never do this without consulting with a physician, as some medications may have detrimental side effects if stopped abruptly.

PHASE 3: THE HEALING PROTOCOL

The following healing protocol has multiple objectives that work synergistically and simultaneously, and is broad enough to encompass other maladies besides Lichen Sclerosis.

The first objective was to help my body detoxify from environmental contaminants such as heavy metals, and toxins from the non-organic products I'd used and foods I'd ingested for most of my life.

The second objective was to aid my body in overcoming internal pathogens such as fungi, bacteria, and viruses that produce their own toxins.

The third objective was to provide my body with the mechanisms to undo the damage that these toxins had caused.

To accomplish all of these objectives, I assembled a collection of supplements and botanicals, each with a specific job to perform.

The elements presented in this book are precisely the way I have used them for my own self-healing, and precisely the way they have been used by the people in my case studies.

The healing protocol takes one year. Generally, healing will become evident within the 3rd to 4th month of the protocol. It is imperative that the full healing protocol be completed. Even if healing appears to have occurred before the end of the protocol, remember that appearances are not the full indicator of what isn't visible so it is highly advised that the full, year-long protocol be completed for optimal healing and health restoration.

The length of time it takes to heal depends upon how long you've been sick. The human body heals itself at a rate of approximately 3 months per every year it has been ill, and that includes the time leading up to diagnosis. Our cells are constantly being replaced. The cells of the human liver are replaced every 4 months.

If your health is not completely restored after a full year on the healing protocol, or if symptoms of any type (not necessarily LS) reappear after completion of the healing protocol, it is advised to start the protocol over from the beginning.

When repeating the protocol, you may stop quarterly to reassess your level of health using body composition analysis, blood work, etc., as well as the return of any symptoms. Should symptoms of any type arise, continue the protocol, stopping quarterly to reassess healing. If you are symptom-free, the protocol is complete, and your body will continue to heal on its own.

Do not become discouraged if after completing the healing protocol symptoms of some sort arise. The body heals itself in mysterious ways. It is thought that the body heals itself in reverse, sort of backtracking, starting with the most recent symptoms and/or disease, and then working its way back in time. Depending upon the symptoms that reappear, you will know how far back in the illness timeline your body has healed.

When I first put together the protocol, it lasted only 8 months. When I stopped the protocol after eight months, I developed the beginning of an eye infection, except that it never progressed beyond the initial stage. This was a symptom that had begun in 1994, so I believed that my body had, in 8 months, healed the damage done to it over the previous 16 years. Once this symptom developed, I continued the protocol for another 4 months, which led to a full year on the healing protocol, after which no symptoms of any type reoccurred.

The healing protocol has been structured for maximum healing. Once it's been given the protocol's building blocks for healing, coupled with continued nutrition, and a lifestyle that restricts potential toxicity, the amazing human body will continue to heal and strengthen itself long after the healing protocol has ended.

THE HEALING PROTOCOL
All Age Groups

1. **Eliminate Medications**
   - Replace Clobetasol, or other prescription cream with organic extra virgin olive oil
   - Phase out the use of other medications (under medical supervision)

2. **Eliminate Environmental Toxins**
   - Use Organic Products
   - Eat Organic Whole Foods
   - Water Purification
   - Air Purification

3. **Restore Body's Regulation of Pathogenic Organisms**
   - Borrelogen™
   - Lymogen™
   - Microbojen™
   - Yeast Ease™
   - L-Lysine
   - Probiotic

4. **Chemical and Heavy Metal Detoxification**
   - Neuro-Antitox II™ Formulas
   - Molybdenum
   - Dry Skin Brushing
   - Healing Soaks
   - Detox Tea

5. **Inflammation Reduction**
   - Omega-3 Fish/Krill Oil
   - Evening Primrose Oil

6. **Endocrine Modulation and Cellular Restoration**
    - TPP® Protease
    - Evening Primrose Oil
    - B-Complex/B12 Vitamins
    - Vitamin C
    - Vitamin D$_3$
    - Vitamin E
    - Calcium
    - CoQ10/Ubiquinol
    - Multi-Vitamin (iron-free for menopausal women only)

7. **Lifestyle Modification**
    - Organic Lifestyle
    - Diet and Exercise

8. **Healing Protocol Schedule – All ages**
   Weeks 1 & 2 – Botanicals
    - Neuro-Antitox II CNS/PNS™
    - Neuro-Antitox II Cardio™
    - Neuro-Antitox II Musculo-Skeletal™
    - Yeast Ease™

Follow age group dosage instructions. Take nutraceuticals 6 days per week, with one day off.

Weeks 1 & 2 – Supplements (follow dosage for age group)
- Multivitamin
- B-Complex 50/B12
- Vitamin C
- Vitamin D$_3$
- Vitamin E
- Calcium
- TPP® Protease
- Probiotic
- Molybdenum
- L-Lysine

- Evening Primrose Oil
- Omega-3 Fish Oil or Krill Oil
- CoQ10/Ubiquinol

Detox Tea

- 1-2 cups per day
- 1 Cup during healing soak

Healing Soak

- 3-4 days per week, you decide which days

1st QUARTER SCHEDULE *(months 1-3)*
For three months, take the following:

Botanicals (follow dosage for age group)

- Neuro-Antitox II™ CNS/PNS
- Neuro-Antitox II™ Cardio
- Neuro-Antitox II™ Musculo-Skeletal
- Yeast Ease™
- *Borrelogen*™

Follow age group dosage instructions. Take 6 days per week, with one day off.

Supplements (follow dosage for age group)

- Multivitamin
- B-Complex 50/B12
- Vitamin C
- Vitamin D_3
- Vitamin E
- Calcium
- TPP® Protease
- Probiotic
- Molybdenum
- L-Lysine
- Evening Primrose Oil
- Omega-3 Fish Oil or Krill Oil
- CoQ10/Ubiquinol

Detox Tea

- 1-2 cups per day
- 1 Cup during healing soak

Healing Soak

- 3-4 days per week, you decide which days

2nd QUARTER SCHEDULE *(months 4-6)*
For 3 months take the following:

Botanicals (follow dosage for age group)

- Neuro-Antitox II™ CNS/PNS
- Neuro-Antitox II™ Cardio
- Neuro-Antitox II™ Musculo-Skeletal
- Yeast Ease™
- *Lymogen*™

The only difference in the protocol is that Lymogen™ has replaced Borrelogen™.

Supplements (follow dosage for age group)

- Multivitamin
- B-Complex 50/B12
- Vitamin C
- Vitamin D_3
- Vitamin E
- Calcium
- TPP® Protease
- Probiotic
- Molybdenum
- L-Lysine
- Evening Primrose Oil
- Omega-3 Fish Oil or Krill Oil
- CoQ10/Ubiquinol

Detox Tea

- 1-2 cups per day
- 1 Cup during healing soak

Healing Soak

- 3-4 days per week, you decide which days

3rd QUARTER SCHEDULE *(months 7-9)*
For 3 months take the following:

Botanicals (follow dosage for age group)

- Neuro-Antitox II™ CNS/PNS
- Neuro-Antitox II™ Cardio
- Neuro-Antitox II™ Musculo-Skeletal
- Yeast Ease™
- *Microbojen*™

The only difference in the protocol is that Microbojen™ has replaced Lymogen™.

Supplements (follow dosage for age group)

- Multivitamin
- B-Complex 50/B12
- Vitamin C
- Vitamin D_3
- Vitamin E
- Calcium
- TPP® Protease
- Probiotic
- Molybdenum
- L-Lysine
- Evening Primrose Oil
- Omega-3 Fish Oil or Krill Oil
- CoQ10/Ubiquinol

Detox Tea

- 1-2 cups per day
- 1 Cup during healing soak

Healing Soak

- 3-4 days per week, you decide which days

4th QUARTER SCHEDULE *(months 10-12)*
For 3 months take the following:

Botanicals (follow dosage for age group)

- Neuro-Antitox II™ CNS/PNS
- Neuro-Antitox II™ Cardio
- Neuro-Antitox II™ Musculo-Skeletal
- Yeast Ease™
- *Borrelogen*™
- *Lymogen*™
- *Microbojen*™

The only difference in the protocol is that Borrelogen™, Lymogen™, and Microbojen™ are combined.

Supplements (follow dosage for age group)

- Multivitamin
- B-Complex 50/B12
- Vitamin C
- Vitamin D_3
- Vitamin E
- Calcium
- TPP® Protease
- Probiotic
- Molybdenum
- L-Lysine
- Evening Primrose Oil
- Omega-3 Fish Oil or Krill Oil
- CoQ10/Ubiquinol

Detox Tea

- 1-2 cups per day
- 1 Cup during healing soak

Healing Soak

- 3-4 days per week, you decide which days

BEGINNING THE HEALING PROTOCOL

Once all of the vitamins, supplements, and nutraceuticals are in place, actually beginning the protocol can seem intense, complex, and overwhelming. There are so many things to take at certain times you may feel like you need a roadmap.

When I began the healing protocol, I literally had a chart that was the length of the refrigerator. But once I got into the groove, I didn't need to refer to my charts. It's just that it was something new, quite different than anything else I'd ever done. To help the reader grasp how all the different parts of the healing protocol come together, I've condensed my original charts, and include them here as examples. The reader is free to design their own charts that best fit their schedule. For instance, based upon my personal schedule, Sundays were my days off from taking nutraceuticals. I did the healing soaks every other day, three days per week, on Monday, Wednesday, and Friday. I used a timer so I'd know when I could eat or brush my teeth before or after the nutraceuticals, or taking TPP™ Protease an hour before or after eating.

Nothing is written in stone. I tried to take the nutraceuticals when I'd first get up in the morning, 15 minutes before lunch, and 15 minutes before dinner. But sometimes I had to take them later in the morning, afternoon, or evening. To take TPP™ Protease I'd set the timer for 1 hour after meals, with the third and last one just before I went to bed.

When traveling for the day, I'd use a small travel bag to carry the nutraceuticals, along with a small glass and child-safe containers of vitamins and supplements. The nutraceuticals are shipped in small, individual bubble-wrap bags that are perfect when traveling with the nutraceuticals.

And, yes, I traveled with my nutraceuticals and all of the vitamins and supplements. When it was time to take my supplements or nutraceuticals, I sometimes pulled over onto the side of the road or into a store parking lot, or else sat in a restaurant. Nothing stood in the way of my fight to regain and keep my health; not then or now.

Following are the charts to health. The first chart outlines the preliminary two weeks of vitamins, supplements, and nutraceuticals that prepare the body for the full protocol, while the remaining four charts outline all four quarters of the year-long healing protocol.

TWO WEEK PRELIMINARY CHART

1st Two Weeks of Protocol Example

	SUNDAY MORNING	MONDAY MORNING	TUESDAY MORNING	WEDNESDAY MORNING	THURSDAY MORNING	FRIDAY MORNING	SATURDAY MORNING
Take Daily Vitamins & Supplements	Take Daily Vitamins & Supplements	Vitamins & Supplements Neuro-Antitox II™ • CNS/PNS • Musculo/Skeletal • Cardio Yeast Ease™	Vitamins & Supplements Neuro-Antitox II™ • CNS/PNS • Musculo/Skeletal • Cardio Yeast Ease™	Vitamins & Supplements Neuro-Antitox II™ • CNS/PNS • Musculo/Skeletal • Cardio Yeast Ease™	Vitamins & Supplements Neuro-Antitox II™ • CNS/PNS • Musculo/Skeletal • Cardio Yeast Ease™	Vitamins & Supplements Neuro-Antitox II™ • CNS/PNS • Musculo/Skeletal • Cardio Yeast Ease™	Vitamins & Supplements Neuro-Antitox II™ • CNS/PNS • Musculo/Skeletal • Cardio Yeast Ease™
AFTERNOON	AFTERNOON	Vitamins & Supplements Neuro-Antitox II™ • CNS/PNS • Musculo/Skeletal • Cardio Yeast Ease™ Detox Tea	Vitamins & Supplements Neuro-Antitox II™ • CNS/PNS • Musculo/Skeletal • Cardio Yeast Ease™ Detox Tea	Vitamins & Supplements Neuro-Antitox II™ • CNS/PNS • Musculo/Skeletal • Cardio Yeast Ease™ Detox Tea	Vitamins & Supplements Neuro-Antitox II™ • CNS/PNS • Musculo/Skeletal • Cardio Yeast Ease™ Detox Tea	Vitamins & Supplements Neuro-Antitox II™ • CNS/PNS • Musculo/Skeletal • Cardio Yeast Ease™ Detox Tea	Vitamins & Supplements Neuro-Antitox II™ • CNS/PNS • Musculo/Skeletal • Cardio Yeast Ease™ Detox Tea
Take Daily Vitamins & Supplements Detox Tea	EVENING	Vitamins & Supplements Neuro-Antitox II™ • CNS/PNS • Musculo/Skeletal • Cardio Yeast Ease™ Healing Soak & Detox Tea	Vitamins & Supplements Neuro-Antitox II™ • CNS/PNS • Musculo/Skeletal • Cardio Yeast Ease™ Healing Soak & Detox Tea	Vitamins & Supplements Neuro-Antitox II™ • CNS/PNS • Musculo/Skeletal • Cardio Yeast Ease™	Vitamins & Supplements Neuro-Antitox II™ • CNS/PNS • Musculo/Skeletal • Cardio Yeast Ease™	Vitamins & Supplements Neuro-Antitox II™ • CNS/PNS • Musculo/Skeletal • Cardio Yeast Ease™ Healing Soak & Detox Tea	Vitamins & Supplements Neuro-Antitox II™ • CNS/PNS • Musculo/Skeletal • Cardio Yeast Ease™
EVENING	Take Daily Vitamins & Supplements						

1st QUARTER CHART

1st Quarter (3 months) of Protocol Example

	SUNDAY MORNING	MONDAY MORNING	TUESDAY MORNING	WEDNESDAY MORNING	THURSDAY MORNING	FRIDAY MORNING	SATURDAY MORNING
Take Daily Vitamins & Supplements		Vitamins & Supplements Neuro-Antitox II™ • CNS/PNS • Musculo/Skeletal • Cardio Yeast Ease™ Borrelogen™	Vitamins & Supplements Neuro-Antitox II™ • CNS/PNS • Musculo/Skeletal • Cardio Yeast Ease™ Borrelogen™	Vitamins & Supplements Neuro-Antitox II™ • CNS/PNS • Musculo/Skeletal • Cardio Yeast Ease™ Borrelogen™	Vitamins & Supplements Neuro-Antitox II™ • CNS/PNS • Musculo/Skeletal • Cardio Yeast Ease™ Borrelogen™	Vitamins & Supplements Neuro-Antitox II™ • CNS/PNS • Musculo/Skeletal • Cardio Yeast Ease™ Borrelogen™	Vitamins & Supplements Neuro-Antitox II™ • CNS/PNS • Musculo/Skeletal • Cardio Yeast Ease™ Borrelogen™
AFTERNOON	AFTERNOON	AFTERNOON	AFTERNOON	AFTERNOON	AFTERNOON	AFTERNOON	AFTERNOON
Take Daily Vitamins & Supplements Detox Tea		Vitamins & Supplements Neuro-Antitox II™ • CNS/PNS • Musculo/Skeletal • Cardio Yeast Ease™ Borrelogen™ Detox Tea	Vitamins & Supplements Neuro-Antitox II™ • CNS/PNS • Musculo/Skeletal • Cardio Yeast Ease™ Borrelogen™ Detox Tea	Vitamins & Supplements Neuro-Antitox II™ • CNS/PNS • Musculo/Skeletal • Cardio Yeast Ease™ Borrelogen™ Detox Tea	Vitamins & Supplements Neuro-Antitox II™ • CNS/PNS • Musculo/Skeletal • Cardio Yeast Ease™ Borrelogen™ Detox Tea	Vitamins & Supplements Neuro-Antitox II™ • CNS/PNS • Musculo/Skeletal • Cardio Yeast Ease™ Borrelogen™ Detox Tea	Vitamins & Supplements Neuro-Antitox II™ • CNS/PNS • Musculo/Skeletal • Cardio Yeast Ease™ Borrelogen™
EVENING	EVENING	EVENING	EVENING	EVENING	EVENING	EVENING	EVENING
Take Daily Vitamins & Supplements		Vitamins & Supplements Neuro-Antitox II™ • CNS/PNS • Musculo/Skeletal • Cardio Yeast Ease™ Borrelogen™ Soak & Detox Tea	Vitamins & Supplements Neuro-Antitox II™ • CNS/PNS • Musculo/Skeletal • Cardio Yeast Ease™ Borrelogen™	Vitamins & Supplements Neuro-Antitox II™ • CNS/PNS • Musculo/Skeletal • Cardio Yeast Ease™ Borrelogen™ Soak & Detox Tea	Vitamins & Supplements Neuro-Antitox II™ • CNS/PNS • Musculo/Skeletal • Cardio Yeast Ease™ Borrelogen™	Vitamins & Supplements Neuro-Antitox II™ • CNS/PNS • Musculo/Skeletal • Cardio Yeast Ease™ Borrelogen™ Soak & Detox Tea	Vitamins & Supplements Neuro-Antitox II™ • CNS/PNS • Musculo/Skeletal • Cardio Yeast Ease™ Borrelogen™

2ND QUARTER CHART

2nd Quarter (3 months) of Protocol Example

	MONDAY MORNING	TUESDAY MORNING	WEDNESDAY MORNING	THURSDAY MORNING	FRIDAY MORNING	SATURDAY MORNING
SUNDAY MORNING Take Daily Vitamins & Supplements	Vitamins & Supplements Neuro-Antitox II™ • CNS/PNS • Musculo/Skeletal • Cardio Yeast Ease™ Lymogen™	Vitamins & Supplements Neuro-Antitox II™ • CNS/PNS • Musculo/Skeletal • Cardio Yeast Ease™ Lymogen™	Vitamins & Supplements Neuro-Antitox II™ • CNS/PNS • Musculo/Skeletal • Cardio Yeast Ease™ Lymogen™	Vitamins & Supplements Neuro-Antitox II™ • CNS/PNS • Musculo/Skeletal • Cardio Yeast Ease™ Lymogen™	Vitamins & Supplements Neuro-Antitox II™ • CNS/PNS • Musculo/Skeletal • Cardio Yeast Ease™ Lymogen™	Vitamins & Supplements Neuro-Antitox II™ • CNS/PNS • Musculo/Skeletal • Cardio Yeast Ease™ Lymogen™
AFTERNOON Take Daily Vitamins & Supplements Detox Tea	Vitamins & Supplements Neuro-Antitox II™ • CNS/PNS • Musculo/Skeletal • Cardio Yeast Ease™ Lymogen™ Detox Tea	Vitamins & Supplements Neuro-Antitox II™ • CNS/PNS • Musculo/Skeletal • Cardio Yeast Ease™ Lymogen™ Detox Tea	Vitamins & Supplements Neuro-Antitox II™ • CNS/PNS • Musculo/Skeletal • Cardio Yeast Ease™ Lymogen™ Detox Tea	AFTERNOON	AFTERNOON	AFTERNOON
EVENING Take Daily Vitamins & Supplements Soak & Detox Tea	Vitamins & Supplements Neuro-Antitox II™ • CNS/PNS • Musculo/Skeletal • Cardio Yeast Ease™ Lymogen™ Soak & Detox Tea	Vitamins & Supplements Neuro-Antitox II™ • CNS/PNS • Musculo/Skeletal • Cardio Yeast Ease™ Lymogen™	Vitamins & Supplements Neuro-Antitox II™ • CNS/PNS • Musculo/Skeletal • Cardio Yeast Ease™ Lymogen™ Soak & Detox Tea	Vitamins & Supplements Neuro-Antitox II™ • CNS/PNS • Musculo/Skeletal • Cardio Yeast Ease™ Lymogen™ Detox Tea	Vitamins & Supplements Neuro-Antitox II™ • CNS/PNS • Musculo/Skeletal • Cardio Yeast Ease™ Lymogen™ Soak & Detox Tea	EVENING

3rd QUARTER CHART

3rd Quarter (3 months) of Protocol Example

	SUNDAY	MONDAY	TUESDAY	WEDNESDAY	THURSDAY	FRIDAY	SATURDAY
MORNING	Take Daily Vitamins & Supplements	Vitamins & Supplements Neuro-Antitox II™ • CNS/PNS • Musculo/Skeletal • Cardio Yeast Ease™ Microbojen™	Vitamins & Supplements Neuro-Antitox II™ • CNS/PNS • Musculo/Skeletal • Cardio Yeast Ease™ Microbojen™	Vitamins & Supplements Neuro-Antitox II™ • CNS/PNS • Musculo/Skeletal • Cardio Yeast Ease™ Microbojen™	Vitamins & Supplements Neuro-Antitox II™ • CNS/PNS • Musculo/Skeletal • Cardio Yeast Ease™ Microbojen™	Vitamins & Supplements Neuro-Antitox II™ • CNS/PNS • Musculo/Skeletal • Cardio Yeast Ease™ Microbojen™	Vitamins & Supplements Neuro-Antitox II™ • CNS/PNS • Musculo/Skeletal • Cardio Yeast Ease™ Microbojen™
AFTERNOON	Take Daily Vitamins & Supplements Detox Tea	Vitamins & Supplements Neuro-Antitox II™ • CNS/PNS • Musculo/Skeletal • Cardio Yeast Ease™ Microbojen™ Detox Tea	Vitamins & Supplements Neuro-Antitox II™ • CNS/PNS • Musculo/Skeletal • Cardio Yeast Ease™ Microbojen™ Detox Tea	Vitamins & Supplements Neuro-Antitox II™ • CNS/PNS • Musculo/Skeletal • Cardio Yeast Ease™ Microbojen™ Detox Tea	Vitamins & Supplements Neuro-Antitox II™ • CNS/PNS • Musculo/Skeletal • Cardio Yeast Ease™ Microbojen™ Detox Tea	Vitamins & Supplements Neuro-Antitox II™ • CNS/PNS • Musculo/Skeletal • Cardio Yeast Ease™ Microbojen™ Detox Tea	Vitamins & Supplements Neuro-Antitox II™ • CNS/PNS • Musculo/Skeletal • Cardio Yeast Ease™ Microbojen™
EVENING	Take Daily Vitamins & Supplements Soak & Detox Tea	Vitamins & Supplements Neuro-Antitox II™ • CNS/PNS • Musculo/Skeletal • Cardio Yeast Ease™ Microbojen™ Soak & Detox Tea	Vitamins & Supplements Neuro-Antitox II™ • CNS/PNS • Musculo/Skeletal • Cardio Yeast Ease™ Microbojen™	Vitamins & Supplements Neuro-Antitox II™ • CNS/PNS • Musculo/Skeletal • Cardio Yeast Ease™ Microbojen™ Soak & Detox Tea	Vitamins & Supplements Neuro-Antitox II™ • CNS/PNS • Musculo/Skeletal • Cardio Yeast Ease™ Microbojen™	Vitamins & Supplements Neuro-Antitox II™ • CNS/PNS • Musculo/Skeletal • Cardio Yeast Ease™ Microbojen™ Soak & Detox Tea	Vitamins & Supplements Neuro-Antitox II™ • CNS/PNS • Musculo/Skeletal • Cardio Yeast Ease™ Microbojen™

4th QUARTER CHART

4th Quarter (3 months) of Protocol Example

	SUNDAY MORNING	MONDAY MORNING	TUESDAY MORNING	WEDNESDAY MORNING	THURSDAY MORNING	FRIDAY MORNING	SATURDAY MORNING
Take Daily Vitamins & Supplements	Vitamins & Supplements Neuro-Antitox II™ • CNS/PNS • Musculo/Skeletal • Cardio Yeast Ease™ Borrelogen™ Lymogen™ Microbojen™	Vitamins & Supplements Neuro-Antitox II™ • CNS/PNS • Musculo/Skeletal • Cardio Yeast Ease™ Borrelogen™ Lymogen™ Microbojen™	Vitamins & Supplements Neuro-Antitox II™ • CNS/PNS • Musculo/Skeletal • Cardio Yeast Ease™ Borrelogen™ Lymogen™ Microbojen™	Vitamins & Supplements Neuro-Antitox II™ • CNS/PNS • Musculo/Skeletal • Cardio Yeast Ease™ Borrelogen™ Lymogen™ Microbojen™	Vitamins & Supplements Neuro-Antitox II™ • CNS/PNS • Musculo/Skeletal • Cardio Yeast Ease™ Borrelogen™ Lymogen™ Microbojen™	Vitamins & Supplements Neuro-Antitox II™ • CNS/PNS • Musculo/Skeletal • Cardio Yeast Ease™ Borrelogen™ Lymogen™ Microbojen™	Vitamins & Supplements Neuro-Antitox II™ • CNS/PNS • Musculo/Skeletal • Cardio Yeast Ease™ Borrelogen™ Lymogen™ Microbojen™
AFTERNOON	AFTERNOON	AFTERNOON	AFTERNOON	AFTERNOON	AFTERNOON	AFTERNOON	AFTERNOON
Take Daily Vitamins & Supplements Detox Tea	Vitamins & Supplements Neuro-Antitox II™ • CNS/PNS • Musculo/Skeletal • Cardio Yeast Ease™ Borrelogen™ Lymogen™ Microbojen™ Detox Tea	Vitamins & Supplements Neuro-Antitox II™ • CNS/PNS • Musculo/Skeletal • Cardio Yeast Ease™ Borrelogen™ Lymogen™ Microbojen™ Detox Tea	Vitamins & Supplements Neuro-Antitox II™ • CNS/PNS • Musculo/Skeletal • Cardio Yeast Ease™ Borrelogen™ Lymogen™ Microbojen™ Detox Tea	Vitamins & Supplements Neuro-Antitox II™ • CNS/PNS • Musculo/Skeletal • Cardio Yeast Ease™ Borrelogen™ Lymogen™ Microbojen™ Detox Tea	Vitamins & Supplements Neuro-Antitox II™ • CNS/PNS • Musculo/Skeletal • Cardio Yeast Ease™ Borrelogen™ Lymogen™ Microbojen™ Detox Tea	Vitamins & Supplements Neuro-Antitox II™ • CNS/PNS • Musculo/Skeletal • Cardio Yeast Ease™ Borrelogen™ Lymogen™ Microbojen™ Detox Tea	Vitamins & Supplements Neuro-Antitox II™ • CNS/PNS • Musculo/Skeletal • Cardio Yeast Ease™ Borrelogen™ Lymogen™ Microbojen™ Detox Tea
EVENING	EVENING	EVENING	EVENING	EVENING	EVENING	EVENING	EVENING
Take Daily Vitamins & Supplements	Vitamins & Supplements Neuro-Antitox II™ • CNS/PNS • Musculo/Skeletal • Cardio Yeast Ease™ Borrelogen™ Lymogen™ Microbojen™ Soak & Detox Tea	Vitamins & Supplements Neuro-Antitox II™ • CNS/PNS • Musculo/Skeletal • Cardio Yeast Ease™ Borrelogen™ Lymogen™ Microbojen™	Vitamins & Supplements Neuro-Antitox II™ • CNS/PNS • Musculo/Skeletal • Cardio Yeast Ease™ Borrelogen™ Lymogen™ Microbojen™ Soak & Detox Tea	Vitamins & Supplements Neuro-Antitox II™ • CNS/PNS • Musculo/Skeletal • Cardio Yeast Ease™ Borrelogen™ Lymogen™ Microbojen™	Vitamins & Supplements Neuro-Antitox II™ • CNS/PNS • Musculo/Skeletal • Cardio Yeast Ease™ Borrelogen™ Lymogen™ Microbojen™ Soak & Detox Tea	Vitamins & Supplements Neuro-Antitox II™ • CNS/PNS • Musculo/Skeletal • Cardio Yeast Ease™ Borrelogen™ Lymogen™ Microbojen™

Chapter 11
A Chapter Ends

Now that the healing protocol has been completed, what comes next?

I feel fortunate that this story has had a happy ending. More than four years have passed without the return of Lichen Sclerosis. Not a flare-up, no itching, no burning, no white patches, no skin tearing, no nothing. I've also never had any recurrences of previous medical issues either.

My life today is *normal* and I enjoy all of the activities that I did before I had LS. But I am committed to my totally organic lifestyle; using only 100% organic products, 100% organic ingredients and eating only 100% organic food, most of it raw. I eat raw egg yolks in fruit shakes and drink 30 ounces of raw A2 cow and/or goat milk every day as well as 16 ounces or more of filtered water. This is a lifestyle that I intend to continue for the rest of my life because if I falter or slip back into my former non-organic ways, my body might travel down the same road to Lichen Sclerosis, or worse. But it doesn't mean I still do everything exactly as I did during the healing protocol. Staying healthy is an on-going learning experience that continuously evolves. Over time, I've added, changed, cut back, or eliminated many of the ingredients I took during the healing protocol. By now, choosing organic foods and using only organic and non-toxic products has become second nature; a new and established way of life.

The way I conduct my life continuously evolves as my research into maintaining my health continues. For example, I used to put a complete raw egg in my fruit shake. But I've learned that while eating raw egg yolk is nutritionally beneficial, eating raw egg whites, especially on a regular basis, can create a biotin deficiency. That's because raw egg whites contain avidin, an antimicrobial protein that binds with the biotin in the raw egg and prevents biotin from being absorbed into the body. Biotin is a B-complex vitamin (Vitamin K) critical for cell growth and processing fats and sugars. Cooking egg whites frees biotin by neutralizing avidin, making cooked egg white a very healthy food. So now I separate the yolk from the white and use the yolk in my fruit shake while saving the raw white for other cooking uses.

And we no longer eat scrambled or hard boiled eggs. That's because raw egg yolk contains healthy, large molecule cholesterol, but cooking egg yolk oxidizes the cholesterol, making it unhealthy. When cooking eggs, I make sure the whites are cooked, but the yolk remains runny.

When I initially switched from commercial cereal to organic cereal, I'd buy it in bulk. Now I never buy cereal because it is processed food. We also went from commercial granola bars to the organic version, but not only are they another processed, dead food, but despite being organic, they are also loaded with five different forms of organic sugar (tapioca syrup, invert cane sugar, molasses, and evaporated cane juice listed twice) making them an unhealthy product, despite being organic, that I no longer purchase.

Subscribing to health newsletters keeps me abreast of the ever-changing rules and regulations regarding foods and products, as well as new studies that reveal potential health hazards or health breakthroughs, and enable me to modify my lifestyle accordingly.

While I've eliminated many of the supplements I used during the healing protocol, I've added new supplements to my daily regimen that were not part of the healing protocol, but contain healing and chemical/heavy metal detoxification properties. I think of it as an on-going mini-healing protocol I can use every day. Below is the list of what I use now:

SPIRULINA

Spirulina is a nutrient-dense super food made up of high-alkaline fresh-water algae that grows on, and is harvested from, pristine natural ponds and man-made enclosed environments. It's impossible to overdose on it and it is 100% non-toxic. Spirulina contains nearly every vitamin, mineral, carotenoid, essential fatty acid, protein, and amino acid the human body needs and I think of it as a whole-food multi-vitamin that is immediately bio-available and readily assimilated in the body.

CHLORELLA

Chlorella is another super food algae that is not only nutrient-dense, but also has powerful detoxifying properties. It acts like a sponge as it neutralizes and binds with toxins of many types, including chemicals such as DDT and PCB, heavy metals of lead, cadmium, and especially mercury, enabling the body to eliminate them. These amazing properties of chlorella are found in its cell wall membranes, but we can't digest these cellular membranes unless they have been broken. Broken cell wall chlorella's power in detoxification extends to diseases including cancer. Not only can chlorella help the body cope with the toxic effects of chemotherapy, it also has been shown to help in suppressing abnormal cell proliferation while promoting the repair of damaged tissue, as well as increasing immune cells.

Taking supplemental spirulina and chlorella are *not* magic bullets or quick fixes. As has already been discussed throughout this book, the human body works slowly but steadily, and the effects of nutrient-dense organic food, vitamins, supplements, and nutraceuticals usually are visible 3-4 months after they've been initiated. After the healing protocol, supplementation with spirulina and chlorella will further stimulate the body's natural healing and detoxification capacity.

Nutrients found in spirulina and chlorella combined include:

SPIRULINA/CHLORELLA NUTRITIONAL ANALYSIS PER 10 GRAMS (2 teaspoons)			
Vitamins	**Value**	**Minerals**	**Value**
Vitamin E	1 IU	Calcium	100 mg
Vitamin A	18 mg	Iron	15 mg
Thiamine (B1)	.31 mg	Zinc	0.3 mg
Riboflavin (B2)	.35 mg	Phosphorus	90 mg
Niacin (B3)	1.48mg	Magnesium	40 mg
Pyridoxine (B6)	80 µg	Copper	0.12 mg
Vitamin B12	32 µg	Sodium	60 mg
Folacin	1 µg	Potassium	160 mg
Pantothenic Acid	.01 mg	Manganese	0.5 mg
Inositol	6.4 mg	Chromium	0.028 mg
		Germanium	0.006 mg
		Selenium	0.002 mg
Essential Amino Acids	**Value**	**Non-Essential Amino Acids**	**Value**
Isoleucine	350 mg	Alanine	470 mg
Leucine	540 mg	Arginine	430 mg
Lysine	290 mg	Aspartic Acid	610 mg
Methionine	140 mg	Cystine	60 mg
Phenylalanine	280 mg	Glutamic Acid	910 mg
Essential Amino Acids	**Value**	**Non-Essential Amino Acids**	**Value**
Threonine	320 mg	Clycine	320 mg
Tryptophane	90 mg	Histidine	100 mg
Valine	400 mg	Proline	270 mg
		Serine	320 mg
		Tyrosine	300 mg

SPIRULINA/CHLORELLA NUTRITIONAL ANALYSIS PER 10 GRAMS (2 teaspoons)			
Essential Fatty Acids	Value	Natural Pigments	Value
Myristic	1 mg	Phycocyanin (Blue)	1000-2000 mg
Palmitic	244 mg	Chlorophyll (Green)	115 mg
Palmitoleic	33 mg	Carotenoids (Orange)	37 mg
Heptadecanoic	2 mg	Beta-Carotene	18 mg
Stearic	8 mg		
Oleic	12 mg		
Linoleic	97 mg		
Gammalinolenic	135 mg		
Others	14 mg		

Essential Amino Acids Found in Spirulina and Chlorella

The essential amino acids found in spirulina and chlorella take a form that is much faster and easier for the body to assimilate than the essential amino acids found in meat or soy protein. Essential amino acids are ones that our body cannot manufacture and which must come from food. The following are eight essential amino acids found in spirulina and chlorella:

- **Isoleucine** - Required for growth, intelligence development, nitrogen equilibrium, and non-essential amino acid synthesis

- **Leucine** – A stimulator of brain function and muscular energy levels

- **Lysine** – A building block for blood antibodies, strengthens the circulatory system, and maintains normal cell growth

- **Methionine** – A fat and lipid metabolizing (lipotropic) amino acid that helps maintain liver health and acts as an anti-stress factor

- **Phenylalanine** – Essential for the production of thyroxin by the thyroid gland

- **Threonine** – Essential for intestinal health and digestion

- **Tryptophane** – Maximizes the body's use of B vitamins; improves nerve health and emotional stability

- **Valine** – Stimulates mental capacity and muscle coordination

Non-Essential Amino Acids Found in Spirulina

Non-essential amino acids simply means that our body can synthesize them itself if they are not provided in food. The non-essential amino acids found in spirulina include:

- **Alanine** – Strengthens cellular walls

- **Arginine** – Helps to detoxify blood and is essential to sexual health

- **Aspartic Acid** – Aids in the transformation of carbohydrates into cellular energy

- **Cystine** – Aids in pancreatic health

- **Glutamic Acid** – A principal fuel of brain cells

- **Glycine** – Promotes cellular energy and oxygen use

- **Histidine** – Strengthens nerve relays, especially in auditory organs

- **Proline** – A precursor amino acid in the production of glutamic acid

- **Serine** – Essential in the formation of myelin, the fatty sheaths that act as insulators surrounding brain nerve fibers

- **Tyrosine** – Slows cellular aging and is involved with hair and skin coloration, including sunburn protection

Pigments Found in Spirulina and Chlorella

While our daily requirements are generally focused on vitamins, minerals, protein, and fats, our health also depends upon pigments found in the foods we eat. While Kermit the Frog wants us to "think green," we also need the rainbow of colors that nature provides us in fruits and vegetables.

- **Phycocyanin** - Essential to healthy liver function and the digestion of amino acids

- **Chlorophyll** – The most abundant pigment on earth, sometimes referred to as "green blood" because it is essential in the formation of hemoglobin and healthy red blood cells

- **Carotenoids** - The carotenoids in spirulina and chlorella provide the non-toxic precursors needed to assimilate and synthesize vitamins, especially vitamin A. The human body can never overdose on carotenoid vitamin A

Many companies offer raw spirulina and chlorella powders, but I look for the kind that contain broken cell wall, are USDA Certified Organic, and I avoid anything grown in China because of the pollution there. Even though many companies now offer combined spirulina and chlorella tablets, I prefer raw powders simply because they have not been subjected to manufacturing processes to make them into tablets. The raw powders provide flexibility and can be dispensed from a salt/pepper shaker and sprinkled on food, or measured in spoons or cups. Buying the powders in bulk is expensive but also significantly less costly than manufactured tablets. But the choice is yours.

OLIVE LEAF

Olive leaf is nature's non-toxic immune system builder that works at the cellular level to strengthen immune response. Olive leaf has the ability to penetrate infected cells and stop viruses from replicating. Along with an array of polyphenol compounds listed below, including three highly active free radical scavenger antioxidants, olive leaf also has a wide array of antioxidant nutrients, healing properties, and the flavonoids hesperidin, rutin, apgenin, quercetin and kaempferol. The following are the polyphenols and other ingredients found in Olive Leaf:

- **Oleuropein** – This phenol possesses antimicrobial properties and inhibits micro-organisms such as viruses, retroviruses, rhinoviruses, myxoviruses, Herpes Simplex type I and II, Herpes Varicella-Zoster (shingles), many strains of influenza and para-influenza viruses, bacteria, fungi, and parasites. It also acts as a modulator of host-cell gene expression by inhibiting cell-to-cell transmission of infection.

- **Hydroxytyrosol** – This antioxidant polyphenol is associated with preventing and/or reducing harmful effects of inflammatory diseases.

- **Tyrosol** – Tyrosol is a phenolic antioxidant that is integral in protecting cells against free radicals.

Olive leaf has been shown to be effective in reducing symptoms of:

- Fibromyalgia
- Chronic Fatigue Syndrome
- Cardiovascular disease
- Ulcerative colitis
- Irritable Bowel Syndrome (IBS)
- Hypertension

Drug Interactions

Olive leaf can have negative impact on the following drug types:

- Diabetic/Hypoglycemic
- ACE inhibitors
- Hypertension
- Anticoagulants
- Antiplatelet (Statins)

There are already several key immune modulating supplements in the healing protocol, and while olive leaf is synergistic and could be included, it is not part of the protocol. Instead, it can be used as a cellular healing and immune building supplement *after* the healing protocol has been completed.

Olive leaf can be an allergen for sensitive individuals. Consult with a health care provider before administering to children.

How to Take Olive Leaf:

Organic olive leaf can be taken powdered in capsule form, or as a liquid extract. Take 7 days per week.

Olivus 500 mg Olive Leaf Extract Capsules

- Children under 6: See Homeopathic Rule of Thumb. Give with meals.
- Children ages 6-12: Give 1/2 capsule 1x per day with meals.
- Teen to Adult: Take 2 capsules per day with meals.

Ingredients: Olive leaf, oleuropein

Olivus 500 mg Olive Leaf Extract Tincture

- Children under 6: See Homeopathic Rule of Thumb. Add drops to water, juice, or any hot or cold liquid once per day.
- Children ages 6-12: 1/2 eyedropper once per day in water, juice, or any hot or cold liquid
- Teen to Adult: Take 1 eyedropper 1x per day in water, juice, or any hot or cold liquid.

Ingredients: Olive leaf extract, oleuropein, alcohol

Olivus 500 mg Olive Leaf Extract Elixir

- Children under 6: See Homeopathic Rule of Thumb. Add drops to water, juice, or any hot or cold liquid; give once per day.

- Children ages 6-12: 1/2 eyedropper in water, juice, or any hot or cold liquid; give once per day.

- Teen to Adult: 1 eyedropper per day in water, juice, or any hot or cold liquid.

Ingredients: Olive leaf extract, oleuropein, organic Manuka honey

VITAMINS AND SUPPLEMENTS

I used to buy raw organic whole food vitamins by Garden of Life, but since I've begun making my own vitamins, and added organic raw milk and other whole foods to my diet that provide micronutrients, I only need to purchase a handful of ready-made vitamins and only take half of the recommended dosages.

- Multivitamin – 4 capsules (750mg each) per day of a 50/50 mix of organic spirulina and chlorella powders that I encapsulate

- Vitamin C - One 750mg capsule per day of organic rose hip powder that I encapsulate

- Vitamin Code Raw D3 5000 IU (organic) - 2 capsules per day during winter only

- Calcium - 2 capsules (500mg each) per day of crushed organic eggshell. I boil empty shells from organic eggs, then powder the shells in a coffee grinder, after which I encapsulate them. Eggshells are 95% calcium bicarbonate, which is the most bioavailable form of calcium.

- Dr. Mercola's Ubiquinol (the active form of CoQ10) – 2 capsules per day

- Olivus® Organic Olive Leaf Extract – 1 capsule per day **or** 1 capsule (750mg) per day of organic powdered olive leaf that I encapsulate

- Dr. Mercola's Krill Oil – 2 capsules per day (not for people with shellfish allergies)

- Health From The Sun Organic Evening Primrose Oil 500 mg – 2 soft gels per day

- Nutritional Yeast Maxi Flake (organic) –1/3 cup on salad every night (high in B-complex and B12 vitamins)

- Spirulina/Chlorella Powder (organic) – 2 tablespoons on nightly salads in addition to 4 "multivitamin" 750 mg capsules per day for a total of 4500 mg. I encapsulate the powders.

NUTRACEUTICALS

I always keep a supply of various Jernigan Nutraceuticals on hand as they are useful for many remedies. Ways in which I or my case studies have used these botanicals include:

- **Cold and flu remedy** - An eyedropper full of Borrelogen under the tongue in the morning, one of Lymogen in the afternoon, and an eyedropper full of Microbojen in the evening until symptoms are gone.

- **Rash, hives, poison ivy, or shingles** - An eyedropper full of Virogen under the tongue in the morning, one of Lymogen in the afternoon, and an eyedropper full of Microbojen in the evening until symptoms are gone. Silphitrin can also be taken orally and/or applied topically 3 times per day. For viral infections such as shingles, 600 mg of L-Lysine can be taken twice a day as well.

- **Muscle and joint aches** - An eyedropper full of Neuro-Antitox II Musculo-Skeletal under the tongue three times a day until symptoms are gone. Silphitrin can also be taken orally and/or applied topically 3 times per day.

- **Broken bones and sprains** – Take one eyedropper full of Neuro-Antitox II Musculo-Skeletal under the tongue three times a day until bones and sprains are healed. Silphitrin can be taken orally 3 times per day and/or applied topically several times a day as well.

- **Eye infections** – One eyedropper each of Neuro-Antitox II CNS/PNS, Virogen, and Microbojen under the tongue three times per day until symptoms are gone. Thankfully I no longer get eye infections.

The empty washed botanical bottles are great for storing small amounts of organic extra virgin olive oil, organic vanilla, and many other liquids that need the application of only a few drops.

HEALING SOAKS

My husband and I soak occasionally after a day of very hard physical work or exercise, or on rare occasions when we experience symptoms of the onset of a cold, or feeling "under the weather."

DETOX TEA

One bag each of Yogi and Triple Leaf detox teas in 8 oz of hot water, with the juice from a slice or two of organic ginger root. I drink this occasionally, but especially when I plan to do a healing soak.

PERSONAL CARE

There are *no commercial personal care products* in my home.

- **Facial Cleanser** - Organic extra virgin olive oil is excellent as a cleanser for removing dirt and grease before bathing. It's also a great hand cleanser.

- **Exfoliating** – To exfoliate I wet my face, then make a scrub using lather from Soap for Goodness Sake's Extra Virgin Olive Oil soap, then add a tablespoon of organic corn meal, rub the mixture in my palms, then gently scrub my face with it. Then I rinse with clean water.

- **Moisturizer** – Organic virgin coconut oil (the same one I use for cooking) is a fabulous moisturizer that seems to make fine lines disappear instantly. While organic extra virgin olive oil used to be a favorite of mine, I've really come to appreciate organic virgin coconut oil. Coconut oil is solid, but will liquefy at a room temperature of 76°. I've slowly melted it in a pot on the stove at 76°, allowed it to cool slightly, then poured it into small glass jars. I keep one in the car, one in the bathroom, and one on my night table to use as a night cream for face, hands, elbows, and any dry skin area.

  Organic virgin coconut oil also works very well as a massage oil, and as a personal lubricant.

- **Bathing** – Soap for Goodness Sake Organic Extra Virgin Olive Oil soap continues to be my favorite soap for bathing. Now that I have no medical issues, I've begun to branch out into more of their soap line and occasionally use other soaps with the fewest ingredients. *Less is more.*

- **Shampoo** – Whatever Soap For Goodness Sake soap I use for bathing, I also use to wash my hair. It is pointless to use two separate products.

- **Toothpaste** – I continue to use Soap For Goodness Sake Spearmint Tooth Powder.

- **Mouthwash** – None. While brushing my teeth with tooth powder, I also brush my tongue as far back into the throat as possible. This removes odor-causing bacteria on the tongue, but it takes practice to control the gag-reflex.

- **Deodorant** – None. What works very well for me is applying organic white vinegar to my armpits using a cotton ball soaked in the vinegar. The vinegar acts as a natural astringent. After allowing the vinegar to dry, I gently wipe the area with a barely damp cloth to remove any lingering vinegar scent, followed by a powder puff dusting of organic non-GMO corn starch.

- **Shaving** – Organic Babassu Shaving Soap by Soap for Goodness Sake is the only shave cream my husband or I use.

- **Ano-Genital Area** – During the healing protocol, after bathing, I applied a few drops of Olio Beato Organic Extra Virgin Olive Oil to my LS-affected skin to help keep it rejuvenated. Six months after completing the healing protocol I switched to applying organic virgin coconut oil. A year after completion of the healing protocol I no longer needed to apply anything to my skin.

When I was diagnosed with LS, I had also suffered from anal tearing and slight bleeding from bowel movements, as well as occasional hemorrhoids. Initially I'd inserted small pieces of a Vitamin E suppository but soon switched to inserting ¼ inch blobs of organic Nutiva virgin coconut oil during the full healing protocol, and drinking more water. I no longer need to do this because I no longer tear and bleed during bowel movements and no longer have hemorrhoids.

- **Bio-Identical Hormones** – I no longer take bio-identical estriol hormone for vaginal lubrication. My body now produces its own lubrication in the amount appropriate for my age.

Organic extra virgin olive oil and organic virgin coconut oil now play many roles in my life and both are incredibly soothing and healing for burned skin either from too much sun exposure or from cooking mishaps.

I believe my skin and hair are healthy as a result of my inner health. A healthy appearance comes from the inside, not the other way around, so applying wrinkle reducers, facial masks, skin rejuvenators, etc., is a waste of time and money. It's more important to feed the body with good nutrition, and maybe then you won't need all those other products.

HOME MAINTENANCE

My lifestyle is very simple, using the purest, most basic things. In many cases I've stepped back in time to when things were much less toxic.

Food

- Only 100% organic raw food is allowed in our home. It comes from local organic farms, farmers' markets, food co-ops, health food stores, online organic food websites, or I grow it myself.

- We eat as much raw food as possible; otherwise it's steamed or baked. We rarely broil or grill and frying is not an option.

- Food that I prepare is made from scratch, using organic ingredients. We don't buy processed food.

- Milk and cream are strictly organic and raw (goat, Jersey or Guernsey cow) from local sources.

- Eggs are from organic free-range chickens we raise ourselves.

- Organic pasture butter (no margarine, organic or otherwise) I've made myself from organic raw milk, or I buy organic Guernsey cow butter from a local farm. My third choice is Woodstock Farms organic butter.

- We use Nutiva organic virgin coconut oil for cooking.

- Organic extra virgin olive oil for cold foods and salads.

- Organic unfiltered apple cider vinegar and organic balsamic vinegar for homemade salad dressings that include Himalayan pink salt, organic pepper, nutritional yeast, and a 50/50 mix of spirulina and chlorella.

Food Storage Containers

- Glass jars, bottles, containers (1950's glass refrigerator storage dishes)
- Stainless steel pots and nesting bowls
- CorningWare dishes
- Bulk food-grade plastic containers may be free upon asking at health food stores and food co-ops, or purchased online

Dining Implements

- Good china or ceramic plates
- Stainless steel utensils
- Glass, china, or ceramic glasses, cups and mugs
- Organic cotton or unbleached paper napkins

Cooking Materials

- Stainless steel pots and pans
- Glass bowls, bread pans, cake pans
- CorningWare dishes (made in USA)
- Stainless steel utensils
- High heat silicon spatulas
- Convection oven
- Cooktop

Do NOT Use These Cooking Techniques or Tools

- Microwave ovens
- Non-stick pans
- Aluminum foil
- Plastic wrap
- Plastic non-food-grade storage containers
- Pan release spray

- Canned food (only glass containers are acceptable)

HOUSEHOLD CLEANERS AND DISINFECTANTS

My home is also a lot healthier now. With absolutely NO commercial detergents, cleansers, scrubs, or the like, I've made my own 100% non-toxic cleaning supplies using individually, or in varying combinations the following ingredients to clean my stove, cooktop, bathroom fixtures, shower, windows, mirrors, carpeting, and anything else that needs cleaning.

- Organic extra virgin coconut oil soap
- Baking soda
- Hydrogen peroxide
- White vinegar

Instead of expensive dishwasher rinse aids, simply fill the rinse aid compartment with white vinegar. It leaves dishes and silverware sparkling clean. It's also non-toxic to pipes, septic systems, ground water, and sewer systems. White vinegar also gets windows and mirrors spotless without streaks.

Soap for Goodness Sake's Organic Extra Virgin Coconut Oil remains my one and only laundry and dish detergent and general purpose household cleaner. It cleans and disinfects rugs, countertops, and toilets. Apply a tablespoon of grated soap to toilet water, soak until the water turns milky, add white vinegar and a tablespoon of baking soda, scrub with a brush, and voila, the toilet is clean. For stubborn stains, before scrubbing add white vinegar and 1/2 teaspoon of baking soda which will make the mixture foam.

A sponge mop has replaced the Swiffer. To wash and disinfect floors, add one part white vinegar to two parts hot water, then apply a bit of elbow grease to the sponge mop. My floors have never been cleaner, there are no toxic fumes, and I no longer have to worry about pets walking across the floor while it's still damp.

ORGANIC FABRICS

- Organic hemp or organic cotton towels and washcloths
- Organic cotton sheets, pillowcases, blankets, and mattress covers
- Organic wool blankets
- Organic cotton, wool, or silk clothing

AIR PURIFICATION

- Open windows
- Lots of green, leafy plants

WATER PURIFICATION

- Aquasana under counter water filtration system
- Well water spin-down filter
- Glass bottles
- Non-BPA stainless steel storage containers

BUG REPELLANT

Bug repellant is important where I live. Blood sucking mosquitoes, black flies, horse/deer flies, and other insects are a nuisance during the warm months. I used to suffer through them because I have always refused to put products containing DEET or any other toxin on my skin or on my clothing. However, I found a wonderful product that repels all of the insects listed above, and many more. It's a natural repellent to help protect your pets, and yourself, I might add, from fleas, ticks, mosquitoes, flies, and no-seeums. It has a nice lemony scent, too. It's *Dr. Mercola Natural Flea and Tick Defense For Dogs and Cats.*

Ingredients (both active and inert):

- Purified water   93.5%
- Lemon Grass Oil   4.0%
- Cinnamon Oil   1.0%
- Sesame Oil   1.0%
- Castor Oil   0.5%

Always test a small skin area first for sensitivity. Do not use if sensitivity occurs, or there is a known allergic reaction to any of the listed ingredients.

To apply to yourself or to pet, generously spray some into your palm, rub your palms together, then rub it into hair or pet fur, until damp. Repeat spraying into the palm of hand and generously rub onto face (avoid eyes, nose, mouth), ears, behind ears, neck, exposed arms, exposed legs, and any other part of body that is exposed. Remember to apply generously so that all exposed areas are quite dampened. The product dries quickly but lasts for hours. Insects, such as mosquitoes, might continue to hover, but they won't land or bite. Other insects might hover initially, and then disappear.

Most of the people I have recommended this product to swear by it and I know of only one person who claims it does not work for them.

CAPSULE FILLING MACHINE

Buying capsules or tablets of vitamins and supplements is expensive and it's much cheaper to purchase ingredients in bulk, along with empty vegetarian capsules, and use a capsule filling machine. Spirulina and chlorella supplements are an example: I buy organic spirulina and organic chlorella powder in 5 pound bulk bags and mix the two together. I like the powders sprinkled on my salad, but not a lot at one time. Plus, I only like the flavor on my salad and don't like it in smoothies, fruit shakes, or in any other food. I prefer to take it throughout the day, but it's inconvenient to take along when dining out. Thus encapsulating the powders resolves all of these issues. Buying the powders in bulk I can make enough multivitamins to last 2-3 years and still have enough spirulina and chlorella powder for other uses.

Making my own capsules has worked well for me and I like to sit at the table after dinner, with the TV on so I can listen to a program while churning out my own vitamins. The capsules I prefer to use come in two sizes: 00 (large, approximately 750mg) and 0 (small, approximately 500mg). The manually operated capsule filling machines also come in the same capsule sizes. The machines usually cost under $20 each and empty capsules come in quantities ranging from 100 to 1,000 and, along with the capsule filling machines, can be purchased at quantity wholesale prices.

I use the machines to encapsulate many things now, including organic white willow bark (nature's original natural aspirin), spirulina and chlorella powders, olive leaf powder, rose hip powder, and many others. Now I make my own filled capsules for pennies, and they contain nothing but the 100% organic raw ingredients of my choosing.

Please note: The capsules are intended for dry ingredients only.

Staying healthy is an ongoing learning experience. As a result, how I conduct my life so that I remain healthy continuously evolves.

Sources:

Natural Ways to Health, "Spirulina's Nutritional Analysis." www.naturalways.com/spirulina-analysis.htm

Chapter 12
The Politics of Health

"A man is truly ethical only when he obeys the compulsion to help all life which he is able to assist, and shrinks from injuring anything that lives."

Dr. Albert Schweitzer

Those of us living in the U.S. have been poisoned steadily since before we were born. We've been fed food laden with pesticides, baby powdered, bathed, clothed, and bedded in chemicals because manufacturers have sold us their toxic products through glitzy packaging and seductive advertising. They've known about the toxicity of their products for years; if they didn't, why would they try so hard to hide what's really in their products? Why use blanket terms like *fragrance*, *spices*, and *seasoning*? Why disguise a chemical no one wants to ingest with a less threatening name? If genetically engineered foods are so good for us, why wouldn't a company be proud to name it? Why fight so hard not to label GMO food? Why such a rush to alter the ingredients when a foreign government forces them to prove their safety before allowing their product into their markets?

Isn't it telling that many soft drinks destined to be sold outside the U.S. are bottled and packaged in other countries because those countries refuse to drink high fructose corn syrup? So why is it in just about every sweet drink in the US?

Other countries refuse American foods containing genetically modified ingredients, so products destined for those countries are reformulated and made without those ingredients. Hazardous chemicals banned by other countries won't be found in their products, but they're allowed here in the U.S.

Here in the USA, our government has allowed us to become the dumping ground for every toxic chemical, waste, and genetically engineered product that other countries neither want nor allow. We have been and are being used as guinea pigs, and our health has been treated cavalierly by one conglomerate after another. It's time to wake up! We *must* put an end to this situation, not only for ourselves, but for our children and for future generations. It's time we all reclaimed our own health.

As if dumping toxic waste into our drinking water and claiming that fluoride is beneficial for our teeth isn't bad enough, in December 2012, the Department of Energy proposed appalling legislation that would end the 2000 ban to sell radioactive metal waste to recyclers who would then turn it into "consumer goods." The Department of Energy claims that the radiation from these metals would be "negligible." This is the same theory behind chemicals in our products and food, but when these chemicals are in every product and food item we buy, the human toxic burden is no longer "negligible."

No amount of radiation poisoning is "negligible," especially when you consider that this radiation-emitting material could end up surrounding us via eyeglasses, dental bridges and implants, medical implants, baby spoons, and jewelry. After reading the Department of Energy's "Programmatic Environmental Assessment for the Recycle of Scrap Metals Originating from Radiological Areas" draft proposal, I took a look around my house. It's overwhelming to think that pots and pans, silverware, kitchen and bath faucets, appliances, light fixtures, buttons and zippers on clothing, safety pins, scissors, paper clips, push pins, electrical wiring, ceiling fan, woodstove, Venetian blinds, pens, doorknobs and hinges, screen door, belt buckle, purse latch, computer components, flashlights, cans, lids, and much more could one day all be emitting radiation if the DOE's proposal is approved. In addition, many of these goods would end up contaminating landfills.

Why would a government agency propose such a thing? One reason is to get rid of the ever increasing stockpile of radioactive metal waste. But an even bigger reason to foist radioactive material onto the public is the agency's estimated gain of $40 million per year at our health expense.

Rather than banning the use of glyphosate due to its toxicity, instead in 2013 the Environmental Protection Agency chose to *double* the *allowable* level of this poison in food crops! Why would an agency that was created to protect us from chemical harm do this? It should come as no surprise that key positions in the EPA are held by former top level employees of the chemical company that invented glyphosate.

We've been deluged with messages over the years that have been carefully crafted and unrelenting, telling us about better living through chemistry, and that every symptom can be cured with a simple pill or cream. We have relinquished our responsibility for our own health, leaving it up to doctors, drug manufacturers, and insurance companies to take care of us.

But there's a serious flaw in that mindset. Why would they want to make us well if it would cut their profits to do so? The health care industry has evolved into nothing more than a disease maintenance machine that keeps us alive but not in good health so they can milk every last penny until we are discarded as no longer useful.

Despite common belief, we are *not* living longer. Published in 2011, a study of 17 industrialized European countries, plus the U.S., Canada and

Australia, showed life expectancy in the U.S. to be *"a pervasive pattern of shorter lives and poor health"* that crossed all socioeconomic lines. Life expectancy in the U.S. not only came in last, but with each passing decade, the mortality gap widens between the U.S. and all other industrialized nations. Today's generation is developing illnesses 15 years earlier than previous generations. That's right; 30 is the new 45.

Why am I not surprised?

In the documentary, Sweet Remedy, Dr. Russell Blaylock, a renowned neurosurgeon, and the author of *Excitotoxins: The Taste That Kills*, summed it up during a lecture on flavor additives:

"We're seeing a chemical dumbing down of society because of all these different toxins that affect brain function. There are a lot more people that have a lower IQ, but a lot fewer people of higher IQ. Everyone is sort of mediocre. That leaves them dependent on government because they can't excel. We have these people of lower IQ who are totally dependent, and we have [a] massive population who are going to believe everything they are told because they can't think clearly; and very few people of very high IQ, who have very good cognitive function, who can figure this all out. And this is what they want. So you can piece together why they'll spend hundreds of millions of dollars of propaganda money to dumb down society."

In the summer of 2010, the Environmental Working Group conducted an independent study in which they cleaned and prepared foods in the way they are typically eaten. From the results of this study, they released their downloadable list of "The Dirty Dozen and the Clean Fifteen" which shows which non-organic fresh fruits and vegetables are the most highly contaminated with pesticide residue, and which non-organic fresh fruits and vegetables have the least amount of contaminants. The list was compiled so that people wanting to reduce their consumption of toxins and make their dollars go further would be able to make educated choices about which non-organic fruits and vegetables to buy and which to avoid in favor of an organic version.

But no good deed goes unpunished. In response to the Environmental Working Group's list, The Alliance for Food and Farming (a lobbying group for Big Agra and pesticide manufacturers) received a $180,000 federally-funded grant from the California Department of Food and Agriculture (CDFA) and the U.S. Department of Agriculture to counter statements from "activist groups [on] unsafe levels of pesticides," and made the absurd claim that the Environmental Working Group was trying to tell the public to eat less fruits and vegetables.

It's true that organic food is sometimes more expensive than non-organic food. But why is that? There are many reasons. Organic farming means using crop rotation, organic feed, only natural fertilizers, planting heirloom seeds, employing natural predators instead of pesticides, and so on. But a big reason organic food costs more than non-organic food is simply because the government subsidizes non-organic farming at a 2010 rate of $20 billion per year. The U.S. Farm Bill does *not* subsidize organic farms.

In Europe, a program called REACH (Registration, Evaluation, Authorization, and restriction of Chemicals) took effect at the end of 2010, which forces manufacturers to submit their personal care products to independent government approved laboratories and prove that the ingredients are safe and non-toxic before they are allowed to bring them to market. As a result, manufacturers have not only replaced many chemical ingredients with truly natural ones, they also now have much shorter lists of ingredients.

Will this ever happen in the United States? With all the political talk about growing obesity in this country, the overloaded healthcare system, and the concern about the health of the current generation, doesn't it make you wonder why OUR government doesn't demand that our food supply be grown organically? Why hasn't OUR government demanded that all of the chemicals in our products be tested for toxicity and replaced with only natural, organic, non-synthetic ingredients? Why hasn't OUR government demanded the reduction of manufacturing pollutants in our air and water?

Medicinal herbs have become illegal in the European Union. The pharmaceutical and agricultural industries have used trade law to enable this coup, and they've managed to convince policy makers that food and traditional medicines are trade issues rather than human rights issues.

In the U.S., similar strategies are being used. The U.S. Food and Drug Administration has been focusing on the natural supplement market for more than two years, despite the absence of any harm to the public from the use of these supplements; natural non-toxic supplements that provide the vitamins, minerals, enzymes, amino acids, and proteins our body needs, and in many instances manufactures itself. Many of the natural supplement makers that I contacted for permission to describe their product's health benefits were currently, or had been scrutinized by the USFDA for a year or longer. They have had to restate health potential, and re-label products in order to be "in compliance" with the USFDA guidelines. To be "in compliance" means that any health claim made by a manufacturer would then classify the supplement as a "drug" that would then fall under the control of the USFDA. As a result, research on, and potential benefits of these supplements that had been described by manufacturers prior to 2011 can no longer be stated. Legislation is in the works to further straightjacket the vitamin and supplements industry. It's not to our advantage that The Food and Drug Administration is funded by self-policing industries and many FDA employees come from these industries. As a result, the only purpose the FDA seems to serve now is to "protect" us from all things truly natural, healthy, and nutritious.

It doesn't matter what political party is in charge. Our government is owned by Big Pharma, Big Chem, Big Agra, Big Oil, etc. Major corporations such as chemical giant Monsanto infiltrate the upper echelons of our government, paying millions of dollars to sway decision makers, as well as offering them key positions when they leave office with salaries in the millions of dollars. Many key players in Washington are former employees of Big Industry and they're the ones writing rules, regulations, and laws that benefit their industry, not we the people.

The same topics have been discussed from one presidency to the next. Childhood cancer rates rising 500%, obesity, the exploding cost of healthcare. The President and members of Congress are the ones who make laws and policy. If they really wanted to reduce cancer, obesity, severely cut back the cost of healthcare and have a healthier population, they'd make laws so that our food and products were non-toxic. But that's not likely to ever happen, regardless of how many new faces are elected. And here are examples of why not.

Donald Rumsfeld, who served in various White House positions under different presidents, had been President of Searle Inc., the chemical company that manufactured Aspartame (aka NutraSweet, Equal, etc.). There were exhaustive tests conducted on aspartame, and independent studies found it to cause cancerous brain tumors time and time again. For ten years Searle fought to have aspartame approved as a food additive. The FDA read the reports, conducted their own independent testing, concluded that aspartame did cause brain tumors, and refused to approve aspartame. But guess what? Ronald Reagan was elected, Donald Rumsfeld became a key player on his staff, and an executive order took away the authority of the head of the FDA and then removed him from office. A new puppet was put into place, and suddenly aspartame was approved.

During the Bush administration, before being appointed as Attorney General, John Ashcroft's senatorial re-election campaign received record donations from Monsanto, a multinational chemical company that makes genetically modified sterile seeds, which prevent farmers from using their own seeds from their own crops to plant the next year's crops, forcing them to buy new seeds from Monsanto every year. Not only that, but Monsanto sues farmers for patent infringement if their non-GMO crops become contaminated by Monsanto's genetically modified crops via wind or insects.

Before that, during the Clinton administration, Robert Shapiro, CEO of Monsanto, became part of President Clinton's advisory board. Here are some other examples of how corporations own the U.S. government, and how decisions are made in their favor, rather than ours:

- Margaret Miller, Monsanto lab supervisor, was instrumental in overseeing a report to the FDA on the safety of GMO crops. Soon after that report was submitted to the FDA, she left Monsanto to become FDA Branch Chief where her responsibilities included reviewing and approving the report she'd written while at Monsanto.

- Linda Fisher, Monsanto VP of Government & Public Affairs, became EPA Deputy Administrator.

- Michael Taylor, an attorney for King & Spaulding, whose major client was Monsanto, became USFDA Deputy Commissioner for Policy. As Monsanto's attorney, he advised Monsanto to refuse labeling on genetically modified foods. As FDA Deputy Commissioner, he oversaw the FDA decision to NOT require GMO (genetically modified organism) food labeling. After leaving the FDA post, he became Monsanto's Vice President for Public Policy. In 2005, 70% of processed food in the supermarket contained GMO's. Today it's nearly 100%. Under President Obama, in 2009, Michael Taylor was named Senior Advisor to the FDA Commissioner and in 2010, he was appointed to the newly created post of Deputy Commissioner for Foods where one of his responsibilities is to "ensure that food labels contain clear and accurate information on nutrition," but you can be sure no Monsanto GMO ingredients will be listed.

- As an attorney, former First Lady and Secretary of State Hillary Clinton worked for a law firm that was counsel Monsanto.

Even the Supreme Court has been tainted with industry insiders with an agenda. Supreme Court Justice Clarence Thomas was counsel for Monsanto. When lawsuits against Monsanto's genetically modified alfalfa were brought before the Supreme Court, Supreme Court Justice Clarence Thomas did not recuse himself. Not surprisingly the lawsuits were decided in favor of Monsanto.

Our government is nothing more than a revolving door between industry insiders and Washington, DC, which may as well be referred to as Monsanto's "branch office." Long gone are the days when the Presidents of the United States would surround themselves with the best independent minds in the country. The current trend is to pluck top corporate executives and place them into positions of policy and power. Of course they are going to promote what is best for their home industry, rather than what's best for the country. All the rhetoric of cleaning house of lobbyists, making government more transparent, and whatever else a candidate will spout in order to be elected is just that—rhetoric. Is it any wonder that Congress is so ineffective?

Increasingly our right to choose raw and unadulterated foods, grown by farmers who use sustainable and organic practices, are being taken away under the guise of "public safety." Meanwhile, giant factory egg farms, with numerous violations in which they have had to recall over ½ million eggs due to salmonella contamination are allowed to remain in business, still producing the eggs sold in your supermarket!

Nearly every state in the union, in conjunction with the FDA, the FBI, and local law enforcement agencies, are raiding small farmers for selling raw milk and cheese. They threaten farmers with fines and imprisonment if they don't conform, forcing them to spill gallons of raw milk and toss raw cheese at a loss of hundreds of thousands of dollars to the farmers. And these are raw products that have never made anyone sick, farms with no complaints lodged against them. Meanwhile, major factory farms owned by conglomerates such as Cargill are allowed to continue their operations pumping out ground turkey contaminated with salmonella and beef contaminated with E.coli, with nothing more than a slap on the wrist and fines that are considered nothing more than the cost of doing business.

Here's another example of why we're at risk: in 1998, the U.S. Department of Agriculture (USDA) implemented Microbial Testing for E.coli and salmonella so that if a plant repeatedly failed the tests, it would be shut down. But this isn't what happened. That's because the Meat and Poultry Association took the USDA to court, and the court ruled that the USDA didn't have the authority to shut down meat processing plants. Only Congress can give that authority to the USDA, and it still hasn't happened. When a little boy died from hemorrhagic E.coli three days after eating contaminated beef, Kevin's Law was introduced, giving the USDA the authority to shut down plants that repeatedly produce contaminated meat. It should come as no surprise that Kevin's Law has never been passed.

In the U.S., the organic market has been growing steadily at a rate of 20% annually. Smelling a dollar to be made, Big Food is quickly finding a way to crack one of the fastest growing market segments in the food industry. But rather than turning to organic methodology, they're simply buying their way into it. One by one, like pieces on a chessboard, small organic farms and businesses are being claimed by Big Food, or else they're destroyed by Big Food's partners in crime, the FDA, the FBI, and local police departments. Big Food influences the laws and rules governing organic farming by twisting the arm of federal agencies. Big Food insiders now sit on the boards that oversee organic regulations. As a result, the organic label has been watered down to include a growing list of non-organic and synthetic ingredients. And once Big Food overtakes organic farms and products, those products that were once 100% natural and organic, no longer are.

A case in point is Ben & Jerry's, the ice cream company that was purchased by Unilever in 2000. When Ben & Jerry opened their ice cream store in Vermont, they used only pure, natural, and fair trade ingredients. In 2010, a class action lawsuit was filed against Ben & Jerry's in the U.S. District Court for the Northern District of California by consumers who allege that the ice cream maker has misrepresented its products as "all natural," despite the presence of artificial ingredients, such as alkalized cocoa, partially hydrogenated soybean oil, corn syrup and corn syrup solids, maltodextrin, anhydrous dextrose, and vanillin (artificially produced vanilla flavor). This isn't how the original ice cream was made, but that's how Unilever makes it now.

This means we all *must* carefully read the labels of every product we purchase, even if it is labelled as "organic." We can't assume that any product that used to be 100% natural or organic still is, especially after Big Food gets its hands on it. For example, Kashi, a maker of all natural cereal was purchased by Kellogg in 2000. In the Cornucopia Institute's 2012 "Cereal Crimes" study in which nearly every brand of cereal was tested, Kashi brand contained 100% GMO ingredients. Kashi promises its products will be non-GMO by 2018. But who wants to wait that long?

Corporate money and power are being used against consumers, as well as against the farmers who want to grow food the way Mother Nature intended. And that's just the tip of the iceberg. Things like this are happening in every manufacturing sector. Instead of eliminating wasteful spending on government officials' pet projects, Federal spending has been reduced, and the budgets of the EPA, along with the FDA's food safety budget have been slashed. The ripple effect is that food safety inspections from the government level, all the way down to local levels will be cut drastically. This is an obvious gain for Big Food, Big Pharma, Big Chem, and Big Industry in general, and a huge loss for the American people. It means there's absolutely no one left to protect us.

If this weren't bad enough, the biotech industry is out of control, and their key players are also in place in Washington, DC, where they're writing the laws governing our food supply to favor that of the biotech industry. An example is that in 2011 genetically modified alfalfa was given the green light to be released into the wild anywhere, and everywhere. This is especially harmful to organic farming since many of their animals, especially dairy, depend upon alfalfa. Carried by wind, GMO alfalfa pollen travels a great distance. This means it will be nearly impossible to prevent organic alfalfa crops from being contaminated by GMO alfalfa. Ditto for genetically modified grass seed, which will wind contaminate the pastures of organic farms. Since organic rules prohibit organic farmers from using genetically modified crops, it may well lead to the destruction of organic farming. It appears that if the biotech industry can't control those who do not want to be forced to plant their "frankenfood," then they will destroy them. There's no one at the government level trying to stop the biotech industry from wreaking havoc on organic farming and the products we need to remain healthy.

In 2013 the U.S. wheat supply was found to be contaminated by an experimental GMO wheat crop grown in 1999. Japan and other countries which do not allow genetically modified crops boycotted U.S. grown wheat. Japan buys 40% of all U.S. grown wheat and refused U.S. wheat shipments until it was assured the wheat was non-GMO tested.

Increasingly our right to choose what we put into and onto our bodies is being taken away, and chemically concocted foods with little or no nutritional value, and chemically laden products are foisted upon us. With government vaccine mandates, parents are losing the right to decide what's best for their children. With every passing year, more of our rights as individuals are being diminished. Rather than us, it's big corporations and their money that are running the government. Everything is being done to favor the health care industry, the food industry, the oil industry, and the chemical companies. The people we elect set the tone of the country, and if they really wanted to fix things in our favor, they would. Sadly, whenever I hear people speak so proudly of "our democracy," I'm afraid they're living in the past. Instead of government for the people and by the people, it's now government of industry, for industry, and by industry.

Today, people are kept on too many prescription drugs to care, and they're too busy with their latest techno-gadgets to notice what's going on around them. It may be the information age, but Big Industry is making sure that the information pertaining to them is harder and harder to find. If you go to a manufacturer's website to look at a commercial non-organic product, you can see the enticing photographs and read the advertising propaganda, but you'll be hard pressed to find an actual ingredients list. What are they hiding and why? By contrast, most organic websites are proud to list their ingredients.

Industry whistleblowers used to be regarded as heroes and were protected. Now they are considered domestic terrorists and prosecuted.

Non-pharmaceutical cures for diseases are being suppressed, and doctors providing non-invasive, herbal remedies are being harassed or even threatened with closure and imprisonment. Meanwhile thousands of people are permanently harmed by drugs with horrific side effects and death, and yet the pharmaceutical companies that make these drugs are not held accountable.

The more I think about it, the more the science fiction books are becoming, or have already become reality. Plots where humans are recycled as food for the masses; where good, clean water is the hardest thing on the planet to find and people are killing each other to get it; where a man-made virus turns humans into cannibalistic, light sensitive mutants; or where an incurable man-made strain of bacteria creates an apocalypse where no human remains uninfected and disease is the accepted norm. Take a good look around you. Diseases that didn't exist 50 years ago are prevalent now, there are increasing strains of "resistant" super bugs, and our air, water and soil are polluted.

Can the tide be turned? I think so if we keep fighting! Public outcry managed to ban cigarette commercials on television and in public places, and fears about secondary smoke made it illegal to smoke in public places in many cities and states. Public outcry can actually change things and protests against the Vietnam War helped to end it.

If we organize and stay informed by subscribing to independent health and nutrition eNewsletters, most of which are free, and stay abreast of health issues via watchdog group websites such as the Environmental Working Group and Jeffrey Smith's Institute for Responsible Technology to name but a few. And sign petitions to Congress and write to your state's senators and representatives demanding the freedom to choose whether or not to be vaccinated, to have healthier foods, non-toxic products, and the right to choose organics and other healthy products. Some states are formulating initiatives for labeling GMO ingredients. Proposition 37 in California, which would demand that GMO ingredients be labeled, was narrowly voted down, but other states are writing similar initiatives. If you live in those states, vote yes! If possible, contribute to the organic farm defense fund.

And remember, don't just get mad, get even! Vote with your dollars! Buy organic foods from organic websites. Health food stores, and food co-ops are also good sources for organic food. To find organically grown foods from local farmers, Local Harvest provides a search by state for the names and locations of family farms and farmer's markets (www.localharvest.org). Not only will the food taste better, it'll also be more nutritious. You'll also help support an individual who is growing things in a way that will sustain the land, not pollute and destroy it. Also try to grow some of your own food if it's possible. Potted vegetables such as tomatoes, cucumbers, yellow squash and zucchini, even lettuce will grow very well on sunny decks, patios, and balconies.

When shopping, be sure to read every label and buy only products that contain no toxic ingredients. Use only truly natural and 100% organic products and don't be afraid to ask a manufacturer or producer what's in their products, where they get the ingredients, and how those ingredients are made. If they refuse to answer or are vague, it may be wise to avoid that product.

Big Industry does everything it can to suppress the opposition by using money and power. They threaten hospitals and universities with loss of funding and grant money. The independent work of brilliant researchers, doctors, and scientists, which prove catastrophic flaws in Big Industry's methodology and products, can end up buried so they never become public knowledge. Their work can be discredited and their careers destroyed. Big Industry sees to it that these brilliant voices are silenced and exiled to intellectual Siberia.

Unfortunately, the broadcast, print and web media also cave under duress, with investigative journalists' jobs threatened and newspaper, magazine, and television broadcasters threatened with lawsuits if they speak out against Big Industry, and the same Big Industry that provides the advertising revenue is what keeps the newspapers, magazines, and television companies afloat.

Books written by impartial researchers, doctors, and scientists, which show the depths to which Big Industry will stoop to cover up their deception, are buried under negative reviews by industry insiders posing as consumers who've read the books. But don't pay any attention to those fake reviews! The information and books we need are out there, so find them, buy them, and read them.

Big Industry in conjunction with government agencies may have taken away your health, but you can regain it. Fight back and don't buy their products. Hurt them where it counts the most...in their bottom line.

Appendices

Appendix A
Lichen Sclerosis Case Studies

Case No. 1 – A 60-year-old woman

I consider myself to be my first case study. When I was diagnosed with Lichen Sclerosis, I was 60 years old and had symptoms of LS for approximately 2 years prior to diagnosis. As a result, my perineum was white, wrinkled, and the skin would tear and bleed during intercourse. My anus would sometimes tear and bleed when moving my bowels. There was also a second white spot of LS between my left labia majora and labia minora. Other maladies that presented before the LS diagnosis included a chronic crack in the inside of my left nostril, an inflamed and cracking bellybutton, itchy red welts and rashes under my breasts, loss of tooth dentine, inflammation of the eyelids, and chronic, extremely viral eye infections. Within two weeks of switching to organic soaps for bathing, washing my hair, and laundering all clothing, bedding, linens, or anything else that would come into contact with my skin, the welts and rashes under my breasts began to subside. Within two months of switching to a 100% organic diet and undergoing the healing protocol, my perineum began healing. Within three months, my perineum was smooth, with no cracking, and the white spot was shrinking and becoming blotched with pink. My anus also stopped cracking during bowel movements. A visit with the gynecologist after only four months on the healing protocol confirmed that the LS spot between my left labia had vanished. My doctor confirmed that my perineum was "smooth and supple," and that the Lichen Sclerosis was dissipating. I ended the healing protocol after eight months. A ten-month gynecological exam revealed a smooth, supple, and pink perineum and I was discharged as a Lichen Sclerosis patient. However, two months after discontinuing the healing protocol, I developed a mild eye infection, but unlike in the past, it did not progress. I continued the healing protocol for another four months, bringing it to a total of one year of following it. After a full year on the healing protocol, LS has been eliminated along with the inflamed eyelids, eye infections, nostril and bellybutton cracking, and skin rashes. In short, I am completely disease-free. The only reminders that I ever had LS are a smaller right labia minora and a biopsy scar.

Case No. 2 – A 6 ½-year-old girl

C. was age 6 ½ when her parents asked for my help. She lives outside the United States and had suffered with Lichen Sclerosis almost since birth. As a baby, she always had what they thought was severe diaper rash. As the child grew, it became evident that there was an ongoing rash, blistering, and bruising, but their doctor dismissed it as nothing to be concerned about. Varying diagnoses called it diaper rash to be treated with diaper cream, or else as a yeast infection to be treated with medication. The bruising was somehow determined to be self-inflicted. The little girl finally was diagnosed with Lichen Sclerosis at the age of 6 and her dermatologist said it was the worst case she had ever seen. Her perineum was white and wrinkled, and the skin so thin that it would tear and bleed when wiped after urinating. Moving her bowels and urinating were so painful that the child would refuse to go to the bathroom. She received a prescription for Clobetasol.

In addition to the LS, C had white spots on her wrists, the tops of her hands, her ankles, and tops of her feet, which the dermatologist diagnosed as contact dermatitis. Her parents disagreed with the dermatologist and believed the white spots on her extremities were LS. C also had plantar warts on the bottoms of her toes, which are caused by a strain of the human Papilloma virus, or HPV. Her doctor had recommended putting duct tape on the warts to starve them of oxygen, but within two weeks, the warts had grown to twice their original size, making it very painful for the little girl to walk.

C also had chronic gum and ear infections, for which she received repeated doses of antibiotics. Severe LS flare-ups always followed the courses of antibiotics.

When I began working with C's parents in 2010, the child's condition had worsened. Her labial skin was so thin that the veins were visible and it was peeling, leaving raw, red skin exposed. The child would go to bed with a pillow between her legs to try to make the burning subside. During the flare-ups, she could not sleep through the night, and the burning and itching were nearly constant, lasting almost a week. Then they'd subside, only to begin again. C did not react well to the Clobetasol, and she'd cry and beg not to have it applied because it burned her skin.

After talking with her parents, I had them discontinue the Clobetasol and instead gently bathe the affected areas with organic olive oil soap, and then apply a thin layer of 100% organic extra virgin olive oil. This was to be done every time the child urinated or moved her bowels, and she described the sensation of the oil on her skin as cool and soothing.

I recommended that her parents eliminate all commercial personal care products in favor of the Soap for Goodness Sake Organic Extra Virgin Olive Oil Soap for bathing their daughter. Her hair was washed separately in a sink using the same soap, and organic white vinegar was used as a rinse for the child's naturally curly hair. I further recommended that all of the child's bedding, clothing, and anything else that would come into contact with her skin be washed with Soap For Goodness Sake Organic Extra Virgin Coconut Oil Soap, which her mother grated by hand. Even her regular toothpaste was exchanged for Soap for Goodness Sake Tooth Powder.

In addition, I recommended that all food the child ate be 100% organic. Because sugar had always seemed to trigger a flare-up, C was given only minimal amounts of sugar on very rare or special occasions.

The child was somewhat cooperative at the start of the protocol, but quickly began to complain about taking the supplements and nutraceuticals. To entice their daughter, she was given her favorite fruit after cooperating. Within a couple of weeks, when her itching and flare-ups had subsided, C refused to participate in the protocol and suffered a major flare-up. After that setback C willingly followed the healing protocol to the end without complaint, even reminding her parents when it was time to take her supplements and nutraceuticals.

After just three months on the year-long healing protocol, C's pediatric dermatologist discharged her as an LS patient; 8 months into the protocol, her pediatrician also discharged her as an LS patient.

In addition, C's white spots on her wrists, hands, ankles, and feet disappeared, her ano-genital area skin has returned to normal, and her plantar warts are gone. She no longer has chronic gum or ear infections. There is no physical evidence that she ever had Lichen Sclerosis and she now leads a normal, healthy 10-year-old's life having sleep-overs with friends, occasionally eating "forbidden" foods without incident, riding a bicycle, swimming, and taking tennis lessons for the first time in her life.

Appendix B
Non-LS Case Study

Case No. 3 – A 62-year-old man

I include Mr. JW, even though he did not have any form of Lichen Sclerosis. I believe it is important to include him as a case study because many people who have LS also have other auto-immune symptoms. Typically they have a growing number of minor ailments before a major disease is diagnosed. Including this gentleman indicates that the healing protocol can work for many ailments and different genders.

When he began the healing protocol, he was 62-years old. For 2 years, he had suffered from increasing muscle pain and weakness, aching joints, hands and spine, a loss of stamina, brain fog, frequent headaches, insomnia, chronic fatigue, a metallic taste in his mouth, chronic gingivitis, stomach acid, dizziness, loss of motivation, and a general feeling of malaise. His wife reported that he would moan in his sleep when changing position in bed.

Multiple visits to doctors and a wide range of testing revealed no obvious cause for his deteriorating health, and the medical establishment offered no other relief than over-the-counter pain medications, which did nothing as his symptoms progressed.

Besides his overall pain and malaise, for at least 20 years he'd lived with a fungus that manifested as shiny oval pale-pink spots and covered his chest and abdomen. When he sweated, the spots became bright red. A dermatologist had prescribed an ointment that made the spots fade, but when he stopped using it, the spots reappeared. When the prescription ran out, he didn't refill it, thinking it was pointless. He recalled neither the name of the fungus nor the name of the ointment.

After only 8 months on the full healing protocol, his dental hygienist confirmed that he no longer had gingivitis. In addition, he no longer suffered from headaches and regained his stamina and muscle strength. Within a year of starting the healing protocol, his brain fog was gone, his joints no longer ache, and he's returned to his hobby of wood turning and furniture design. He now excels at both running and bicycling, which he could barely do before beginning the healing protocol. Previous to using the protocol, he struggled to keep up with his group. A year later, he not only outperformed the group, but also joined a second biking group with individuals half his age. He now participates in long distance rides (85-100 miles within 7-8 hours). His chronic fatigue has been eliminated, along with his insomnia, and after a full year on the healing protocol, his chest fungus was gone. He says he feels like he's 25 years old.

In 2011, he had unexplained tingling and numbness in his lip, then developed what he thought was a cold sore on his lip. Then, blisters began to appear on his temple, near his eye, and inside his mouth. He was diagnosed with shingles. His doctor prescribed pain medication and the usual prescription medications for shingles, which did not stop the outbreak, and blisters continued to spread on the right side of his face, in his hair, and affected his ear and his hearing. At that point, he stopped taking the shingles medication and switched to 1200 mg of L-Lysine once a day, along with 1 dropper each, three times a day, of Jernigan's Virogen, Lymogen, and Microbojen. He also spread a thin layer of Manuka Honey on the blisters. Within 24 hours of taking the botanicals, L-Lysine, and applying the honey, further blistering had ceased and his blisters began scabbing over. At a follow-up visit, his doctor said "Your body is *really* holding it together!"

Once the blisters healed and the scabbing was gone, he applied aconite oil to the area of numbness around his lip and wherever else the blisters had appeared. From diagnosis to full recovery: 4 weeks.

Appendix C
Recommended Reading

Excitotoxins: The Taste that Kills, Russell L. Blaylock, M.D., Health Press, 1997.

The Fluoride Deception, Christopher Bryson, Seven Stories Press, 2004.

Corrupt to the Core: Memoirs of a Health Canada Whistleblower, Shiv Chopra, KOS Publishing, 2009.

The Case Against Fluoride: How Hazardous Waste Ended Up in Our Drinking Water and the Bad Science and Powerful Politics that Keep It There, Paul Connett, Ph.D., Chelsea Green Publishing Company, 2010.

The Milk Book: How Science Is Destroying Nature's Nearly Perfect Food, William Campbell Douglas, MD, Rhino Publishing S.A. 1994.

Nourishing Traditions: The Cookbook that Challenges Politically Correct Nutrition and the Diet Dictocrats, Sally Fallon and Mary G. Enig, Ph.D., New Trends Publishing, 2001.

The Hundred-year Lie: How to Protect Yourself from the Chemicals That Are Destroying Your Health, Randall Fitzgerald, Penguin Group, 2007.

Beating Lyme Disease, David A Jernigan, D.C., Somerleyton Press, 2nd edition, 2008.

Vaccine Safety Manual for Concerned Families and Health Practitioners, 2nd Edition: Guide to Immunization Risks and Protection, Neil Z. Miller, New Atlantean Press, 2nd edition, 2010.

Selling Sickness: How the World's Biggest Pharmaceutical Companies Are Turning Us All Into Patients, Ray Moynihan, Alan Cassells, Nation Books, 2005.

Confessions of an Rx Drug Pusher, Gwen Olsen, iUniverse, 2009.

The World According to Monsanto, Marie-Monique Robin, The New Press, 2010.

The Untold Story of Milk, Ron Schmid, ND, New Trends Publishing, 2009.

In Bad Taste: The MSG Symptom Complex, George R. Schwartz, M.D., Health Press, 1999.

The Seeds of Deception: Exposing Industry and Government Lies About the Safety of the Genetically Engineered Foods You're Eating, Jeffrey M. Smith, Yes! Books, 2003.

Genetic Roulette: The Documented Health Risks of Genetically Engineered Foods, Jeffrey M. Smith, Yes! Books, 2007.

$29 Billion Reasons to Lie About Cholesterol, Justin Smith, Troubador Publishing, Ltd., 2009

What Your Doctor Doesn't Know About Nutritional Medicine May Be Killing You, Ray D. Strand, M.D., Thomas Nelson, [pub], 2002.

Death by Prescription: The Shocking Truth Behind an Overmedicated Nation, Ray D. Strand, M.D., Thomas Nelson, [pub], 2003.

Sacred Spark, Rev. Lisa K. Sykes, Fourth Lloyd Productions, 2009.

Callous Disregard: Autism and Vaccines - The Truth Behind a Tragedy, Andrew J. Wakefield, Skyhorse Publishing, 2010.

Devil in the Milk: Illness, Health and the Politics of A1 and A2 Milk, Keith Woodford, Chelsea Green Publishing, 2009.

The Cholesterol Myth: Believe It to Your Peril, Dr. R. L. Wysong, Inquiry Press, 2010.

Appendix D
Recommended Videos

Cori Brackett, **Sweet Misery: A Poisoned World**, directed by Cori Brackett, California: Cinema Libre Studio, 2005. DVD.

Kristin Canty, **Farmageddon: The Unseen War on American Family Farms**, directed by Kristin Canty, Massachusetts: Kristin Marie Productions LLC, 2011. DVD.

Michael Connet, **Professional Perspectives on Water Fluoridation**, Fluoride Action Network, 2011. DVD.

Ana Sofia Joanes, **Fresh: New Thinking About What We're Eating**, directed by Ana Sofia Joanes. Maryland: Ripple Effect Productions, 2009. DVD.

Robert Kenner, **Food, Inc.**, directed by Robert Kenner. California: Magnolia Home Entertainment, 2009. DVD.

Leslie Manookian, Kendall Nelson and Chris Pilaro, **The Greater Good**, directed by Kendall Nelson and Chris Pilaro, California: BNB Pictures Production, 2011. DVD.

Don McCorkell, **A River of Waste: The Hazardous Truth About Factory Farms,** directed by Don McCorkell, California: Cinema Libre Studio, 2009. DVD.

Marie-Monique Robin, **The World According to Monsanto**, directed by Marie-Monique Robin, France: Image & Compagnie Productions, 2008. DVD.

Jeffrey Smith, **Genetic Roulette: The Gamble of Our Lives**, directed by Jeffrey Smith, Iowa: Institute for Responsible Technology, 2012. DVD.

Justin Smith, **$tatin Nation: The Great Cholesterol Cover-Up**, directed by Justin Smith, London: Rethink Productions, Ltd., 2012. DVD.

Bertram Verhaag, **Scientists Under Attack: Genetic Engineering in The Magnetic Field of Money**, directed by Bertram Verhaag, Germany: DENKmal-Films Ltd., 2010. DVD.

Appendix E
Healing Protocol Products

Jernigan Nutraceuticals
www.jernigannutraceuticals.com

Borrelogen™
Lymogen™
Microbojen™
Yeast Ease™
Neuro-Antitox II Cardio™
Neuro-Antitox II CNS/PNS™
Neuro-Antitox II Musculo-Skeletal™
Molybdenum™

TPP™ Protease by Transformation Enzymes
www.naturalhealinghouse.com

Product Password: health
Coupon Code for 5% Discount: health

Soap For Goodness Sake LLC
www.soapforgoodnesssake.com

Organic Extra Virgin Olive Oil Soap
Organic Extra Virgin Coconut Oil Soap
Organic Bassasu Shaving Soap
Tooth Powder

Vitamins

- Garden of Life Vitamin Code Raw Vitamins
   www.amazon.com
   www.vitaminshoppe.com
   www.luckyvitamin.com
   Various online retailers

- Whole Food Multivitamin Plus
   www.mercola.com

- Children's Chewable Multivitamins
  www.mercola.com

- Various online Vitamin Retailers
  www.amazon.com
  www.vitaminshoppe.com
  www.luckyvitamin.com
  www.wildearthmarket.com

Supplements

- **Fish Oil - Carlson Labs**
  www.amazon.com
  www.luckyvitamin.com
  www.vitaminshoppe.com
  Various online retailers

- **Salmon Oil**
  www.vitalchoice.com

- **Krill Oil**
  www.vitalchoice.com
  www.mercola.com

- **Krill Oil for Kids**
  www.mercola.com

- **CoQ$_{10}$/Ubiquinol**
  www.mercola.com
  Various online retailers

- **L-Lysine Amino Acid** (powder by Carlson Labs)
  www.amazon.com
  www.luckyvitamin.com
  www.vitaminshoppe.com
  www.wildearthmarket.com
  Various online retailers

- **L-Lysine Amino Acid** (capsules by Source Naturals)
  www.amazon.com
  www.luckyvitamin.com
  www.vitaminshoppe.com
  Various online retailers

- **Molybdenum**™
  www.jernigannutraceuticals.com

- **Probiotics**
  Transformation Enzymes Probiotic 42.5™
  www.naturalhealinghouse.com (code "health" for $5 off)

  Nutri-West Total Probiotics™
  www.amazon.com
  Various online retailers

- **Detox Tea** (Yogi & Triple Leaf)
  www.amazon.com
  www.luckyvitamin.com
  www.vitaminshoppe.com
  Supermarkets, food co-ops, health food stores
  Various online retailers

- **Raw Ginger Root** (organic preferred)
  Supermarkets, food co-ops, health food stores

- **Epsom Salts and Hydrogen Peroxide**
  Supermarkets, food co-ops, pharmacies, health food stores
  Various online retailers

- **Organic Extra Virgin Olive Oil**
  www.organicoil.com/olive-oil.aspx
  www.amazon.com
  Supermarkets, food co-ops, health food stores

Appendix F
Post Healing Protocol Products

- **Organic Spirulina Powder**
  www.nuts.com
  www.livesuperfoods.com
  Various online retailers

- **Organic Chlorella Powder**
  www.nuts.com
  www.livesuperfoods.com
  Various online retailers

- **Olive Leaf Extract Capsules & Liquid**
  www.olivus.com

Appendix G
Other Products

Powder Supplies (Box and/or Puff)
- Rachels Supply
  www.rachelssupply.com/powpuff.htm

Popcorn Popper
- Back to Basics™ or other brand stainless steel stove-top popcorn popper
  www.Amazon.com

Essential Oils
- Mountain Rose Herbs
  www.mountainroseherbs.com/aroma/ess.html

- Young Living Essential Oils
  www.youngliving.com

Omron Pedometer
- Omron Web Store
  http://omronwebstore.com/detail/OMR+HJ-112

Organic Fabrics
- Hemp Towels and Washcloths
  www.soapforgoodnesssake.com

- Organic Cotton and Wool Bath and Bedding
  www.lifekind.com

Nutiva Organic Virgin Coconut Oil
- Amazon
  www.amazon.com
  Various online retailers

Capsule Filling Machines & Empty Vegetarian Capsules

- Capsule Connection
  www.capsuleconnection.com

- Cap-M-Quik
  www.cap-m-quik.com

- Wonder Labs
  www.wonderlabs.com

Water Bottles

- Klean Kanteen
  www.kleankanteen.com

- Go Green Travel Green
  http://gogreentravelgreen.com

- Good Life Bottles
  www.goodlifebottles.com

- Safe Water Bottle Review
  http://safewaterbottlereview.com/

Water Filters

- Aquasana Water Filters
  www.aquasana.com

- Aquaspace Water Systems
  www.aquaspace.com

- Berkey Water Filters
  www.berkeyfilters.com
  www.pleasanthillgrain.com

Stainless Steel Storage Containers – BPA- and BPS- Free

- Life Without Plastic
  www.lifewithoutplastic.com

- LunchBots
  www.lunchbots.com

- PlanetBox
  www.meals.planetbox.com

Bulk Food-Safe Plastic Storage Containers

I buy organic herbs, beans, nutritional yeast, chlorella, spirulina, and more in bulk. Buying bulk saves money, but finding inexpensive storage containers that are air tight and moisture-proof can be challenging.

Many bulk organic food items are shipped to retail organic food stores in bulk plastic buckets that are considered food safe. The containers are made of high-density polyethylene and are marked on the bottom as **HDPE 2**. Once these stores have emptied the contents, they will recycle the containers. It has been my experience that if I ask, these stores are usually happy to save the containers and give them to me at no cost.

I also request that the containers not be cleaned because once I received pre-washed buckets that had a strong chemical smell that no amount of washing could remove and I refused to use it.

If free buckets aren't available, they can be purchased online from 1 gallon to 6 gallon sizes. Also available is a wrench for easy lid opening, air tight and waterproof Gamma-seal screw-on replacement lids, dry packs and oxygen absorbers for long-term storage.

The HDPE 2 food safe buckets, snap on or Gamma-seal lids, dry packs, and oxygen absorbers are available on-line at:

- Pleasant Hill Grain (buckets, Gamma-seal lids, snap-on lid openers)
  www.pleasanthillgrain.com

- Amazon (buckets, Gamma-seal lids, snap-on lid wrench, dry packs, oxygen absorbers)
  www.amazon.com

- USA Emergency Supply (buckets, Gamma-seal lids, snap-on lid wrench, dry packs, oxygen absorbers)
  www.usaemergencysupply.com

- Various online sellers

Stainless Steel Cookware - BPA & BPS-Free

eBay has been my source for Revere Ware stainless steel pots and loaf pans made around the 1940s, and sell on eBay for a fraction of new stainless cookware. These older pots and pans have withstood the test of time and are very heavy because the stainless steel and copper cladding is thicker than that of modern-day stainless steel copper clad cookware. Look for Revere Ware pots marked Clinton, Illinois (the original manufacturing plant) or Rome, New York (the 2nd manufacturing plant). A pot marked as "Patent 2272609 – Made Under Process Patent 2363973" is most desirable because it is one of the earliest pots manufactured at the Clinton, Illinois plant.

- www.ebay.com

Stainless Steel Cooking Utensils - BPA & BPS-Free

- Lee Valley Tools Ltd.
  www.leevalley.com

China Dishes, Glass Storage Containers and Cookware

eBay has been my source for CorningWare cookware, Pyrex pie and cake pans, Glasbake bundt pans, and Food Saver glass storage containers made between the 1940s and 1950s. These early glass cooking and storage containers are made of thick glass and seem almost indestructible. These items sell on eBay for a fraction of what they would cost new.

- www.ebay.com

Appendix H
Organic Food Websites

The following websites are just a start, and there are many organic food websites on the Internet. But sites below offer the best product, prices (including shipping), coupons, discounts, and customer service. Sometimes the best prices are found at small organic farms such as Billy The Kid Nuts (pecans), and Dixon Ridge Farms (walnuts).

Bulk sellers and companies such as Amazon.com carry many of the products from the vendors listed below, and it pays to shop around for the best prices.

If you live outside the U.S., you should be able to find similar websites wherever you reside.

Cereal/Granola Bars
- Nature's Path
  www.naturespath.com

Chocolates
- Mama Ganache Artisan Chocolates
  www.mama-ganache.com

Coconut Oil – Nutiva Virgin
- Amazon
  www.amazon.com

  Various on-line retailers
  Food Co-ops and healthfood stores

Condiments
- Amy's Kitchen
  www.amys.com

Cookies, Crackers, Snacks
- Late July
  www.latejuly.com

Dairy
- Organic Valley
  www.oranicvalley.coop

- Stonyfield
  www.stonyfield.com

- Woodstock Farms
  www.woodstock-farms.com

Desserts – Gluten-Free & Vegetarian
- Amy's Kitchen
  www.amys.com

Flour
- Jaffe Bros
  www.organicfruitsandnuts.com

- Nuts.com
  www.nuts.com

- To Your Health Sprouted Flour Co.
  www.organicsproutedflour.net

Fruits & Vegetables - Frozen
- Woodstock Farms
  www.woodstock-farms.com

Grains, Beans, Seeds
- Pleasant Hill Grain
  www.pleasanthillgrain.com

- Purcell Mountain Farms
  www.purcellmountainfarms.com

Herbs & Spices
- Frontier Coop
  www.frontiercoop.com

- Mountain Rose Herbs
  www.mountainroseherbs.com

- Starwest Botanicals
  www.starwest-botanicals.com

- Stony Mountain Botanicals
  www.wildroots.com

Raw Honey - Y.S. Organic Bee Farms
- Amazon
  www.amazon.com

- The Natural
  www.thenaturalonline.com
  Various online retailers

Meats/Poultry
- Applegate Farms
  http://store.applegatefarms.com

- Organic Prairie
  http://store.organicprairie.com

- U.S. Wellness Meats
  www.grasslandbeef.com

- Yankee Farmers Market
  http://yankeefarmersmarket.stores.yahoo.net/

Nuts
- Billy The Kid Nuts
  www.billythekidnuts.com

- Braga Farms
  http://stores.buyorganicnuts.com

- Dixon Ridge Farms
  www.dixonridgefarms.com

- Jaffe Bros.
  www.organicfruitsandnuts.com

- Nuts.com
  www.nuts.com

Olive Oil – Extra Virgin
- Olio Beato
  www.organicoil.com/olive-oil.aspx

Pasta & Semolina Flour
- Purcell Mountain Farms
  www.purcellmountainfarms.com

- A.G. Ferrari Foods
  www.agferrari.com

Raisins
- Braga Farms
  http://stores.buyorganicnuts.com

Raw Food
- Raw Guru
  www.rawguru.com

Salt
- Salt Works Himalayan Pink Salt
  www.saltworks.us/wholesale-bulk-gourmet-sea-salt.asp

Seafood
- Rushing Waters Fisheries
  www.rushingwaters.net

- Vital Choice
  www.vitalchoice.com/shop/pc/home.asp

Wild Rice
- North Bay Trading
  www.northbaytrading.com/

Appendix I
Coupons and Discounts

Organic product manufacturers are just as marketing savvy as mainstream industry. You can write or email a manufacturer and tell them how much you like their product, and more often than not, they will send you coupons as a goodwill gesture.

- **Food Co-ops** - Food co-ops offer members special member-only discounts and provide coupons throughout the year. Health food stores may offer a modest annual membership fee that guarantees members-only specials, and/or discounts. They also may offer a price break for ordering products in bulk.

- **Buy in Bulk** - It also pays to approach a store and request items in bulk, and also ask for a discount. For example, at my local food co-op, organic Greek yogurt by the case of twelve would cost $19.55. Bought individually, those 12 containers would cost $23.88

- **Organic Food Websites** - Organic food websites offer coupons just as mainstream food manufacturers do. By signing up for their newsletters or email alerts, you'll get email notification for special discounts on food or shipping. Many also offer downloadable coupons. Check their websites for coupons, promotions, and specials.

- **Coupon Websites** - Also sign up for coupons at Coupons.com. Occasionally this site will carry coupons for Organic Valley, Stonyfield Farms, and other organic food companies. But beware as most of the coupons are from Big Food companies and are to be avoided.

- **Amazon** - Amazon.com is a very good source for organic products. Multi-packs of Nature's Path granola bars and their cereals can be purchased through Amazon.com at a discounted price and free Super Saver shipping. Also use automatic shipping which reduces the price even further. I always check Amazon first for Nutiva Organic Virgin Coconut Oil, Y.S. Organic Honey, and many other products, and in many instances, free super-saver shipping is available.

- **Barter** - And finally, in 2011, I volunteered my time working on an organic farm in exchange for free produce and raw goat milk. The following year I converted my lawn, which had never been subjected to synthetic fertilizer or toxic weed killer, to an organic vegetable garden. Recently my family has taken on the challenge of organically raising chickens for eggs, some of which we barter, along with my homemade organic loaves of bread, in exchange for locally grown organic hay, raw milk, raw cream, raw yogurt, and vegetables.

There are many ways to obtain organic food at a reduced cost if you're willing to shop carefully and be creative.

Appendix J
Health Information

A great health resource is the Internet. The following alphabetical list of health news resources is by no means complete, nor is it listed by preference. There are many credible and informative internet health sites, too many to list here.

HEALTH RESOURCES	
Resource	**Website**
AlterNet	www.alternet.org
Coalition for Mercury-free Drugs	http://mercury-freedrugs.org
Confessions of an R_X Drug Pusher	www.gwenolsen.com
Dr. Mercola Newsletter	www.mercola.com
Environmental Working Group	www.ewg.org
Fluoride Action Network	www.fluoridealert.org
Institute for Responsible Technology	www.responsibletechnology.org
National Vaccine Information Center	www.nvic.org
Natural News	www.naturalnews.com
Organic Consumers Association	www.organicconsumers.org
S.A.N.E VAX, Inc.	sanevax.org
The Cornucopia Institute	www.cornucopia.org
The Linus Pauling Institute	http://lpi.oregonstate.edu/
The Weston A. Price Foundation	www.westonaprice.org
Truth About Gardasil	truthaboutgardasil.org
Truth About Splenda	www.truthaboutsplenda.com

About the Author

Ginny Chandoha lived and worked for 30 years in New York City and its metropolitan area. Her career took many twists and turns, beginning as an executive secretary at an oil conglomerate and ending as director of human resources for a scholarly book publisher. In between, her accomplishments include being editorial assistant and contributing editor for travel trade publications, computer systems manager for a major Madison Avenue advertising agency, as well as a computer services manager for a premier Wall Street financial institution. She once owned a computer services company that provided on-site corporate training. In addition, her short stories have been published in four different books.

She lives in northern New England with her husband, two cats, and chickens.

Index

A

Agent Orange, 104, 111
Agglutinin, 160
AIR, 188
   Building products, 193
   Fresheners, 188
   Perfume, 192
   Purification, 194
ANTIBIOTICS, 293
   Used in food-producing animals, 133
ARTIFICIAL COLORS, 81, 138
   Blue 1, 81
   Blue 1 Lake, 81
   Blue 2, 81
   Red 33, 22
   Red 40, 22
   Yellow 5, 24
   Yellow 5 Lake, 81
   Yellow 6, 25, 81
   Yellow 6 Lake, 81
Artificial flavor, 138
ARTIFICIAL SWEETENERS, 69
   AminoSweet, 69
   Aspartame, 69, 70, 71, 75, 118, 167, 168, 434
   High fructose corn syrup (HFCS), 71
   Neotame, 69
   NutraSweet, 69
   Splenda, 69, 473
   Sweet N Low, 69
   Symptoms, 70
Automobile emissions, 195
Avidin in egg whites, 406

B

Becker, Dr. Karen, 327
Blaylock, Dr. Russell, 273, 279, 431

Blepharitis, 2, 9
Body Composition Analysis, 6, 7, 309, 314, 389
Borrelogen, 378, 391, 394, 395, 397, 416, 458
Bug repellant, 424
Butter vs margarine, 233

C

Canola oil, 224
Capsule filling machine. *See* ENCAPSULATION
Caramel color, 138
Carrageenan, 163
Case Studies, 446
    Non-LS, 450
Center For Food Safety, 118
Cervarix. *See* VACCINES
Chemicals ingested per year, 62
CHOCOLATE, 79
    Mama Ganache Artisan Chocolates, 82, 220, 467
    Polyglycerol Polyricinoleate (PGPR), 80
CHOLESTEROL, 237, 265, 297, 317
    Gap junctions, 319
    HDL/LDL Ratios, 320
    Lipoprotein a Lp(a), 319
    Low cholesterol problems, 322
    Rhabdomyolysis (muscle weakness), 323
    Statin usage problems, 323
Cleaners and disinfectants, 423
CLOBETASOL PROPIONATE, 22, 184, 329
    Ingredients, 15
    vs Organic Extra Virgin Olive Oil, 381
Coalition for Mercury-free Drugs, 294
COCONUT OIL, 33, 35, 36, 44
    Virgin, 44
    Lauric acid, 19, 44, 45
    Moisturizer, 37, 38, 44
Cooking Oils, 232
Cookware, 465
Cornucopia Institute, 439, 473
Coupons and Discounts - Appendix I, 471

D

D'Adamo, Dr. Peter J.
    Eat Right For Your Type, 217
DDT, 105, 111, 192
Deodorant, 419
Detox Tea, 367
Diet, 217
Dodds, Dr. Jean, 327

E

Electrolytes, 43, 244, 245, 246, 314
ENCAPSULATION
    Calcium, 415

Capsule filling machine, 426
Multivitamin, 415, 416
Olive leaf, 415
Vitamin C, 415
Where to buy supplies, 463
Epsom salts, 369
Essential oils, 30
Exercise, 239

F

Fabrics, organic, 424, 462
Facial cleanser/exfoliation, 418
Factory farming, 126
Fibromyalgia, 63, 71, 201, 252, 301, 413
FISH, 141
    Antibioitics, 146
    Diseases of, 142
    Disinfectants, 146
    Fraud, 149
    Fungicides, 146
    GMO, 148
    Organic, 147
    Salmo fan, 146
    Salmon Nutritional Content, 145
    Sodium tripolyphosphate (STPP), 147
Flavonoids, 41
Flu. *See* VACCINES
FLUORIDE, 173
    All sources, 184
    Fluorosis, 175, 176, 179
    Hydrogen Fluoride, 174
    In food, 183
    In pharmaceuticals, 183
    Silicon Tetrafluoride, 176
    Sodium Fluoride, 181
    Sodium Fluorosilicate, 182
    State fluoridation map, 185
    Symptoms of fluoride toxicity, 179, 180
Fluoride Action Network, 185
FOOD
    Additives, 67
    Defined, 60
    Evolution, 58
    Raw, 227
    Science, 66
Food websites - Appendix H, 467
Fragrance, 18, 189, 190, 191
FRUIT JUICE, 74
    De-aeration, 79

Flavor packs, 79
Orange juice, 78

G

Gap junctions. *See* CHOLESTEROL
Gardasil. *See* VACCINES
Garden of Life, 415
Ginger root, 370
Glutathione, 228, 241, 282
Glyphosate, 102, 106, 107, 108, 109, 110
GMO, 96
    Arctic Apple, 112
    GMO-free food companies, 118
    GMO-free shopper's guide, 118
    Micronutrient reduction, 107
Gum Acacia, 81

H

HEALING PROTOCOL, 386
    1st Quarter Schedule, 394
    2nd Quarter Schedule, 395
    3rd Quarter Schedule, 396
    4th Quarter Schedule, 397
    Beginning the protocol, 398
    Chart - 1st Quarter, 401
    Chart - 2nd Quarter, 402
    Chart - 3rd Quarter, 403
    Chart - 4th Quarter, 404
    Chart - Preliminary 2-week, 400
    Outline, 391
    Phase 1, 386
    Phase 2, 387
    Phase 3, 388
    Product websites, 458
    Two-week preliminary preparation, 376
Healing Soak, 369
HEAVY METALS, 195
    Aluminum, 197
    Mercury, 196
    Testing. *See* PRELIMINARY TESTING
Herxheimer reaction, 330
Hilleman, Dr. Maurice, 268, 281
Himalayan pink salt, 125, 220, 230, 245, 421, 470
Hippocrates, 217, 239
Homeopathic Rule of Thumb, 337
Honey, 87
Hs-CRP. *See* PRELIMINARY TESTING
Human papilloma virus (HPV). *See* VACCINES

Hydrogen Peroxide, 370, 387, 460

I

Independent organic GMO-free companies, 118
INFANT FORMULA, 160, 163, 164, 165, 166
    Crypthecodinium Cohni Oil. *See* Martek Biosciences Corporation
    Ingredients, 163
    Mortierella Alpina Oil. *See* Martek Biosciences Corporation
Irvin, Rick, 14
Irradiation, 119

J

Jernigan, Dr. David A., 248, 250, 373
Jobs, Steve, 308

K

KiGGS – The German Health Interview and Examination Survey for Children and Adolescents, 288
King, Dr. Paul G. *See* Coalition for Mercury-free Drugs

L

LABELING, 114
    100% Organic, 114
    Made with organic ingredients, 115
    Natural, 114
    Organic, 115
    Synthetic ingredients in organics, 117
Lauric Acid, 19, 44, 45
Lymogen, 378, 391, 395, 396, 397, 416, 451, 458

M

Makeup, chemicals absorbed per year, 62
Manuka Honey, 415, 451
Martek Biosciences Corporation, 166
MEAT, 130
    Ammonia hydroxide, 62
    Cured, 136
    E.coli, 130
    Glue, 139
    Pink slime, 131
    Polycyclic aromatic hydrocarbons (PAHs), 137
    Processed, 135
Microbojen, 378, 391, 396, 397, 416, 417, 451, 458

MICROWAVE, 121
    PFOA, 123
    Popcorn lung, 123
    Radiolytic compounds, 121
    Swiss Macrobiotic Institute, 122
MILK, 150
    A1 and A2 beta-casein, 155
    Artificial sweeteners, 167
    Goat vs Cow, 161
    IgF-1 growth factor, 151
    Nutrients in raw milk, 154
    Oakhurst Dairy lawsuit, 152
    Organic Pastures Dairy pathogen testing, 158
    Raw vs Pasteurized, 160
    rBGH, 151
    rBST, 152
    Substitutes, 163
    The Milk Cure, 157
    Ultra-pasteurization, 153
Mitchell, Dr. Roby, 253
Moderation, everything in, 65
MSG, 83
    Syndrome, 86

N

National Vaccine Injury Compensation Program (NVICP), 269
Natural flavor, 138
NUTRACEUTICALS, 372
    Borrelogen, 378
    Lymogen, 378
    Microbojen, 378
    Neuro-Antitox II Cardio, 377
    Neuro-Antitox II CNS/ PNS, 376
    Neuro-Antitox II Musculo-Skeletal, 376
    Remedies, 416
    Yeast Ease, 377
NVIC, 272, 279, 473
NVICP, 269

O

Olive leaf nutrients, 412
OLIVE OIL, 31, 38
    Extra Light, 39
    Extra Virgin, 39
    Extra Virgin Nutrients, 41
    Moisturizer, 38, 44
    Olio Beato, 38
    Pomace, 40

Replacing Clobetasol with, 381
Virgin, 39
Olsen, Gwen, 262, 266, 454
Omega-3 Fatty Acids, 43
Omega-6 Fatty Acids, 43
Organic,
Who owns, 115

P

PARABENS
Butylparaben, 21
Concentrations found in breast cancer tumors, 21
Ethylparaben, 21
Isobutylparaben, 21
Methylparaben, 19
Paraben, 20
Propylparaben, 20
Paracelsus, 178, 220
Peanut Butter Cups, 82
Pedometer, 242
Perfume, 192
PERSONAL CARE PRODUCTS
Common ingredients, 16
PESTICIDES, 89
Average annual consumption, 62
Bt Toxin, 90
Consumption by children, 116, 117
DDT, 105, 111, 192, 407
Dirty Dozen & Clean Fifteen, 95
Glufosinate. *See* Agent Orange
Glyphosate. *See* Glyphosate
Neutralizing Systems, 95
Top 10 Contaminated Foods, 91
Phytosterols, 42, 77
Pink slime, 62, 131, 132
POULTRY, 127
Chicken life cycle, 127
Egg layers, 128
Meat bird guidelines, 128
USFDA 2013 Organic Guidelines, 129
PRELIMINARY TESTING, 314
Body Composition Analysis, 314
Cholesterol levels, 317
Heavy metals, 316
Hs-CRP, 324
Lyme Testing, 315
Thickened blood, 325
Vitamin & Mineral Testing, 316
Probiotics, 354

Problem-Reaction-Solution strategy, 291
Products, where to buy - Appendix G, 462
PTFE, 193, 226

R

rBGH, 105, 151, 152, 153, 230
rBST, 105, 152, 153, 230

S

SaneVax.org, 272, 473
Scented candles, 192
Schwartz, Dr. George R., 83
Schweitzer, Dr. Albert, 428
Seborrheic keratoses, 2
Shelf life, 126
SLS
    Sodium Lareth Sulfate, 25
    Sodium Lauryl Sulfate, 25
Smith, Jeffrey M., 97, 442, 454, 457
SOAP, 26, 27
    Cetaphil, 27
    Dove, 26
    Glycerin, 27
    Saponification, 31
    Soap for Goodness Sake, 30, 31, 33, 37, 418, 419, 423, 448, 453
Soybean oil, 106
SPIRULINA/CHLORELLA, 407
    Nutritional analysis, 408
Sprouted flour, 238, 468
Storage containers, food safe, 422
Sublingual, 29, 30, 341, 379, 380
Supplements, 352
SV-40 monkey kidney virus, 281
Symptoms of toxicity, 200

T

Thickened blood. *See* PRELIMINARY TESTING
Thyroid conditions, 24, 138, 175, 180, 201, 228, 235, 289, 332, 348, 410
Titer, 278
Tooth powder, 33, 37, 419, 448, 458
Toxic body burden, 55, 66
Toxiniophobe, 48
TPP Protease, 334, 352, 353, 392, 458
Traditional Chinese Medicine (TCM), 251, 267, 300

Trevisan, Dr. Giusto, 249
Triclosan, 24, 36, 354

U

Ubiquinol, 324, 392, 393, 394, 415, 459

V

VACCINES, 268
  Cervarix, 283
  Decline in infectious diseases, 286
  Flu, 276
  Gardasil, 283, 284, 285, 286, 473
  Gardasil adverse reactions, 284
  Human Papilloma virus (HPV), 283, 333
  Ingredients, 280
  SV-40 Monkey Kidney Virus, 281
VAERS, 270, 273, 274, 284, 285
Virogen, 378, 416, 417, 451
Vital Choice, 149, 470
Vitamin D Council, 347
VITAMINS and SUPPLEMENTS, 327
  B12, 339
  B-complex, 339
  C, 341
  Calcium, 350
  CoQ10/Ubiquinol, 365
  D3, 343
  D3 Optimum Serum Levels, 346
  D3 Serum Test 25(OH)D, 345
  E, 348
  Evening Primrose Oil, 359
  Homeopathic Rule of Thumb, 337
  L-Lysine, 357
  Molybdenum, 356
  Multivitamins, 338
  Omega-3 Fish/Krill Oil, 362
  Probiotics, 354
  Synthetic, 335
  TPP Protease, 334, 352, 353, 392, 458

W

Wakefield, Dr. Andrew, 268, 273, 290
Walls, Michael, 14
WATER, 168
  Bottled, 186
  BPA-free water bottles, 187

Chemicals found in, 171
Chlorination, 170
Chlorine induced skin conditions, 171
Filtration systems, 171
Wild rice, 220
Wulzen factor, 236
Wysong, Dr. Randy L., 60, 126, 256, 298

X

Xylitol, 33

CPSIA information can be obtained at www.ICGtesting.com
Printed in the USA
BVOW05s1447190116

433361BV00007B/93/P